Biennial Review of Infertility

Catherine Racowsky • Peter N. Schlegel
Bart C. Fauser • Douglas T. Carrell
Editors

Biennial Review of Infertility

Volume 2
2011

Springer

Editors
Catherine Racowsky, Ph.D.
Harvard Medical School
Brigham and Women's Hospital
Department of Obstetrics and
Gynecology Boston, MA, USA
cracowsky@partners.org

Peter N. Schlegel, M.D.
New York Presbyterian Hospital
Weill Cornell Medical Center
Department of Urology
New York, NY, USA
pnschleg@med.cornell.edu

Bart C. Fauser, Prof. Ph.D.
University Medical Center Utrecht
Department of Reproductive Medicine
Utrecht, The Netherlands
b.c.fauser@umcutrecht.nl

Douglas T. Carrell, Ph.D., H.C.L.D
Andrology and IVF Laboratories
Departments of Surgery (Urology)
Obstetrics and Gynecology and
Physiology
University of Utah School of Medicine
Salt Lake City, UT, USA
douglas.carrell@hsc.utah.edu

ISBN 978-1-4419-8455-5 e-ISBN 978-1-4419-8456-2
DOI 10.1007/978-1-4419-8456-2
Springer New York Dordrecht Heidelberg London

Library of Congress Control Number: 2011928231

Printed on acid-free paper

Springer is part of Springer Science+Business Media (www.springer.com)

We dedicate this book to Robert G. Edwards for his vision, creativity, and determination in the development of in vitro fertilization as a successful therapeutic option for infertility patients and for his enormous influence in the ethics and politics that challenge our field.

Preface

The initial volume of *Biennial Review of Infertility* was published in 2009. In the preface to that volume we shared our vision that this series would serve as a forum for evidence-based reviews of cutting-edge topics in the field of infertility, written by experts in the field and accessible and applicable to clinicians and researchers alike. We also began a tradition of highlighting and providing contrasting reviews to emerging and controversial topics. We are very pleased with the response we have had to *Biennial Reviews of Infertility*, Volume 1, and are excited now to present Volume 2.

The exponential growth of technologies and of data generated in research studies can be both breathtaking and daunting. The expansion in the number of manuscripts relevant to understanding infertility is growing not only due to growth in the number of researchers, but also due to emerging technologies, newly developing fields of study, and broad collaboration between diverse specialties. This volume includes discussion of cutting-edge topics such as epigenetics, proteomics, and the role of the environment in infertility, along with evidence-based discussion of routine clinical procedures. Together, these diverse topics are likely to benefit a wide spectrum of healthcare professionals involved in the study and treatment of infertility by providing both broad perspective and pointed practical advice.

We have all recently felt great excitement with the announcement of the awarding of the Nobel Prize in Medicine to Dr. Robert G. Edwards for his contributions to the development of in vitro fertilization as a therapy to millions of infertile patients. Dr. Edward's influence has been huge, not only in the science underpinning infertility, but also in the ethical and political arenas that impact our field. His contributions and the interface of these disciplines in our daily practices bring us to reflect on the advances we have made in understanding and treating infertility, and on the challenges that lay ahead. Such reflection can aid and inspire us in our quest to discover new insights through our studies for improved care of our patients. We hope that this volume of *Biennial Review of Infertility* can serve as a valuable reference and tool to implement "best practices" and to aid in the development of more accurate diagnoses and more effective treatments of infertility.

Boston, MA, USA	Catherine Racowsky
New York, NY, USA	Peter N. Schlegel
Utrecht, The Netherlands	Bart C. Fauser
Salt Lake City, UT, USA	Douglas T. Carrell

Contents

Part I Female Infertility

1 **Autoimmunity and Female Infertility: Fact vs. Fiction** 3
Lawrence N. Odom, Amy M. Cline, and William H. Kutteh

2 **Minimal Stimulation IVF** 11
Ahmad O. Hammoud and Mark Gibson

3 **Current Understanding of Anti-Müllerian Hormone** 19
Dimitrios G. Goulis, Marina A. Dimitraki, and Basil C. Tarlatzis

4 **The Role of Obesity in Reproduction** 35
Barbara Luke

5 **Endometrial Receptivity in Natural and Controlled Ovarian-Stimulated Cycles** 43
José A. Horcajadas, José A. Martínez-Conejero, and Carlos Simón

6 **Current Understanding of Mullerian-Inhibiting Substance** 57
Antonio La Marca, Giovanna Sighinolfi, and Annibale Volpe

7 **Evidence-Based Use of Progesterone During IVF** 79
Elena H. Yanushpolsky

8 **Monozygotic Twinning and Perinatal Outcomes** 91
Kenneth J. Moise Jr. and Ramesh Papanna

9 **Multiple Pregnancy Vanishing Twin Syndrome** 103
Gabriel de la Fuente, Jose Manuel Puente, Juan A. García-Velasco, and Antonio Pellicer

Part II Male Infertility

10 **The Effect of Cancer Therapies on Sperm: Current Guidelines** 117
Akanksha Mehta and Mark Sigman

11 **Environmental Insults on Spermatogenesis** ... 133
Stefan S. du Plessis and Ashok Agarwal

12 **Sperm DNA Damage: Causes and Guidelines for Current Clinical Practice** ... 155
Aleksander Giwercman, Marcello Spanò, and Mona Bungum

13 **The Emerging Role of the Sperm Epigenome and its Potential Role in Development** ... 181
Sue Hammoud and Douglas T. Carrell

Part III Assisted Reproduction Techniques

14 **ART and Epigenetic Disorders: Should We Be Concerned?** ... 197
Christopher N. Herndon and Paolo F. Rinaudo

15 **Novel Approaches of Sperm Selection for ART: The Role of Objective Biochemical Markers of Nuclear and Cytoplasmic Integrity and Sperm Function** ... 211
Gabor Huszar and Denny Sakkas

16 **The Role of the Oocyte in Remodeling of Male Chromatin and DNA Repair: Are Events During the Zygotic Cell Cycle of Relevance to ART?** ... 227
Liliana Ramos and Peter de Boer

17 **Proteomic/Metabolomic Analysis of Embryos: Current Status for Use in ART** ... 245
Mandy G. Katz-Jaffe and Susanna McReynolds

18 **Ultrasound-Guided Embryo Transfer** ... 255
Robert L. Gustofson and William B. Schoolcraft

Part IV Evolving Controversies in Contemporary Reproductive Medicine

19 **IMSI as a Valuable Tool for Sperm Selection During ART** ... 263
Monica Antinori, Pierre Vanderzwalmen, and Yona Barak

20 **Thoughts on IMSI** ... 277
Gianpiero D. Palermo, Jennifer C.Y. Hu, Laura Rienzi, Roberta Maggiulli, Takumi Takeuchi, Atsumi Yoshida, Atsushi Tanaka, Hiroshi Kusunoki, Seiji Watanabe, Queenie V. Neri, and Zev Rosenwaks

Index ... 291

Contributors

Ashok Agarwal, PhD, HCDL Center for Reproductive Medicine, Cleveland Clinic, Cleveland, OH, USA

Monica Antinori, MD Infertility Unit, RAPRUI Day Hospital, Rome, Italy

Yona Barak, PhD Dr. Yona Barak Laboratories Ltd, Rosh HaAyin, Israel

Mona Bungum, PhD Reproductive Medicine Centre, Skåne University Hospital, Malmö, Sweden; Department of Clinical Sciences, Lund University, Malmö, Sweden

Douglas T. Carrell, PhD, HCLD Andrology and IVF Laboratories, Departments of Surgery (Urology), Obstetrics and Gynecology and Physiology, University of Utah School of Medicine, Salt Lake City, UT, USA

Amy M. Cline, MD, PhD Division of Reproductive Endocrinology, Department of Obstetrics and Gynecology, The University of Tennessee Health Science Center, Memphis, TN, USA

Peter de Boer, PhD Department of Obstetrics and Gynecology, Radboud University Nijmegen Medical Center, Nijmegen, The Netherlands

Gabriel de la Fuente, MD IVI Madrid & Rey Juan Carlos University, Madrid, Spain

Marina A. Dimitraki, MD Section of Reproductive Medicine, First Department of Obstetrics and Gynecology, Medical School – Aristotle University of Thessaloniki, Thessaloniki, Greece

Stefan S. du Plessis, PhD Division of Medical Physiology, Stellenbosch University, Tygerberg, South Africa

Juan A. García-Velasco, MD, PhD IVI Madrid & Rey Juan Carlos University, Madrid, Spain

Aleksander Giwercman, MD, PhD Reproductive Medicine Centre, Skåne University Hospital, Malmö, Sweden; Department of Clinical Sciences, Lund University, Malmö, Sweden

Mark Gibson, MD Utah Center for Reproductive Medicine, Department of Obstetrics and Gynecology, University of Utah School of Medicine, Salt Lake City, UT, USA

Dimitrios G. Goulis, MD, PhD Section of Reproductive Medicine, First Department of Obstetrics and Gynecology, Medical School – Aristotle University of Thessaloniki, Thessaloniki, Greece

Robert L. Gustofson, MD Colorado Center for Reproductive Medicine, Lone Tree, CO, USA

Ahmad O. Hammoud, MD, MPH Utah Center for Reproductive Medicine, Department of Obstetrics and Gynecology, University of Utah, School of Medicine Salt Lake City, UT, USA

Sue Hammoud, BS Andrology and IVF Laboratories, Department of Surgery (Urology), University of Utah School of Medicine, Cairns Laboratory, Huntsman Cancer Institute, Salt Lake City, UT, USA

Christopher N. Herndon, MD Division of Reproductive Endocrinology and Infertility, Department of Obstetrics, Gynecology and Reproductive Sciences, University of California San Francisco, San Francisco, CA, USA

José A. Horcajadas, PhD Fundación IVI-Instituto Universitario IVI-University of Valencia, Valencia, Spain

Gabor Huszar, MD Sperm Physiology Laboratory, Department of Obstetrics, Gynecology and Reproductive Sciences, Yale University School of Medicine, New Haven, CT, USA

Jennifer C.Y. Hu, MSc The Ronald O. Perelman and Claudia Cohen Center for Reproductive Medicine, Weill Cornell Medical Center, New York, NY, USA

Mandy G. Katz-Jaffe, PhD Colorado Center for Reproductive Medicine, Lone Tree, CO, USA;
National Foundation for Fertility Research, Lone Tree, CO, USA

Hiroshi Kusunoki, PhD Faunal Diversity Science, Graduate School of Agriculture, Kobe University, Kobe, Japan

William H. Kutteh, MD, PhD Division of Reproductive Endocrinology, Department of Obstetrics and Gynecology, The University of Tennessee Health Science Center, Memphis, TN, USA

Antonio La Marca, MD, PhD Mother-Infant Department, Section of Obstetrics and Gynecology, University of Modena and Reggio Emilia, Modena, Italy

Barbara Luke, ScD, MPH Department of Obstetrics, Gynecology, and Reproductive Biology, Michigan State University, East Lansing, MI, USA

Susanna McReynolds, PhD National Foundation for Fertility Research, Lone Tree, CO, USA

Roberta Maggiulli, MSc Genera Center for Reproductive Medicine, Valle Giullia Clinic, Rome, Italy

José A. Martínez-Conejero, PhD Fundación IVI-Instituto Universitario IVI-University of Valencia, Valencia, Spain

Akanksha Mehta, MD Division of Urology, Rhode Island Hospital, Warren Alpert Medical School at Brown University, Providence, RI, USA

Kenneth J. Moise Jr., MD Department of Obstetrics and Gynecology, Division of Maternal-Fetal Medicine, Baylor College of Medicine and the Texas Children's Fetal Center, Texas Children's Hospital, Houston, TX, USA

Queenie V. Neri, BSc, MSc Candidate The Ronald O. Perelman and Claudia Cohen Center for Reproductive Medicine, Weill Cornell Medical Center, New York, NY, USA

Lawrence N. Odom, MD Division of Reproductive Endocrinology, Department of Obstetrics and Gynecology, The University of Tennessee Health Science Center, Memphis, TN, USA

Gianpiero D. Palermo, MD The Ronald O. Perelman and Claudia Cohen Center for Reproductive Medicine, Weill Cornell Medical College, New York, NY, USA

Ramesh Papanna, MD, MPH Department of Obstetrics and Gynecology, Division of Maternal-Fetal Medicine, Baylor College of Medicine and the Texas Children's Fetal Center, Texas Children's Hospital, Houston, TX, USA

Antonio Pellicer, MD, PhD IVI Valencia & Valencia University, Valencia, Spain

José Manuel Puente, MD IVI Madrid & Rey Juan Carlos University, Madrid, Spain

Liliana Ramos, PhD Department of Obstetrics and Gynecology, Radboud University Nijmegen Medical Center, Nijmegen, The Netherlands

Laura Rienzi, MSc Genera Center for Reproductive Medicine, Valle Giullia Clinic, Rome, Italy

Paolo F. Rinaudo, MD, PhD Department of Obstetrics, Gynecology and Reproductive Sciences, Division of Reproductive Endocrinology and Infertility, University of California, San Francisco, CA, USA

Zev Rosenwaks, MD The Ronald O. Perelman and Claudia Cohen Center for Reproductive Medicine, Weill Cornell Medical Center, New York, NY, USA

Denny Sakkas, PhD IVF Laboratories, Department of Obstetrics, Gynecology and Reproductive Sciences, Yale University School of Medicine, New Haven, CT, USA

William B. Schoolcraft, MD Colorado Center for Reproductive Medicine, Lone Tree, CO, USA

Giovanna Sighinolfi, MD Mother-Infant Department, Section of Obstetrics and Gynecology, University of Modena and Reggio Emilia, Modena, Italy

Mark Sigman, MD Division of Urology, Rhode Island Hospital, Warren Alpert Medical School, Brown University, Providence, RI, USA

Carlos Simón, MD, PhD Fundación IVI-Instituto Universitario IVI-University of Valencia, Valencia, Spain; Valencia Stem Cell Bank, Centro de Investigaciones Principe Felipe, Valencia, Spain

Marcello Spanò, PhD Laboratory of Toxicology, Unit of Radiation Biology and Human Health, UTBIORAD-TOSS, ENEA Casaccia Research Center, Rome, Italy

Takumi Takeuchi, MD, PhD The Reproduction Center, Kiba Park Clinic, Koto-ku, Tokyo, Japan

Atsushi Tanaka, PhD Saint Mother Hospital, Kitakyushu-City, Fukuoka, Japan

Basil C. Tarlatzis, MD, PhD Section of Reproductive Medicine, First Department of Obstetrics and Gynecology, Medical School – Aristotle University of Thessaloniki, Thessaloniki, Greece

Pierre Vanderzwalmen, PhD IVF Centers Prof. Zech, Bregenz, Austria; Centre Hospitalier Inter Régional Cavell (CHIREC), Braine l'Alleud, Brussels, Belgium

Annibale Volpe, MD Mother-Infant Department, Section of Obstetrics and Gynecology, University of Modena and Reggio Emilia, Modena, Italy

Seiji Watanabe, PhD Department of Anatomical Science, Hirosaki University Graduate School of Medicine, Hirosaki, Japan

Elena H. Yanushpolsky, MD Department of Obstetrics and Gynecology, Brigham and Women's Hospital, Boston, MA, USA

Atsumi Yoshida, MD The Reproduction Center, Kiba Park Clinic, Koto-ku, Tokyo, Japan

Part I

Female Infertility

Autoimmunity and Female Infertility: Fact vs. Fiction

1

Lawrence N. Odom, Amy M. Cline, and William H. Kutteh

Abstract

Several autoimmune factors have been investigated as possible influences on reproductive success of both natural conception and conception by the use of assisted reproductive technologies. In order for a pregnancy to succeed, two immunologically and genetically distinct tissues must coexist. During implantation, local and systemic immune factors, cytokines, and growth factors may interact with adhesion molecules and other matrix-associated proteins, glycoproteins, and peptides. Antiphospholipid antibodies are identified more frequently in women undergoing in vitro fertilization, but their presence does not appear to influence the outcome of pregnancy, miscarriage, or live birth rates. Antithyroid antibodies are commonly found in women of reproductive age, but implantation rates and miscarriage rates are not altered when women have normal thyroid function. Antinuclear antibodies may be a marker for underlying autoimmune disease when coupled with certain signs and symptoms, but low titer antibodies do not influence in vitro fertilization outcome. Antisperm antibodies are more often associated with fertilization failure when found in high titers in seminal plasma, on sperm, or in the mucosal immune system of women. Antiovarian antibodies are uncommon, but most often associated with ovarian hypofunction. Other autoimmune factors are under investigation as markers of in vitro fertilization failure.

Keywords

Antiphospholipid antibodies • Antinuclear antibodies • Antithyroid antibodies • Antiovarian antibodies • Antisperm antibodies • Infertility • In vitro fertilization

W.H. Kutteh (✉)
Division of Reproductive Endocrinology,
Department of Obstetrics and Gynecology,
The University of Tennessee Health Science Center,
Memphis, TN, USA
e-mail: wkutteh@uthsc.edu

C. Racowsky et al. (eds.), *Biennial Review of Infertility: Volume 2*,
DOI 10.1007/978-1-4419-8456-2_1,

1.1 Introduction

Approximately 10–15% of couples desiring children suffer from infertility. Despite thorough investigation, the cause of infertility remains unknown in at least 10% of these couples. "Reproductive autoimmune failure syndrome" was originally described by Gleicher et al. [1] in women with endometriosis, infertility, and increased autoantibodies. Autoimmunity refers to an immune reaction of the body against substances normally present in the body. Since the mention of this reproductive autoimmune failure syndrome, numerous studies have been performed in an attempt to identify specific factors or antibodies associated with pregnancy loss and infertility.

Implantation is one of the most important aspects of pregnancy that these studies have targeted. Implantation represents a critical developmental process in that it requires the interaction of immunologically and genetically distinct tissues. The immune system may influence pregnancy success or failure during any of the critical steps of implantation. First, the blastocyst must hatch from the zona pellucida to attach to the epithelium of the uterus. Second, apposition occurs when L-selectin on the blastocyst interacts with the endometrial surface expressing L-selectin ligand [2]. Next, hCG secreted from the human blastocyst induces troponin expression in human endometrial epithelial cells enriched in pinopodes [3]. Finally, the outer trophoblast layer must breach the epithelium and invade the underlying stroma and vasculature so as to establish a direct contact with maternal blood flow.

Attachment occurs only during the "implantation window," the time period when the epithelium is receptive. This period is from day 19–23 of a 28-day menstrual cycle. The preimplantation embryo must be at a developmental point such that it is capable of attaching to the endometrium of the uterus. Failure of this synchronization precludes success, as demonstrated in human studies of implantation [4].

Implantation is the most important limiting factor in human reproduction. Only 25% of all fertilized ova will generate a live birth and 50% appear to fail at time of implantation. Chromosomal abnormalities alone do not account for this number of pregnancy losses, meaning that a large number of these losses are otherwise normal human embryos. Human preimplantation embryos express major histocompatability antigens theoretically capable of inducing an immune response [5, 6]. The possibility exists that maternal immune responses play a role in the failure of implantation [7, 8].

1.2 Autoimmune Factors Potentially Related to Pregnancy Failure

Recent studies have investigated the role of autoimmune factors in implantation in women undergoing fertility treatment. The most commonly studied antibodies include antiphospholipid antibodies, antithyroid antibodies, antinuclear antibodies, antiovarain antibodies, and antisperm antibodies.

1.2.1 Antiphospholipid Antibodies

Antiphospholipid antibodies are present in an estimated 2–5% of the general population [9] and form a heterogenous group of antibodies that target negatively charged phospholipids via interaction with phospholipid-binding plasma protein [10]. Antiphospholipid antibodies are commonly associated with other autoimmune diseases, such as systemic lupus erythematosus, but can also present in isolation in the form of primary antiphospholipid syndrome [11]. Antiphospholipid syndrome was first described in 1983 in patients with concurrent lupus, the presence of anticardiolipin antibodies, and thrombosis [12]. Since this initial presentation, the criteria for diagnosis have been revised with the most recent revision in 2006. In order for a patient to be diagnosed with antiphospholipid syndrome, at least one of the clinical criteria and one of the laboratory criteria must be met as follows [13].

1.2.1.1 Clinical Criteria

1. Vascular thrombosis: One or more episodes of arterial, venous, or small vessel thrombosis in any tissue or organ.
2. Morbidity in pregnancy
   (a) One or more unexplained deaths of a morphologically normal fetus at or beyond the tenth week of gestation.
   (b) One or more premature births of a morphologically normal neonate prior to the 34th week of gestation secondary to eclampsia or severe preeclampsia or recognized features of placental insufficiency.
   (c) Three or more unexplained consecutive spontaneous miscarriages before the tenth week of gestation.

1.2.1.2 Laboratory Criteria

(Must be present on two or more occasions at least 12 weeks apart):

1. Lupus anticoagulant present.
2. Anticardiolipin antibody; medium or high titer (>40 μg of IgG or IgM phospholipid or >99th percentile) of IgG or IgM isotype.
3. Anti-β2-glycoprotein; medium or high titer (>40 μg of IgG or IgM phospholipid or >99th percentile) of IgG or IgM isotype.

The presence of antiphospholipid antibodies can have a tremendous impact on reproductive success. Antiphospholipids interact with the maternal–fetal interface in multiple aspects and are associated with recurrent spontaneous miscarriage [14] as well as preeclampsia, intrauterine growth restriction, and fetal demise. The involvement of antiphospholipid antibodies with pregnancy is thought to be more of an autoimmune factor than a thrombophilic factor as exhibited by histological studies showing a lack of intravascular or intervillous blood clots in placentas obtained following spontaneous miscarriage [15]. Studies have linked antiphospholipid antibodies with decreased release of hCG from human placental explants, prevention of in vitro trophoblast migration and invasion, inhibition of trophoblast cell adhesion molecules, and activation of complement on the trophoblast surface inducing an inflammatory response [16].

Antiphospholipid antibodies have been found in 15% of patient with recurrent first trimester loss [17] and up to 9% in patients with unexplained infertility and recurrent implantation failure [18]. Treatment of patients with antiphospholipid antibody-associated recurrent pregnancy loss with heparin and low-dose aspirin has been shown to improve live birth rates [14]. Treatment of patients with recurrent pregnancy loss and antiphospholipid antibodies with low molecular weight heparin and aspirin has also been shown to have similar obstetrical outcomes as well as safety parameters compared to treatment with unfractionated heparin and aspirin [19]. However, recent studies have not shown a benefit of treatment with unexplained recurrent pregnancy loss [20].

Several published reports indicate that positive APAs are found more frequently in patients undergoing IVF or who have failed IVF [21]. However, positive antiphospholipid antibodies have not been associated with decreased pregnancy rates in women undergoing IVF [22] and treatment with heparin and aspirin of women undergoing IVF who concurrently test positive for antiphospholipid antibodies does not improve pregnancy or implantation rates [23].

1.2.2 Antithyroid Antibodies

Antithyroid antibodies, specifically thyroglobulin and thyroid peroxidase antibodies, are commonly found in patients with Graves' disease, postpartum thyroiditis, and Hashimoto's thyroiditis. However, antithyroid antibodies have been reported in healthy individuals and are observed more frequently in women during their reproductive years [24]. The prevalence of antithyroid antibodies has been reported in 15–20% of normal pregnant women and women undergoing assisted reproductive techniques compared to 20–25% in women with recurrent miscarriage [25], and on average, 46% of pregnant women with a diagnosis of hypothyroidism [26].

Multiple studies have investigated the role of thyroid autoimmunity in infertility, but the interpretation of the evidence as a whole is difficult secondary to numerous variations in study design.

Some studies have shown a significantly increased relative risk for thyroid autoimmunity among endometriosis [27, 28], which can also be linked to infertility. However, others have failed to show this association [29]. Other studies have shown an association with ovarian causes of infertility, such as polycystic ovarian syndrome. Janssen et al. [30] reported a relative risk of 3.2 (CI 1.9–5.6) of both thyroglobulin and thyroid peroxidase in females with infertility and polycystic ovarian syndrome compared to age-matched controls, suggesting that multifactorial causes as opposed to isolated thyroid autoimmunity may be responsible for infertility.

Another theory is that hypothyroidism resulting from thyroid autoantibodies may be responsible for the increased incidence of infertility in this population. Thyroid hormone receptors have been described in human oocytes where they assist in the stimulation of granulosa cell function [31] and trophoblastic differentiation [32]. Cramer et al. [33] showed an increased risk of in vitro fertilization in women with infertility and elevated levels of thyroid-stimulating hormone, suggesting an association of hypothyroidism with adverse reproductive potential. Studies on the treatment of subclinical hypothyroidism are widely variable [26] and current guidelines on screening patients with infertility for thyroid dysfunction and autoimmunity are conflicted. There are insufficient data to recommend screening asymptomatic infertile women for autoimmune thyroid dysfunction.

1.2.3 Antinuclear Antibodies

Antinuclear antibodies are a group of antibodies that target nuclear and cytoplasmic antigens. These antigens are essential to cell function through playing a role in transcription, translation, and cell cycle regulation [34]. A positive antinuclear antibodies titer is associated with multiple autoimmune disorders such as systemic lupus erythematosus [34]. The role of antinuclear antibodies in infertility is largely undetermined; however, they have been associated with implantation failure secondary to an endometriosis-induced autoimmune reaction [35]. Elevated antinuclear antibody titers were discovered in 27% of patients with endometriosis compared to 18% of patients without endometriosis [36]. Implantation and pregnancy rates have been shown to improve with short-term medication-induced immunosuppression. However, this treatment has not been shown to improve live birth rates [37] and treatment of patients with positive antinuclear antibodies with heparin and aspirin failed to show an improvement in implantation and pregnancy rates [38]. A study performed recently [34] found elevated antinuclear antibody titers in 97 (50%) women with recurrent pregnancy loss and in only 16 (16%) of age-matched controls, but also state that the significance of this finding is yet to be determined.

1.2.4 Antiovarian Antibodies

Antiovarian antibodies include antibodies against a heterogeneous group of antigens, including molecular targets in the zona pellucida, theca interna, granulosa cells, ooplasm [39], and heat shock protein 90-β [40]. Studies have suggested numerous associations of antiovarian antibodies with infertility, such as reduced fertilization rates and pregnancy rates, inhibited response to gonadotropin stimulation, altered egg and embryo development, and possibly implantation failures [39]. One pilot study showed an improvement in pregnancy rate, implantation rate, and live birth rate with prednisolone administration to patients with antiovarian antibodies and at least two previously failed IVF attempts [41]. The authors [41] concluded that corticosteroids are useful in a subset of patients with IVF failure and autoimmunity. Data are still inadequate to provide a solid link between antiovarian antibodies and infertility, but their presence may be linked to ovarian hypofunction.

1.2.5 Antisperm Antibodies

Sperm contain antigens that are foreign to both male and female immune systems. Antisperm antibody production may be induced in the seminal plasma, in male or female serum, or in the

Table 1.1 Associations of autoantibodies with female infertility

Autoantibody	Frequency in infertile women	Infertility association	Known associations
Antiphospholipid	Increased	Unproven	Recurrent pregnancy loss
Antithyroid	No difference	Unproven	Thyroiditis
Antisperm	No difference	Unproven	Fertilization failure
Antinuclear	Slightly increased	Unproven	Autoimmune disease
Antiovarian	Slightly increased	Unproven	Ovarian failure

cervical mucus when sperm are exposed to the immune system [42]. Antisperm antibodies have been identified in 10–15% of men with infertility and in 15–20% of women with unexplained infertility. The prevalence and presumed significance reported depends on the population, source of the specimen (serum, cervical mucus, semen), and method of testing. These antibodies are postulated to interfere with the fecundity process through various mechanisms, such as interference with sperm transport within the female genital tract, alteration of sperm capacitation or acrosomal reaction, interference with fertilization, or inhibition of implantation of the early embryo. Possible sites where sperm-bound antisperm antibodies might interfere with fertilization include sperm binding to zona pellucida, sperm penetration of the zona pellucida, zona reaction, gamete fusion, embryo cleavage, and embryo development [43]. A few retrospective studies have suggested that sperm-bound antisperm antibodies decrease oocyte fertilization rates, implantation rates, or embryo quality; however, these data are not strong enough to recommend generalized screening in the infertility population.

1.3 Conclusion

Failed implantation as a result of early embryo demise is thought to play a tremendous role in pregnancy failure. We have recently demonstrated that the presence of antiphospholipid antibodies, antinuclear antibodies, and/or antithyroid antibodies does not affect the pregnancy outcome in donor oocyte recipients [44]. This suggests that pregnancy loss and infertility may be secondary to other causes such as embryonic defects, defects in uterine receptivity, or multifactorial causes [45].

Unfortunately, the majority of available data on the role of immunity in infertility is hindered by small or poorly conducted studies. This limits the ability to form definitive recommendations for the screening and treatment of autoimmunity in the infertile population. While the existence of two immunologically distinct organisms during pregnancy suggests an essential role of the immune system in fertility, additional studies are needed to suggest treatments and recommendations for immune modulation and screening in patients with infertility (Table 1.1).

Acknowledgments Funding: Frank Ling Research Grant in Obstetrics and Gynecology.

References

1. Gleicher N, El-Roeiy A, Confino E, Friberg J. Reproduction failure because of autoantibodies: unexplained infertility and pregnancy wastage. Am J Obstet Gynecol. 1989;160(6):1376–80.
2. Sugihara K, Kabir-Salmani M, Byrne J, et al. Induction of trophinin in human endometrial surface epithelia by CGbeta and IL-1beta. FEBS Lett. 2008;582(2): 197–202.
3. Fukunda MN, Sugihara K. An integrated view of L-selectin and troponin in human embryo implantation. J Obstet Gynaecol Res. 2008;34:129–36.
4. Milki AA, Hinckley MD, Fisch JD, et al. Comparison of blastocyst transfer with day 3 embryo transfer in similar patient populations. Fertil Steril. 2000;73(1): 126–9.
5. Moffett A, Loke C. Implantation, embryo-maternal interactions, immunology and modulation of the uterine environment – a workshop report. Placenta. 2006;27(Suppl A):S54–5.
6. Porcu-Buisson G, Lambert M, Lyonnet L, et al. Soluble MHC Class I chain-related molecule serum levels are predictive markers of implantation failure and successful term pregnancies following IVF. Hum Reprod. 2007;22(8):2261–6.
7. Yoshinaga K. Review of factors essential for blastocyst implantation for their modulating effects on the

maternal immune system. Semin Cell Dev Biol. 2008; 19(2):161–9.
8. Chaouat G, Ledee-Bataille N, Dubanchet S. Immune cells in uteroplacental tissues throughout pregnancy: a brief review. Reprod Biomed Online. 2007;14(2): 256–66.
9. Petri M. Epidemiology of the antiphospholipid antibody syndrome. J Autoimmun. 2000;15(2):145–51.
10. Galli M, Comfurius P, Maassen C, et al. Anticardiolipin antibodies (ACA) directed not to cardiolipin but to a plasma protein cofactor. Lancet. 1990;335(8705): 1544–7.
11. Cervera R, Piette JC, Font J, et al. Antiphospholipid syndrome: clinical and immunologic manifestations and patterns of disease expression in a cohort of 1000 patients. Arthritis Rheum. 2002;46(4):1019–27.
12. Hughes GR. Thrombosis, abortion, cerebral disease and the lupus anticoagulant. Br Med J. 1983; 287(6399):1088–9.
13. Miyakis S, Lockshin MD, Atsumi T, et al. International consensus statement on an update of the classification criteria for definite antiphospholipid syndrome (APS). J Thromb Haemost. 2006;4(2):295–306.
14. Kutteh WH. Antiphospholipid- antibody associated recurrent pregnancy loss treatment with heparin and low-dose aspirin is superior to low-dose aspirin alone. Am J Obstet Gynecol. 1996;174(5):1584–9.
15. Sebire NJ, Fox H, Backos M, et al. Defective endovascular trophoblast invasion in primary antiphospholipid antibody syndrome-associated early pregnancy failure. Hum Reprod. 2002;17(4):1067–71.
16. Girardi G, Yarilin D, Thurman JM, et al. Complement activation induces dysregulation of angiogenic factors and causes fetal rejection and growth restriction. J Exp Med. 2006;203(9):2165–75.
17. Rai RS, Clifford K, Cohen H, Regan L. High prospective fetal loss rate in untreated pregnancies of women with recurrent miscarriage and antiphospholipid antibodies. Hum Reprod. 1995;10(12):3301–4.
18. Sauer R, Roussev R, Jeyendran RS, Coulam CB. Prevalence of antiphospholipid antibodies among women experiencing unexplained infertility and recurrent implantation failure. Fertil Steril. 2010;93(7):2441–3.
19. Noble LS, Kutteh WH, Lashey N, et al. Antiphospholipid antibodies associated with recurrent pregnancy loss: prospective, multicenter, controlled pilot study comparing treatment with low-molecular-weight heparin versus unfractionated heparin. Fertil Steril. 2005;83(3):684–90.
20. Kaandorp SP, Goddijn M, van der Post JA, et al. Aspirin plus heparin or aspirin alone in women with recurrent miscarriage. N Engl J Med. 2010;362(17): 1586–96.
21. Ghazeeri GS, Kutteh WH. Autoimmunity and assisted reproduction. Infertil Reprod Med Clin North Am. 2002;13:183–201.
22. Hornstein MD, Davis OK, Massey JB, et al. Antiphospholipid antibodies and in vitro fertilization success: a meta-analysis. Fertil Steril. 2000;73(2): 330–3.
23. Kutteh WH, Yetman DL, Chantilis SJ, Crain J. Effect of antiphospholipid antibodies in women undergoing in vitro fertilization: role of heparin and aspirin. Hum Reprod. 1997;12(6):1171–5.
24. Geva E, Amit A, Lerner-Geva L, Lessing JB. Autoimmunity and reproduction. Fertil Steril. 1997;67(4):599–611.
25. Kutteh WH, Yetman DL, Carr AC, et al. Increased prevalence of antithyroid antibodies identified in women with recurrent pregnancy loss but not in women undergoing assisted reproduction. Fertil Steril. 1999;71(5):843–8.
26. Poppe K, Velkeniers B, Glinoer D. The role of thyroid autoimmunity in fertility and pregnancy. Nat Clin Pract Endocrinol Metab. 2008;4(7):394–405.
27. Poppe K, Glinoer D, Van Steirteghem A, et al. Thyroid dysfunction and autoimmunity in infertile women. Thyroid. 2002;12(11):997–1001.
28. Abalovich M, Mitelberg L, Allami C, et al. Subclinical hypothyroidism and thyroid autoimmunity in women with infertility. Gynecol Endocrinol. 2007;23(5): 279–83.
29. Petta CA, Arruda MS, Zantut-Wittmann DE, Benetti-Pinto CL. Thyroid autoimmunity and thyroid dysfunction in women with endometriosis. Hum Reprod. 2007;22(10):2693–7.
30. Janssen OE, Mehlmauer N, Hahn S, et al. High prevalence of autoimmune thyroiditis in patients with polycystic ovary syndrome. Eur J Endocrinol. 2004; 150(3):363–9.
31. Wakim AN, Polizotto SL, Buffo MJ, et al. Thyroid hormones in human follicular fluid and thyroid hormone hormone receptors in human granulosa cells. Fertil Steril. 1993;59(6):1187–90.
32. Maruo T, Matsuo H, Mochizuki M. Thyroid hormone as a biological amplifier of differentiated trophoblast function in early pregnancy. Acta Endocrinol (Copenh). 1991;125(1):58–66.
33. Cramer DW, Sluss PM, Powers RD, et al. Serum prolactin and TSH in an in vitro fertilization population: is there a link between fertilization and thyroid function? J Assist Reprod Genet. 2003;20(6):210–5.
34. Ticconi C, Rotondi F, Veglia M, et al. Antinuclear autoantibodies in women with recurrent pregnancy loss. Am J Reprod Immunol. 2010;64(6):384–92.
35. Tomassetti C, Meuleman C, Pexsters A, et al. Endometriosis, recurrent miscarriage and implantation failure: is there an immunological link? Reprod Biomed Online. 2006;13(1):58–64.
36. Lucena E, Cubillos J. Immune abnormalities in endometriosis compromising fertility in IVF-ET patients. J Reprod Med. 1999;44(5):458–64.
37. Taniguchi F. Results of prednisolone given to improve the outcome of in vitro fertilization-embryo transfer in women with antinuclear antibodies. J Reprod Med. 2005;50(6):383–8.
38. Stern C, Chamley L, Norris H, et al. A randomized, double-blind, placebo controlled trial of heparin and aspirin for women with in vitro fertilization implantation failure and antiphospholipid or antinuclear antibodies. Fertil Steril. 2003;80(2):376–83.

39. Pires ES. Multiplicity of molecular and cellular targets in human ovarian autoimmunicty: an update. J Assist Reprod Genet. 2010;27(9–10):519–24.
40. Pires ES, Khole VV. A block in the road to fertility: autoantibodies to heat-shock protein 90-β in human ovarian autoimmunity. Fertil Steril. 2009;92(4):1395–409.
41. Forges T, Monnier-Barbarino P, Guillet-May F, et al. Corticosteroids in patients with antiovarian antibodies undergoing in vitro fertilization: a prospective pilot study. Eur J Clin Pharmacol. 2006;62(9):699–705.
42. Marshburn PB, Kutteh WH. The role of antisperm antibodies in infertility. Fertil Steril. 1994;61(5):799–811.
43. Kutteh WH. Do antisperm antibodies bound to spermatozoa alter normal reproductive function? Hum Reprod. 1999;14(10):2426–9.
44. Chantilis SJ, Kutteh WH, Blankenship L, et al. Antiphospholipid (APA), antinuclear (ANA), and antithyroid (ATA) do not affect pregnancy outcome in oocyte donation recipients [abstract P-835]. Am Soc Reprod Med. Nov 2008;64th Annual Meeting.
45. Margalioth EJ, Ben-Chetrit A, Gal M, Eldar-Geva T. Investigation and treatment of repeated implantation failure following IVF-ET. Hum Reprod. 2006; 21(12):3036–43.

2 Minimal Stimulation IVF

Ahmad O. Hammoud and Mark Gibson

Abstract

Minimal stimulation IVF was utilized in the early IVF experiences. It is proposed now as a solution for the unwanted consequences and costs of current conventional IVF protocols. Minimal stimulation IVF is thought to be a means to achieve some of the fertility-enhancing effects of IVF while minimizing discomforts, risks (especially of ovarian hyperstimulation syndrome), and costs. An additional benefit is a marked reduction in the likelihood of unused embryos. In aggregate, these advantages should increase the access to and acceptability of IVF for many potential patients. While the per cycle pregnancy rate in minimal stimulation IVF is lower than that of conventional protocols, proponents of this method cite increased patient tolerance and access that allow multiple efforts, with a cumulative success rate that can approach that of a single cycle of conventional IVF (Curr Opin Obstet Gynecol 22:189–192, 2010). Minimal stimulation IVF is now being offered in many fertility clinics both to young patients with good prognosis and to poor responders and women of advanced age as an alternative to conventional protocols. The renewed interest in minimal stimulation IVF is largely a result of improved outcomes in the IVF laboratory that have led to higher likelihoods of viable embryos and better success rates with single embryo transfer.

Keywords

IVF • Hyperstimulation • Gonadotropins • Minimal stimulation • Embryo transfer

A.O. Hammoud (✉)
Utah Center for Reproductive Medicine,
Department of Obstetrics and Gynecology,
University of Utah School of Medicine,
Salt Lake City, UT, USA
e-mail: ahmad.hammoud@hsc.utah.edu

C. Racowsky et al. (eds.), *Biennial Review of Infertility: Volume 2*,
DOI 10.1007/978-1-4419-8456-2_2, © Springer Science+Business Media, LLC 2011

2.1 Classification and Terminology

The field of minimal stimulation IVF is becoming popular and several recent publications have described the success with various stimulation protocols [1–4]. It is not uncommon to refer to minimal stimulation IVF as mild stimulation IVF or low-dose IVF. The various protocols and terminology used in this field make the comparison between studies challenging (Table 2.1). An interested group of experts from the International Society for Mild Approaches in Assisted Reproduction (ISMAAR) met and proposed the following classifications [5].

2.1.1 Natural Cycle IVF

The term Natural cycle IVF should be used when IVF is carried out with oocytes collected from a woman's ovary or ovaries in a spontaneous menstrual cycle without administration of any medication at any time during the cycle. The aim of this cycle is to collect a naturally selected single oocyte at the lowest possible cost.

2.1.2 Modified Natural Cycle IVF

The term Modified natural cycle should be applied when exogenous hormones or any drugs are used when IVF is being performed during a spontaneous cycle with the aim of collecting a naturally selected single oocyte, but with a reduction in chance of cycle cancelation. Modified natural cycle IVF employs hCG triggering of ovulation, with or without concomitant GnRH antagonist for suppression of the endogenous LH surge.

2.1.3 Mild IVF

A mild IVF cycle is defined by use of oral agents (antiestrogens or aromatase inhibitors) and/or low-dose gonadotropins to modestly increase oocyte yields (2–7 oocytes). LH surge suppression with GnRH antagonist and triggering with hCG or GnRH agonist is followed by luteal support.

2.1.4 Conventional IVF

This term is used to define scenarios in which conventional gonadotropin dosing is employed to achieve maximum controlled ovarian hyperstimulation below the threshold for significant risk of OHSS. In all such scenarios, endogenous LH is suppressed with GnRH agonist in long or flare protocols, or with GnRH antogonist, triggering employs hCG or GnRH agonist, and luteal support is given.

2.2 Adoption of Minimal Stimulation IVF

There are currently several proposed indications for minimal stimulation IVF, including young patients with male factor or tubal factor infertility, poor responders, and patients with prior implantation failures [6, 7]. The rationale for its use in poor responders is that comparable oocyte yields

Table 2.1 Different protocols of minimal stimulation IVF

	Ovarian stimulation	Prevention of premature LH surge	Ovulation trigger	Luteal phase support
Natural cycle IVF	None	None	None	None
Modified natural cycle IVF	None	None	hCG	Yes
	Gonadotropins add back	GnRH antagonist	hCG	Yes
Mild IVF	Clomiphene, letrozole, early or late low-dose gonadotropins	GnRH antagonist	hCG, or GnRH agonist	Yes
Conventional IVF	High-dose gonadotropins	GnRH agonist or antagonist	hCG, or GnRH agonist	Yes

are obtained without the costs and intrusiveness of high-dose conventional dosing, but success of this approach for these patients has been mixed [7]. Adoption of minimal stimulation IVF has been slow, particularly in the United States where it is not offered in most centers. The slow acceptance of minimal stimulation IVF is thought in part to be due to reluctance of clinics to use protocols that might adversely affect their published success rates in a competitive marketplace. Other factors include the often smaller margin of profitability, reduced number of embryo available for cryopreservation, and health plans that limit the benefits to a certain number of IVF cycles [6].

2.3 Comparison of Different Protocols for Minimal Stimulation IVF

2.3.1 Modified Natural Cycle IVF

Natural Cycle IVF was the protocol used in the early publications describing IVF [8]. Since then, several changes were introduced to the normal cycle IVF, mainly the control of the LH surge and modified oocyte retrieval methods. Natural IVF cycles have an inherently high cancelation rate because of premature LH surge, premature ovulation, and increased risk of failed oocyte retrieval [4]. Because of the unpredictable nature of the natural LH surge, early natural IVF cycles required intense and frequent monitoring and around the clock availability of the IVF team and laboratory to achieve a successful retrieval [2]. Controlling the timing of ovulation was one of the main achievements that improved the feasibility of natural cycle IVF. This was achieved with the administration of hCG to trigger the ovulation and later the introduction of GnRH antagonist to suppress the endogenous LH surge. Other less known methods to prevent a premature LH surge include endomethacin and clomiphene use [9, 10].

The introduction of hCG injection to trigger ovulation helped reduce the cancelation rates with natural IVF. In a study that included 35 women with infertility and tubal damage and 17 women with reduced ovarian reserve, a total of 202 natural cycle IVFs were performed [4]. All women who participated in this study had normal menstrual function and normal semen parameters in the male partner. The median age was 34 years with a range of 24–40 years. The protocol for natural cycle IVF in this study included initiating follicular scan on day 8 or 9 of a natural cycle, ultrasound monitoring was repeated as appropriate, and hCG 5,000 IU was administered when the follicular diameter reached 16–18 mm. There was no follicular growth documented in 21 cycles. In the 181 cycles where oocyte retrieval was attempted, pregnancy rate per cycle was 12.7% and live birth rate was 8.8%. After four cycles, the cumulative pregnancy rate was 46% and cumulative birth rate was 32% [4]. A subgroup of this cohort received Indomethacin 50 mg three times daily which was administered from Friday until Monday morning to allow delaying hCG administration so that all retrievals could occur on week days. Of these subjects, the rate of oocyte retrieval was 90.4%, oocyte fertilization 71%, and pregnancy rates per cycle 9.6% [4].

McDougall et al. compared modified natural IVF to IVF after stimulation with clomiphene 100 mg daily from day 3–7. The cancelation rate in the modified natural IVF cycle (4/14) was higher than that in the group stimulated with clomiphene (0/16). The clinical pregnancy rate was lower in modified natural IVF group (0%) when compared to that after clomiphene stimulation (18% per transfer) [11]. In a later study, Ingerlev et al. compared modified natural cycle IVF to clomiphene stimulation. This study included good prognosis young patient (<35 years), with unexplained, tubal, or severe male factor infertility and regular cycles. The proportion of cycle that resulted in embryo transfer (53.2%) was higher in the clomiphene group when compared to that in the modified natural cycle IVF group (25.4%). The clinical pregnancy rates in the clomiphene group (18% per cycle and 33.9% per transfer) were higher than those in the modified natural IVF group (3.5 and 13.8%, respectively) [12]. In women with previous poor response (less than four follicles), modified natural cycle IVF had higher implantation rates (14.9%) when compared to the GnRH agonist microflare protocol (5.5%); however, the ongoing pregnancy rates were similar (6.1% in the natural cycle group and 6.9% in microflare protocol) [13].

While natural IVF cycle with utilization of hCG to trigger ovulation is classified as modified natural IVF, true modified natural IVF cycle refers mainly to the utilization of GnRH antagonists to prevent premature LH surge. The administration of gonadotropins helps supplement the natural gonadotropins expected to fall after the administration of GnRH antagonist, which helps maintain the follicular growth and the estradiol levels [14].

Pelinck et al. described a protocol for modified natural IVF cycle as follows: During spontaneous unstimulated cycles, follicular scans were initiated on cycles days 3 or 8, then repeated daily or every other day. A mean follicular diameter of 14 mm was used to determine the need to start the GnRH antagonist to prevent premature LH surge. At the same day, 150 IU of recombinant FSH (rFSH) was also started. The GnRH antagonist and rFSH were continued daily until the day of triggering of ovulation. The follicular growth was monitored with daily or every other day morning follicular scans, LH, and estradiol levels. hCG 10,000 IU was given when a mean follicular diameter of 18 mm and or an estrogen levels of 0.8 nmol/L (218 pg/dL) were reached. Cycle cancelation occurred if there was premature LH surge documented by an elevated LH levels ≥20 IU/L (if the mean follicular diameter was less than 15 mm), or regardless of the follicular diameter, if the LH levels were ≥30 IU/L. Oocyte retrieval occurred 34 h after hCG injection. Analgesia was only given at patient's request. In this protocol, embryo transfer occurred on day 3 and luteal support was provided through hCG injections of 1,500 IU days 5, 8, and 11 after oocytes retrieval [15]. The rate of oocyte retrieval was 76.9% and the rate of 2PN fertilization was 68.2% per oocytes. The rate of transfer was 43.7% per initiate cycle. The success rates of this protocol were initially reported as a birth rate of 13.4% per initiated cycles and 30.8% per embryo transfer [15]. In a later study, the cumulative live birth rate with this protocol after three cycles in a cohort of 350 patients was reported as 20.8% per patient [3]. The same group published a study that looked at the cumulative pregnancy rate after an average of nine cycles of modified natural cycle (using GnRH antagonist) and reported a modest 8% ongoing pregnancy rate per cycle in a cohort of 268 patients aged 18–36 with regular ovulatory function [14]. In patient with previously poor response with conventional IVF, the success of modified natural IVF cycle was reported to be between 0 and 14% [2].

2.3.2 Mild IVF

Mild stimulation IVF can be done using antiestrogens for ovulation induction such as clomiphene or letrozole or using low-dose gonadotropins. Typically, endogenous LH is suppressed by addition of GnRH antagonist once folliculogenesis is underway. Proponents of milder stimulation propose several advantages to this protocol including: the possibilities of a more receptive endometrium and better quality embryos as well as less stress for patient and lower overall costs [16]. This approach may be most effective in young patients with normal ovarian function and good prognosis. Advantages of oral antiestrogen when compared to gonadotropins includes oral administration, lower costs, and wider availability [2].

A mild stimulation cycle using clomiphene can start with 100 mg of clomiphene from day 3 to day 7 of the cycle. Gonadotropins (HMG or rFSH) are given at a dose of 150 IU at day 9 of the cycle. Ultrasound monitoring starts at day 9 of the cycle and then frequently after that. GnRH antagonist is started when the lead follicle reaches 14 mm in diameter and is continued until the day of ovulation induction. hCG is used to trigger ovulation and retrieval occurs 35 h after the hCG injection. Luteal support is given as IM progesterone injection or vaginal suppositories [17].

When compared to conventional IVF, mild IVF using clomiphene (with or without the GnRH antagonist) showed similar clinical pregnancy rate in a retrospective controlled study (37% for minimal stimulation and 41% for conventional IVF) [17]. Weigert et al. compared the success of mild IVF using clomiphene followed by gonadotropins to conventional IVF in a randomized controlled study. The pregnancy rate per initiated cycle in the mild stimulation cycle (35.1%) was not statistically different from that in the conventional IVF group (29.3%) [18]. Another study compared the clomiphene /gonadotropins protocol with the GnRH antagonist to conventional long stimulation IVF, in patients undergoing their first IVF ICSI for male factor infertility. They found similar pregnancy rates in both treatment groups (41.7 and 40%) [19].

An alternative protocol for mild stimulation IVF was developed to alleviate some of the concerns associated with the utilization of GnRH antagonist including a low LH environment and the requirement of a relatively high dose of gonadotropins [9]. This protocol relies on continuation of clomiphene to inhibit the LH surge. A Japanese group reported their experience with this protocol in 44,345 cycles. Clomiphene was administered at a dose of 50 mg daily until the day before triggering ovulation using a GnRH agonist. If the patient was found to have multifollicular growth, gonadotropins were added at a dose of 150 IU every other day (urinary HMG or rFSH) until the day before the GnRH agonist trigger. GnRH agonist was administered when the follicular diameter reached 18 mm or the estradiol level was ≥300 pg/mL. Follicular scans were started at day 8. Oocyte retrieval occurred 32–35 h after the ovulation trigger. The rate of premature LH surge with this protocol was 5.1%. Among this small subset of women with detected LH surges, Oocyte retrieval was scheduled immediately when LH levels indicated an imminent ovulation by reaching its peak value and documentation of a drop in 4 h. Oocyte retrieval was delayed 24 h if LH levels suggested the onset of LH surge by documenting increased levels in 4 h. Luteal phase support was provided using dydrogesterone at a dose of 30 mg daily. The embryo transfer occurred at either the four cells or the blastocyst stages. The use of birth control in the preceding month increased the number of oocytes and embryos available. The live birth rate for the fresh embryo transfer of four cell stage embryos was 5.2%, the frozen four cell embryo transfer 0.2%, and for the frozen blastocyst transfer 5.6% [9].

Aromatase inhibitors have been suggested as another way of reducing the total requirement of gonadotropins in ovarian stimulation protocols for mild IVF [20]. The role of aromatase inhibitors in IVF remains poorly studied. Grabia et al. studied letrozole (2.5 mg) as an alternative to clomiphene in minimal stimulation IVF in good prognosis patients. A clinical pregnancy rate of 27% was reported [21].

Gonadotropins may be used without prior oral agents in low doses with the intent to reduce the costs of medications and avoid complications associated with standard controlled ovarian hyperstimulation. They may be initiated on day 2–3 of cycle or in the second half of the follicular phase, although early starts more consistently achieve multifollicular responses [22]. Fernandez-Shaw et al. reported the efficacy of the low gonadotropins IVF protocol in 79 young women with a good prognosis. Patients with polycystic ovarian syndrome, severe endometriosis, ovarian failure, or elevated early follicular FSH or estradiol were excluded. The stimulation starts similar to the traditional long stimulation protocol utilizing GnRH agonist in the luteal phase of the previous cycle. Pituitary suppression is evaluated on day 3 by vaginal ultrasound and estradiol levels (<50 pg/mL). Gonadotropins were started on day 3 at a low dose of 100 IU rFSH. After 5–6 days of stimulation, the dose is increased if needed. hCG 10,000 IU was given when 1–3 follicles reached 18 mm. Oocyte retrieval was performed 35 h after hCG injection. Luteal support was given in the form of intravaginal micronized progesterone at a dose of 200 mg TID starting the day of oocytes retrieval. The protocol resulted in lower number of embryo when compared to conventional dose gonadotropins (150 IU); however, the pregnancy rates were not different (51.8 vs. 50.7%) [16].

2.4 Minimal Stimulation IVF and Single Embryo Transfer

One goal of minimal stimulation IVF is to reduce the number of multiple pregnancies as well as the cost of care. The overall number of embryos transferred should be, in theory, lower than that during conventional IVF, and if combined with single embryo transfer, the cost saving could be considerable [23]. Heijnen et al. compared, in a randomized controlled study, the success of four cycles of mild IVF (gonadotropins started mid follicular phase) with single embryo transfer to three cycles of conventional IVF with transfer of two embryos [24]. Participants were good prognosis women who either had one birth through IVF or did not have IVF before. The patients were younger than 38 and had regular cycles and BMIs. The duration of stimulation, total dose of medication, number of oocyte retrieved, and number of embryo transferred were lower in the mild IVF group when compared to the conventional IVF group. The rate of live birth per started fresh mild IVF cycle with single embryo transfer (15.8%) was lower when compared with that of conventional IVF with dual embryo transfer (24%). Cumulative pregnancy rate and term delivery were calculated by adding the rates of pregnancy of the fresh and frozen cycle that originated from the same treatments. The 1-year cumulative term live birth rate per couple (43.4%) in the mild IVF group was not inferior to that of the conventional IVF group (44.7%). The proportion of multiple pregnancy rates per couple in 1 year in the mild IVF group (0.5%) was significantly lower than that in the conventional IVF group (13.1%) [24].

2.5 Follicular Flushing

In protocols where few mature follicles are present, optimal yield of oocytes per follicle is critical [25]. Follicular flushing has been advocated as a way to improve the yield of oocytes during oocyte retrieval in the hope of increasing the number of good quality embryos available for transfer. Follicular flushing is thought to have a role in patients undergoing conventional IVF with poor response or in patients undergoing minimal stimulation IVF [26]. The technique of follicle flushing can vary between centers. The most common technique involves the utilization of double lumen needles that can be used to aspirate the follicular fluid. The follicle is then injected with a sterile solution (such as sterile phosphate-buffered saline) and the fluid is reaspirated. The procedure can be repeated. In one study, the optimal number of flushing was found to be four, and beyond this, the yield of oocyte retrieval is low [25]. Another study showed that only 4.3% of oocytes can be retrieved with the second flushing [27].

A recent randomized controlled trial compared follicular flushing to direct follicular aspiration in poor responders to conventional IVF stimulation. Poor responders were defined as patients who on the day of oocytes retrieval had a cumulative follicle count of 4–8 follicle ≥12 mm and at least two follicles ≥16 mm. There was no difference in the total number of oocytes or number of mature oocytes between the study groups. However, retrieval time was two times longer in patients undergoing follicular flushing when compared to direct aspiration technique. Follicular flushing did not improve the fertilization, implantation, or pregnancy rates [28]. Other observational studies did not show any benefit from follicular aspiration in the context of conventional IVF [26, 29].

In the context of minimal stimulation IVF, follicle flushing may be more important because of the expected low number of oocytes retrieved [30]. The competence of oocyte retrieved through flushing in the context of minimal stimulation IVF was studied by Lozano et al. In this study, 271 minimal stimulation IVF cycles were included. The oocytes retrieved were divided into two groups: retrieved with the first aspiration or retrieved through flushing. Embryo morphology and implantation rates were higher in the oocytes retrieved through flushing; however, the fertilization rate and clinical pregnancy rates were comparable in both groups [31, 32].

2.6 Cost Considerations

Cost of fertility treatment and IVF are under strict scrutiny and often cited as the reason for the absence of insurance coverage of fertility care in the United States [33, 34]. Economic considerations remain the main barrier to increased IVF availability and utilization in the United States [35].

Minimal stimulation IVF is thought to reduce the overall cost of fertility treatment. The cost reduction results from the reduced dose of gonadotropins and the presence of fewer embryos which can reduce the variable costs of IVF laboratories and may permit lower fees for IVF procedures (retrieval, fertilization, and culture fees). The cost of natural IVF cycle based on the cost of limited ultrasound scans, oocyte retrieval, cost of embryo transfer, and cost of medication is thought to be 23% of that of conventional IVF [4]. However, with lower pregnancy rates, cumulative costs incurred to achieve likelihoods of pregnancy rivaling those seen with conventional IVF may not offer savings relative to conventional IVF [7]. Another proposed cost reduction with minimal stimulation IVF occurs if associated with single embryo transfer [24, 36]. Although single embryo transfer may be common with minimal stimulation IVF because of limited numbers of oocytes and viable embryos, it is not by any means within the exclusive domain of minimal stimulation IVF and can be employed with the same benefits in conventional IVF. Single embryo transfer results in an overall reduction in the cost of care of infertility patients by reducing multiple pregnancy rates. When minimal stimulation IVF was associated with single embryo transfer, the incremental cost per additional pregnancy leading to live birth in the conventional IVF was €185,000 when compared to minimal stimulation IVF [24]. It is predicted that with increasing success of single embryo transfer, the option of minimal stimulation IVF in good prognosis patient would reduce the number of multiple pregnancies and the overall cost of care [36].

2.7 Conclusion

In conclusion, minimal stimulation IVF is gaining more ground because of increased concern regarding the complications of conventional IVF. Clinical pregnancy rates per cycle are lower with minimal stimulation IVF when compared to conventional IVF. However, with better tolerance of minimal stimulation protocols, cumulative pregnancy rates may be similar. Ideal candidates for minimal stimulation IVF are young patients with good prognosis or patients who failed conventional IVF. Minimal stimulation IVF has the potential of reducing the side effects of IVF as well as the overall cost of care.

References

1. Moragianni VA, Penzias AS. Cumulative live-birth rates after assisted reproductive technology. Curr Opin Obstet Gynecol. 2010;22:189–92.
2. Verberg MF, Macklon NS, Nargund G, et al. Mild ovarian stimulation for IVF. Hum Reprod Update. 2009;15:13–29.
3. Pelinck MJ, Vogel NE, Hoek A, et al. Cumulative pregnancy rates after three cycles of minimal stimulation IVF and results according to subfertility diagnosis: a multicentre cohort study. Hum Reprod. 2006;21:2375–83.
4. Nargund G, Waterstone J, Bland J, Philips Z, Parsons J, Campbell S. Cumulative conception and live birth rates in natural (unstimulated) IVF cycles. Hum Reprod. 2001;16:259–62.
5. Nargund G, Fauser BC, Macklon NS, Ombelet W, Nygren K, Frydman R. The ISMAAR proposal on terminology for ovarian stimulation for IVF. Hum Reprod. 2007;22:2801–4.
6. Heng BC. Reluctance of medical professionals in adopting natural-cycle and minimal ovarian stimulation protocols in human clinical assisted reproduction. Reprod Biomed Online. 2007;15:9–11.
7. Kolibianakis E, Zikopoulos K, Camus M, Tournaye H, Van Steirteghem A, Devroey P. Modified natural cycle for IVF does not offer a realistic chance of parenthood in poor responders with high day 3 FSH levels, as a last resort prior to oocyte donation. Hum Reprod. 2004;19:2545–9.
8. Steptoe PC, Edwards RG. Birth after the reimplantation of a human embryo. Lancet. 1978;2:366.
9. Teramoto S, Kato O. Minimal ovarian stimulation with clomiphene citrate: a large-scale retrospective study. Reprod Biomed Online. 2007;15:134–48.
10. Nargund G, Wei CC. Successful planned delay of ovulation for one week with indomethacin. J Assist Reprod Genet. 1996;13:683–4.
11. MacDougall MJ, Tan SL, Hall V, Balen A, Mason BA, Jacobs HS. Comparison of natural with clomiphene citrate-stimulated cycles in in vitro fertilization: a prospective, randomized trial. Fertil Steril. 1994;61:1052–7.
12. Ingerslev HJ, Hojgaard A, Hindkjaer J, Kesmodel U. A randomized study comparing IVF in the unstimulated cycle with IVF following clomiphene citrate. Hum Reprod. 2001;16:696–702.
13. Morgia F, Sbracia M, Schimberni M, et al. A controlled trial of natural cycle versus microdose gonadotropin-releasing hormone analog flare cycles in poor responders undergoing in vitro fertilization. Fertil Steril. 2004;81:1542–7.

14. Pelinck MJ, Knol HM, Vogel NE, et al. Cumulative pregnancy rates after sequential treatment with modified natural cycle IVF followed by IVF with controlled ovarian stimulation. Hum Reprod. 2008;23:1808–14.
15. Pelinck MJ, Vogel NE, Hoek A, Arts EG, Simons AH, Heineman MJ. Minimal stimulation IVF with late follicular phase administration of the GnRH antagonist cetrorelix and concomitant substitution with recombinant FSH: a pilot study. Hum Reprod. 2005;20:642–8.
16. Fernandez-Shaw S. Perez Esturo N, Cercas Duque R, Pons Mallol I. Mild IVF using GnRH agonist long protocol is possible: comparing stimulations with 100 IU vs. 150 IU recombinant FSH as starting dose. J Assist Reprod Genet. 2009;26:75–82.
17. Williams SC, Gibbons WE, Muasher SJ, Oehninger S. Minimal ovarian hyperstimulation for in vitro fertilization using sequential clomiphene citrate and gonadotropin with or without the addition of a gonadotropin-releasing hormone antagonist. Fertil Steril. 2002;78:1068–72.
18. Weigert M, Krischker U, Pohl M, Poschalko G, Kindermann C, Feichtinger W. Comparison of stimulation with clomiphene citrate in combination with recombinant follicle-stimulating hormone and recombinant luteinizing hormone to stimulation with a gonadotropin-releasing hormone agonist protocol: a prospective, randomized study. Fertil Steril. 2002; 78:34–9.
19. Lin YH, Hwang JL, Seow KM, Huang LW, Hsieh BC, Tzeng CR. Comparison of outcome of clomiphene citrate/human menopausal gonadotropin/cetrorelix protocol and buserelin long protocol–a randomized study. Gynecol Endocrinol. 2006;22:297–302.
20. Mitwally MF, Casper RF. Aromatase inhibition reduces gonadotrophin dose required for controlled ovarian stimulation in women with unexplained infertility. Hum Reprod. 2003;18:1588–97.
21. Grabia A, Papier S, Pesce R, Mlayes L, Kopelman S, Sueldo C. Preliminary experience with a low-cost stimulation protocol that includes letrozole and human menopausal gonadotropins in normal responders for assisted reproductive technologies. Fertil Steril. 2006;86:1026–8.
22. de Jong D, Macklon NS, Fauser BC. A pilot study involving minimal ovarian stimulation for in vitro fertilization: extending the "follicle-stimulating hormone window" combined with the gonadotropin-releasing hormone antagonist cetrorelix. Fertil Steril. 2000; 73:1051–4.
23. Ledger WL. Favourable outcomes from "mild" in-vitro fertilisation. Lancet. 2007;369:717–8.
24. Heijnen EM, Eijkemans MJ, De Klerk C, et al. A mild treatment strategy for in-vitro fertilisation: a randomised non-inferiority trial. Lancet. 2007;369:743–9.
25. Bagtharia S, Haloob AR. Is there a benefit from routine follicular flushing for oocyte retrieval? J Obstet Gynaecol. 2005;25:374–6.
26. Hill MJ, Levens ED. Is there a benefit in follicular flushing in assisted reproductive technology? Curr Opin Obstet Gynecol. 2010;22:208–12.
27. El Hussein E, Balen AH, Tan SL. A prospective study comparing the outcome of oocytes retrieved in the aspirate with those retrieved in the flush during transvaginal ultrasound directed oocyte recovery for in-vitro fertilization. Br J Obstet Gynaecol. 1992;99:841–4.
28. Levens ED, Whitcomb BW, Payson MD, Larsen FW. Ovarian follicular flushing among low-responding patients undergoing assisted reproductive technology. Fertil Steril. 2009;91:1381–4.
29. Knight DC, Tyler JP, Driscoll GL. Follicular flushing at oocyte retrieval: a reappraisal. Aust N Z J Obstet Gynaecol. 2001;41:210–3.
30. Lozano DH, Fanchin R, Chevalier N, et al. Optimising the semi natural cycle IVF: the importance of follicular flushing. J Indian Med Assoc. 2006;104:423–7.
31. Mendez Lozano DH, Fanchin R, Chevalier N, et al. [The follicular flushing duplicate the pregnancy rate on semi natural cycle IVF]. J Gynecol Obstet Biol Reprod (Paris). 2007;36:36–41.
32. Mendez Lozano DH, Brum Scheffer J, Frydman N, Fay S, Fanchin R, Frydman R. Optimal reproductive competence of oocytes retrieved through follicular flushing in minimal stimulation IVF. Reprod Biomed Online. 2008;16:119–23.
33. Philips Z, Barraza-Llorens M, Posnett J. Evaluation of the relative cost-effectiveness of treatments for infertility in the UK. Hum Reprod. 2000;15:95–106.
34. Jain T, Harlow BL, Hornstein MD. Insurance coverage and outcomes of in vitro fertilization. N Engl J Med. 2002;347:661–6.
35. Hammoud AO, Gibson M, Stanford J, White G, Carrell DT, Peterson M. In vitro fertilization availability and utilization in the United States: a study of demographic, social, and economic factors. Fertil Steril. 2009;91:1630–5.
36. Nygren KG. Single embryo transfer: the role of natural cycle/minimal stimulation IVF in the future. Reprod Biomed Online. 2007;14:626–7.

3 Current Understanding of Anti-Müllerian Hormone

Dimitrios G. Goulis, Marina A. Dimitraki, and Basil C. Tarlatzis

Abstract

During the last years, anti-Müllerian hormone (AMH) has been transformed into a "hot issue" of Reproductive Medicine, as it has attracted the attention of many research groups and has found considerable clinical applications. In this review, we have summarized available evidence on possible roles of AMH in women with polycystic ovary syndrome (PCOS). We have arranged the material into three sections. In the first section, we briefly present the AMH as a molecule, in the second we pay special attention on AMH involvement in PCOS pathophysiology and, in the third section, we discuss possible roles of AMH as a predictive factor in women with PCOS undergoing assisted reproduction technologies (ART).

Serum AMH concentrations, being stable and consistent throughout the menstrual cycle, constitute a reliable marker of ovarian reserve; thus, AMH has already found a role in the clinical practice, particularly when combined with classic markers of ovarian reserve such as age, follicle-stimulating hormone (FSH), and antral follicle count (AFC). The significance of AMH in women with PCOS undergoing ART is increasing as well. On top of being a marker of ovarian reserve, AMH has been used for predicting success of ovulation induction and controlled ovarian hyperstimulation protocols, as well as avoidance of ovarian hyperstimulation syndrome (OHSS).

Despite this evidence, many issues remain to be elucidated. AMH physiology is still obscure, especially its exact role in ovarian folliculogenesis, significance of serum and follicular fluid concentrations, and possible extraovarian actions. As far as PCOS is concerned, there is agreement that AMH concentrations are elevated in women with the syndrome as compared to normo-ovulatory women. Nevertheless, it is still not known if this difference is the result of disrupted folliculogenesis, due to increased

D.G. Goulis (✉)
Section of Reproductive Medicine,
First Department of Obstetrics and Gynecology,
Medical School – Aristotle University of Thessaloniki,
Thessaloniki, Greece
e-mail: tarlatzis@hol.gr

C. Racowsky et al. (eds.), *Biennial Review of Infertility: Volume 2*,
DOI 10.1007/978-1-4419-8456-2_3, © Springer Science+Business Media, LLC 2011

number of small antral follicles, or the cause of it, due to AMH inhibition on folliculogenesis. Data on AMH pathophysiology in adolescent girls with PCOS are particularly scarce.

The answers to these questions will broaden the spectrum of AMH clinical applications. Adjustment of overall ART strategy and individualization of protocols according to AMH concentrations seems to constitute possibilities for the near future. More distant applications could include use of AMH in hormonal contraception, given its inhibitory action on follicular development, or even development of AMH-antagonists in the therapeutic approach of women with PCOS.

Keywords

Anti-Müllerian hormone • Müllerian inhibiting substance • Polycystic ovary syndrome • Transforming growth factor-β • Estradiol • AMH receptor, type I • AMH receptor, type II • Gonadotropins • Follicle-stimulating hormone • Human chorionic gonadotropin • Luteinizing hormone • Androgens • Testosterone • Hyperandrogenism • Insulin • Insulin resistance • Hyperinsulinemia • Bone morphogenetic proteins • Inhinins • Inhibin B • Activins • Smads • Ovary • Oocyte • Aromatase • Follicle, primordial • Follicle dominant • Antral follicle count • Granulosa cells • Theca cell • Metformin • Clomiphene citrate • In vitro fertilization • Controlled ovarian hyperstimulation • Ovarian hyperstimulation syndrome

3.1 Introduction

During the last years, anti-Müllerian hormone (AMH) has been transformed into a "hot issue" of Reproductive Medicine, as it has attracted the attention of many research groups and has found considerable clinical applications. A MEDLINE search performed in July 2010 revealed almost 1,200 papers under the medical subheading (MeSH) term "anti-Müllerian hormone." Of them, more than 50 were specifically focused on women with polycystic ovary syndrome (PCOS).

In this review, we have attempted to summarize available evidence on possible roles of AMH in women with PCOS. We have arranged the material into three sections. In the first section, we briefly present the AMH as a molecule. We discuss the gene and the protein, its expression and actions, as well as the controversial issue of serum concentrations during a spontaneous menstrual cycle. The section closes with a reference to current clinical applications of serum AMH measurement.

In the second section, we pay special attention on AMH involvement in PCOS. Aspects of ovarian physiology and PCOS pathophysiology are discussed as well as serum AMH concentrations in women with PCOS. We also present data on correlation of AMH with other important parameters of PCOS, such as gonadotropins, androgens, and indices of insulin resistance.

Finally, in the third section, we discuss possible roles of AMH as a predictive factor in women with PCOS undergoing assisted reproduction technologies (ART). Thus, we present data on two techniques (ovulation induction and controlled ovarian hyperstimulation) as well as one complication (ovarian hyperstimulation syndrome, OHSS), in an attempt to clarify if the outcome/presence of them could be predicted by routine application of serum AMH measurement.

3.2 Anti-Müllerian Hormone

3.2.1 The Gene and the Protein

The human AMH gene has a length of 2,750 basepairs, is divided into five exons, and maps on chromosome 19 p13.3 [1]. Its product, AMH, is a dimeric glycoprotein [2], a member of the transforming growth factor-β (TGF-β) superfamily, that also includes inhibins, activins, bone morphogenetic proteins (BMPs), and a wide range of growth and differentiation factors (GDFs) [3]. The proteins in this family have a broad range of functions in mesenchymal – epithelial interaction, cell growth, extracellular matrix production, and tissue remodeling [4]. They are produced as dimeric precursors and undergo posttranslational processing for activation; cleavage and dissociation is required for biologically active C-terminal fragments to be released [5].

As for other members of the TGF family, AMH signals through membrane receptors, the TGF/activin group of type I receptors (ALK-1, -4 and -5), and the BMP/GDF group of type II receptors (ALK-2, -3 and -6). They all have intrinsic protein kinase activity that catalyzes phosphorylation of proteins on serine and threonine residues. The AMH receptors consist of two nonidentical subunits, each of which has a single membrane spanning region and an intracellular kinase domain [6]. Binding of AMH to its receptor causes it to complex with and phosphorylate a signal-transducing subunit. The activated receptor complex associates with and phosphorylates cytosolic proteins called Smads, which enter the nucleus and activate transcription of specific genes. Smads fall into three different classes, receptor-regulated R-Smads, inhibitory Smads, and the common Smad-4 [6]. The R-Smads-2 and -3 are phosphorylated by the TGF/activin type I receptors ALK-4 and -5, whereas the R-Smads-1, -5, and -8 are phosphorylated by the BMP/GDF type II receptors ALK-2, -3, and -6. The phosphorylated Smads dimerize with the common Smad-4 to form heteromeric complexes that translocate to the nucleus. They act by binding to the Smad-responsive DNA element CAGAC, with a relatively low specificity or with cofactors into a super-complex that can modulate ligand-specific gene expression [7].

3.2.2 Expression

AMH is secreted by the human testis from the sixth week of gestational age (eighth week of amenorrhea) and provokes irreversible Müllerian duct regression, which is completed by the end of ninth week [8]. The AMH receptors are expressed in the fetuses of both sexes at the time when sexual differentiation is triggered. Thus, AMH is one of the earliest Sertoli cell-specific proteins expressed by the gonad [9]. Except for a transient decline in the perinatal period [5, 10, 11], testicular AMH secretion is maintained at high levels until puberty, when Sertoli cell maturation is characterized by a decreasing AMH activity in all species studied [12–20] (Fig. 3.1). The decline of AMH production by Sertoli cells during puberty in the boy is related to the stage of pubertal development. The most significant decrease in serum AMH is observed between stages II and III of pubertal development [21], in coincidence with the increase of intratesticular testosterone concentration [22].

Ovarian granulosa cells, the homologous to testicular Sertoli cells, also produce AMH [23], but with several differences: AMH expression only begins at the perinatal period [19, 24, 25], remains low throughout reproductive life, and becomes undetectable after menopause. Thus, gonadal AMH secretion shows a clear-cut sexual dimorphism in prepubertal ages, when serum AMH concentrations are significantly lower in females; in adults, serum AMH concentrations are similarly low in both sexes [10, 26, 27], whereas show a progressive decline along reproductive life in women [28].

Ovarian AMH expression, observed as late as gestational week 32 [19], seems to be absent in primordial follicles, theca cells, or oocytes [25, 29–31], but is highest in granulosa cells of preantral and small antral follicles (Fig. 3.2). Interestingly, AMH is expressed in follicles that

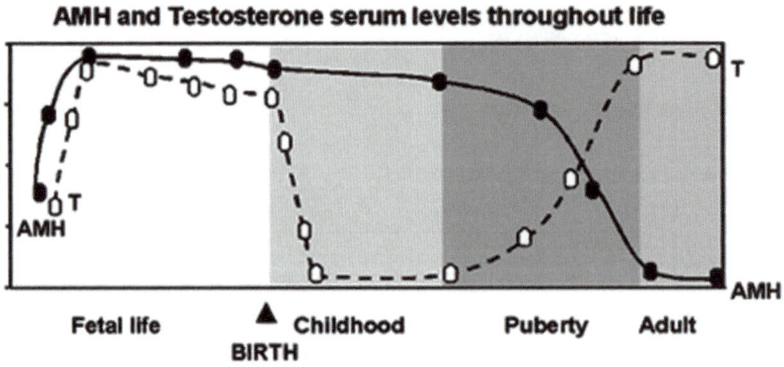

Fig. 3.1 Profiles of serum anti-Müllerian hormone (AMH) and testosterone (T) in the male. The serum AMH concentration is inversely proportional to the serum T concentration in males after the neonatal period (reproduced from Rey [133])

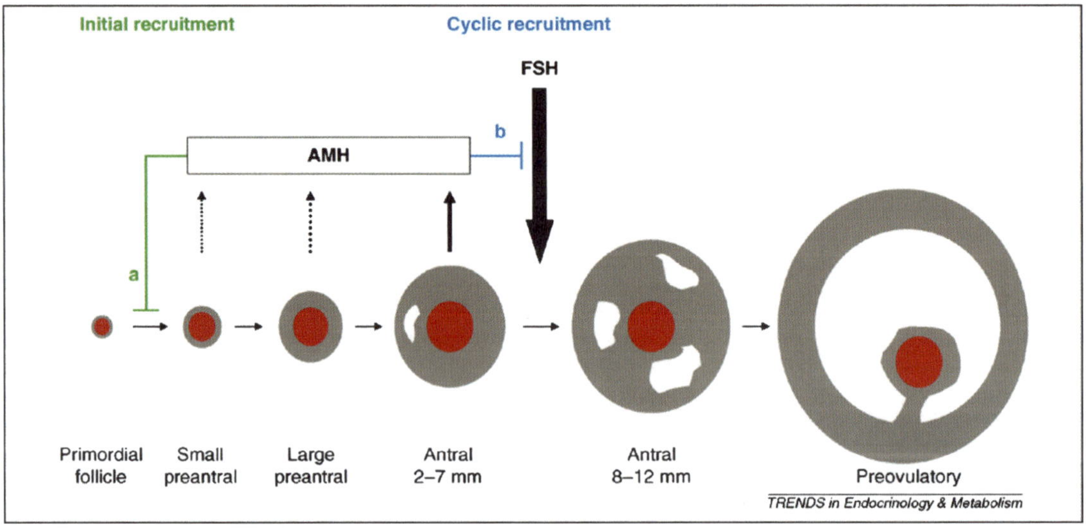

Fig. 3.2 The role of anti-Müllerian hormone (AMH) in the two main compartments of normal ovarian follicle development (the *red center* represents the oocyte, the *grey area* represents the granulosa cell layer, and the *white area* represents follicle fluid in the antrum). AMH is expressed in small and large preantral follicles (*broken arrows*) and in small antral follicles (*unbroken arrow*), and the latter mainly contributes to serum levels. Initial recruitment takes place as a continuous process, whereas cyclic recruitment is driven by a rise in FSH serum levels at the end of a previous menstrual cycle. The inhibitory effects of AMH are shown (**a**) on the initial recruitment of primary follicles from the resting primordial follicle pool and (**b**) on the sensitivity of antral follicles for FSH (reproduced with permission from Broekmans et al. [134])

have undergone recruitment from the primordial follicle pool, but have not been selected for dominance.

The intrafollicular concentrations of AMH become progressively lower with increasing follicle diameters [32]. At the larger antral follicle stage (>8 mm), AMH expression diminishes. Within these follicles, AMH expression is not always evenly distributed, as expression may be highest in the granulosa cells immediately surrounding the antrum and around the oocyte [25, 29–31, 33]. This gradient of AMH expression within a follicle may reflect functional differences between the granulosa cells surrounding the oocyte and the more peripheral ones, such as differences in proliferation capacity and steroidogenic activity [30]. These functional differences may arise under the influence of factors produced by the oocyte, as it has been shown for GDF-9 [34]. Follicles showing signs of atresia also have decreased or no AMH expression; expression is completely lost in corpus luteum.

3.2.3 Actions

In human ovary, possible actions of AMH include inhibition of follicular activation and growth, inhibition of follicle-stimulating hormone (FSH)-dependent growth, inhibition of granulose cells growth, and inhibition of aromatase (Fig. 3.2).

There is evidence that AMH undertakes important intrafollicular functions around the time of normal follicular selection, in the midfollicular phase of the menstrual cycle [32]. Thus, AMH may serve to inhibit recruitment of primordial follicles into the pool of growing follicles to prevent early depletion [31, 34, 35] and decrease follicle sensitivity to gonadotropin stimulation, to control the number of large preantral and small antral follicles that reach the preovulatory stage [35, 36].

As it is well established that follicles are more sensitive to FSH in the absence of AMH, primordial follicles are recruited at a faster rate under these conditions, resulting in premature exhaustion of the primordial follicle pool [37, 38]. In addition, diminished expression of AMH within the follicles reduces the threshold level for FSH, allowing follicles to continue growing and to ovulate in the next cycle [36, 39].

Oocytes upregulate AMH expression in granulosa cells in a manner that is dependent upon the developmental stage of the oocyte [40]. This observation leads to the hypothesis that oocytes in the pool of growing follicles could control the pool of primordial follicles by modulating the expression of the inhibiting factor AMH [41]. In addition, considerable attention has focused on the possible role of AMH in a new signaling pathway between granulosa and theca cells in the developing follicle [42]. Studies suggest a role for AMH even as a coregulator of steroidogenesis in granulosa cells, as AMH concentrations appear to be related to estradiol concentrations in follicular fluid from small antral follicles [43]. Finally, AMH may play a significant physiological role in controlling involution of the normal breast [44].

3.2.4 Serum Concentrations During a Spontaneous Menstrual Cycle

Numerous studies have shown that the AMH assay has high reproducibility in repeated measurements [45] and AMH concentrations, unlike steroids, gonadotropins, and peptides, such as inhibin B, have been reported to be constant throughout the menstrual cycle [46–49]. Indeed, serum AMH concentrations have been measured at different times during the menstrual cycle, suggesting extremely subtle or nonexistent fluctuation [27, 46]. It may be hypothesized that minimal fluctuations in serum AMH concentrations may be consistent with continuous noncyclic growth of small follicles. Thus, AMH may constitute a unique endocrine parameter for the investigation of ovarian function.

In contrast to the above results, some investigators have demonstrated significant cyclical fluctuations in AMH concentrations, with a rapid decrease in the early luteal phase [50, 51]. They report that the changes in AMH concentrations after ovulation are slight, yet statistically significant, and suggest that these changes may influence the circulating gonadotropin and steroid hormone concentrations. Excursions from mean levels of 3–219% have been reported [50, 51].

In the clinical setting, the inter- and intracycle variability in serum AMH concentrations may be considered to be low enough to permit the use of serum AMH as a cycle-independent marker for ovarian reserve and ovarian activity [52]. In addition, AMH concentrations appear to be unmodified in conditions under which endogenous gonadotropin release is substantially diminished, strengthening the concept that AMH levels reflect the continuous, FSH-independent, noncyclic growth of small follicles in the ovary.

3.2.5 Clinical Applications

According to the published evidence, determination of serum AMH concentrations could be useful in the following clinical conditions:

1. In children, for the presence of testicular tissue [10, 53, 54], when serum testosterone concentrations are very low.
2. In the differential diagnosis of patients with intersex disorders [53, 54]. AMH concentrations are an instructive marker [55] in the evaluation of androgen insensitivity syndrome or steroidogenic disorders, particularly in the infant or young male, in whom the normally low and fluctuating testosterone concentrations cannot be detected, unless stimulated with human chorionic gonadotropin (hCG) or luteinizing hormone (LH).
3. In patients with bilateral nonpalpable gonads [56].
4. In females with granulosa cell tumors [57–60], where AMH concentrations can be dramatically elevated.

3.3 Anti-Müllerian Hormone in Polycystic Ovary Syndrome

3.3.1 Pathophysiology

Many studies of ovarian histology have shown that the number of primordial follicles is the same in women with PCOS compared to normo-ovulatory controls, but the number of developing and, subsequently, atretic follicles is doubled [61, 62]. Thus, in women with PCOS, ovaries with polycystic morphology differ from normal ovaries in that follicle development is arrested at the stage where, under normal conditions, dominant follicle selection would have taken place [63–65].

On a histology level, AMH concentrations were found to be, on average, 75 times higher in granulosa cells from polycystic ovaries, compared with concentrations in normal ovaries [42]. Although there is positive correlation between AMH concentrations and follicle number in women with PCOS, it is unclear whether AMH has a regulatory role in follicle development or whether this is a consequence of increased antral follicle number in women with PCOS [66]. In mice, exogenous AMH inhibits FSH-mediated follicle growth [36]. In humans, several investigators have demonstrated higher AMH concentrations in amenorrhoeic compared to oligomenorrhoeic women with PCOS [67]. Alternatively, high AMH values could reflect a more evident impairment in follicular development and granulosa cell function in the ovaries of amenorrhoeic compared to oligomenorrhoeic women with PCOS. Increased ovarian AMH production may exert a paracrine negative control on follicle growth, sufficient to prevent selection of a dominant follicle.

The cause of the increased AMH production in PCOS is unknown. However, the intraovarian hyperandrogenism may be the main culprit for the follicular arrest observed in PCOS, promoting early follicular growth and leading to an excess of 2–5 mm follicles [68]. Insulin is the second candidate for the cause of the increase of AMH concentrations in women with PCOS.

According to recent data, genetic variation of ALK-2 is associated with AMH concentrations and follicle number in women with PCOS, suggesting that this type I receptor for AMH/BMP signaling contributes to the disturbed folliculogenesis in women with PCOS [69].

3.3.2 Serum Concentrations

Based on the observation that AMH is predominantly expressed by small follicles, several studies have concluded that AMH serum concentrations are increased in women with PCOS [36, 70]. AMH measurement has been found to offer a relatively high specificity and sensitivity (92 and 67%, respectively) as a diagnostic marker for PCOS [71]. Furthermore, it seems that AMH concentrations correlate with the extent of ovarian dysfunction in these women, as represented by elevated LH or testosterone levels and an increased follicle number and/or ovarian volume, as established on ultrasound. These elevated serum AMH concentrations in women with PCOS might indicate an increased ovarian reserve [72].

In a longitudinal study [73], serum AMH concentrations were found to decline over time both in PCOS group and in controls. However, the reduction in women with PCOS was lower. These results may indicate a sustained reproductive lifespan in these patients.

It has been shown that metformin administration in women with PCOS is associated with a reduction in AMH concentrations in both serum and antral follicles, suggesting that the measurement of AMH could be used to evaluate the treatment efficacy with insulin sensitizers [66].

3.3.3 AMH and Androgens

Serum AMH has been positively correlated to androgen concentrations [72, 74, 75]. Women with hyperandrogenism and polycystic ovary morphology (PCO) had higher serum AMH concentrations compared to women with PCO and normal androgen concentrations [75].

Androgen production per theca cell is equally increased in anovulatory and ovulatory women with PCOS [76]. However, the total number of follicles found in the anovulatory ovary is higher, resulting in increased total androgen concentrations [77]. This fact may not only explain the higher AMH concentrations in women with PCOS as a whole, but also the significantly higher production of AMH by anovulatory ovaries. Nevertheless, the results of a recent study rather contradict this hypothesis [78]. Although, at the beginning of the study, there was a direct correlation between AMH and androgen concentrations in women with PCOS, after 6 months of androgen suppression with dexamethasone, the AMH concentrations remained unchanged [78]. However, several possibilities exist that the concentration of androgen within the ovary is the determining factor and that a different control mechanism would have to be present in the ovary than in the testis for androgens to cause the rise of AMH, described in women with PCOS.

3.3.4 AMH and Insulin Resistance

PCOS is considered to be a syndrome of preserved [79], if not increased [80], ovarian sensitivity to insulin with systemic resistance to insulin action. Though insulin resistance is amplified by increasing obesity, women with PCOS are more insulin resistant than can be accounted for by their obesity per se [81–83]. Moreover, in women with PCOS, ovarian antral follicle counts and ovarian volume correlate positively with endogenous and exogenous hyperinsulinemia [84, 85]. Hyperinsulinemia may stimulate the development of antral follicles, increase the sensitivity of granulosa cells to FSH, and thus, increase the number of follicles and ovarian volume [86]. Finally, insulin has been shown to promote in vitro secretion of androgens by ovarian theca and stromal tissue [87] and, in women with PCOS, to stimulate testosterone biosynthesis by binding to its own receptor in theca cells [88].

La Marca et al. [89] found no correlation between serum AMH and androgen concentrations, but did observe a direct correlation between AMH and insulin insensitivity, reporting that the raised AMH may be secondary to an effect of insulin on androgen concentrations. In addition, women with PCOS have been reported to have a positive correlation between AMH and the 2-h insulin concentrations [90]. However, other investigators have failed to find a direct correlation between insulin and AMH concentrations [74, 75] and reported that, even when insulin concentrations have been reduced with treatment, a fall in serum AMH has not followed directly [78, 91].

Quantitative ultrasound evaluation of follicle distribution in PCO suggests a possible role for insulin in the dysregulation of folliculogenesis [68]. Some study groups [92] have shown that follicular development in response to the induction of ovulation with gonadotropins is qualitatively different in insulin-resistant women with PCOS. Treatment with the insulin sensitizer metformin reduces the number of antral follicles, ovarian volume, and circulating AMH concentrations [66]. It is most likely that the decrease is simply related to the decrease of follicle number, but the contribution of the improvement of hyperandrogenism, insulin action, or menstrual pattern cannot be excluded. Short-term metformin treatment was reported to result in improvements in hyperandrogenism, menstrual cyclicity, reduction in the number of antral follicles, and insulin resistance [91], while long-term metformin administration is required for a reduction in AMH concentrations [66, 93].

3.3.5 AMH and Gonadotropins

FSH directs the cyclic recruitment and forms the basis of the menstrual cycle by enabling the secretion of the steroid estradiol from the dominant follicle. It has been hypothesized that AMH could be one of the factors involved in determining the responsiveness of ovarian follicles to FSH during cyclic recruitment, playing an inhibitory role in the FSH-dependent follicle growth (Fig. 3.2). AMH also plays a role in the fine-tuning of the FSH threshold for dominant follicle selection. Both in vitro and in vivo studies have shown that large antral follicles are more sensitive to FSH in the absence of AMH [38].

An inverse correlation between AMH and estradiol concentrations in follicular fluid of small antral follicles has been demonstrated, which indicates a close interdependent regulation between AMH production and FSH activity [43]. In addition, FSH has been reported to decrease the expression of AMH and its type II receptors in granulosa cells [30].

Correlation between FSH and AMH concentrations has been observed in several studies [70, 74, 89, 94–96]. Whereas FSH and AMH were negatively correlated in women without PCOS, a positive correlation was found in the PCOS group. This observation leads to speculation on the role of AMH as direct modulator of the FSH sensitivity of individual follicles in PCOS, which in turn may also explain previous data on follicular recruitment and delayed ovarian aging in women with PCOS [73].

It has been demonstrated [97] that exogenous AMH administration reduced aromatase expression and the number of LH receptors in cultured granulose cells. Positive correlation has been reported between AMH and LH in women with PCOS. In these women, increased LH concentrations might be a significant link between disorders of ovulation and the observed increase in serum AMH concentration.

3.4 Anti-Müllerian Hormone in Assisted Reproduction Technologies

3.4.1 Ovulation Induction

There is limited evidence on the clinical relevance of serum AMH concentrations in women in whom clomiphene citrate ovulation induction previously failed [72]. An AMH concentration of 1.2 ng/mL could be used to predict response to clomiphene citrate in obese women with PCOS, with a sensitivity of 71.0% and a specificity of 65.7% [98]. However, the response to clomiphene citrate in obese patients with PCOS seems to be dependent on initial AMH concentrations. In addition, in the same group of women, pregnancy rates and miscarriage rates were similar in patients with moderately and severely elevated AMH serum concentrations [98]. Although, among women with PCOS, those who have the highest concentrations of AMH seem to respond less well to ovulation induction [99], elevated AMH serum concentration is a marker of limited predictive power in these patients, as far as adverse treatment outcome is concerned.

In anovulatory women with PCOS, a gentle increase in serum FSH concentrations reduces the AMH excess, thus relieving the inhibition from the latter on aromatase expression by selectable follicles [100]; this mechanism allows the development of a dominant follicle. In addition, it has been shown [92] that follicular development, as a response to ovulation induction with gonadotropins, is qualitatively different in insulin-resistant women with PCOS. Treatment with the insulin sensitizer metformin reduces the number of antral follicles, ovarian volume, and circulating AMH concentrations [66].

3.4.2 Controlled Ovarian Hyperstimulation

Ovarian hyperstimulation by exogenous FSH has allowed for the investigation of the contribution of different follicular stages on AMH serum concentrations, as it forces many small antral follicles to be transformed into large dominant follicles. Indeed, hyperstimulation results in a remarkable decline in serum AMH concentrations [101, 102]. Under such conditions, serum AMH concentrations correlate with the number of smaller (<12 mm diameter) but not larger (>12 mm) follicles [70, 89, 103, 104]. In addition, a significant reduction has been observed in concentrations of AMH protein in the conditioned medium from granulose cells from women with PCOS, which had been treated with FSH [42].

AMH seems to be a better predictor for oocyte maturation and successful in vitro fertilization (IVF) treatment than traditional markers [105–107]. While FSH mostly reflects the last 2 weeks of follicular maturation, when follicles become gonadotropin sensitive, AMH is mostly representative of the young, postprimordial to preantral follicle pool going through earlier stages of folliculogenesis [41, 108, 109].

More specifically, lower serum AMH concentrations preceding or during ART were strongly associated with reduced oocyte yield and low oocyte quality [106, 107]. In a similar way, higher day 3 serum AMH concentrations were associated with greater number of retrieved oocytes [50, 70, 95, 104, 105, 107, 110–122]. As a confirmation, serum AMH concentrations have been shown to be tenfold lower in the canceled cycles [41]; thus, in prediction of a canceled cycle, AMH seems to be a better marker compared with FSH or inhibin B [123] and an equal one to AFC [52]. For the prediction of nonpregnancy, both serum AMH levels and AFC were shown to be similarly poor performers [124].

A number of investigators have tried to identify threshold AMH concentrations that are able to distinguish between pregnancy and nonpregnancy in an IVF procedure [110, 112, 115, 116]. However, the majority of them indicated that AMH measurement is not useful for predicting this end-point [95, 104, 114, 115, 125–127]. Up to the present, only one study has been published relating serum AMH concentrations to the live birth rate following IVF [122]. In this prospective study of 340 patients, it was demonstrated that the live birth rate dramatically increases with increasing basal AMH concentrations, indicating that serum AMH may definitely be considered a better marker for quantitative than for qualitative aspects of ART [123].

Maximal receiver operating characteristic (ROC) curve inflections, which differentiate between better and poorer delivery chances in women with diminished ovarian reserve, independent of age, were at AMH 1.05 ng/mL (improved odds for live birth 4.6, 95% confidence interval 2.3–9.1), although live births occurred even with undetectable AMH [128]. Pregnancy wastage was very low at AMH concentrations less than 0.04 ng/mL, but significantly increased at AMH 0.41–1.05 ng/mL, resulting in similarly low live birth rates at all AMH concentrations less than 1.05 ng/mL and significantly improved live birth rates at AMH more than 1.06 ng/mL [128].

In a recent study [129], AMH concentrations were measured in follicular fluid collected at the time of oocyte retrieval for IVF from women with PCOS. Although AMH was higher compared to ovulatory women, the concentrations in both small and large follicles were found to be lower in those women who began a pregnancy. This finding indicates that even following a stimulation protocol, it is those women with PCOS producing the relatively lower levels of AMH who have the best outcome. In addition, it has been suggested that there is an association between follicular fluid AMH concentrations and the quality of embryos in patients with PCOS [130].

3.4.3 Ovarian Hyperstimulation Syndrome

Considerable attention has been attracted on the finding that elevated serum AMH concentrations could be associated with greater probability of developing OHSS. A trend, but not statistically significant difference ($p = 0.052$), was reported in day 3–5 AMH concentrations between those women who developed OHSS and those who did not [113]. Inconsistent with these findings, however, another study noted sixfold higher serum AMH concentrations in women with OHSS [131]. A recent study [132] has clearly demonstrated that basal AMH measurement works as well as the AFC and estradiol levels on the day of hCG in the identification of women who will develop OHSS.

3.5 Conclusions

In this review, we have attempted to summarize available evidence on possible roles of AMH in women with PCOS. Serum AMH concentrations, being stable and consistent throughout the menstrual cycle, constitute a reliable marker of ovarian reserve; thus, AMH has already found a role in the clinical practice, particularly when combined with classic markers of ovarian reserve such as age, FSH, and AFC. The significance of AMH in women with PCOS undergoing ART is increasing as well. On top of being a marker of ovarian reserve, AMH has been used for predicting success of ovulation induction and controlled ovarian hyperstimulation protocols, as well as avoidance of OHSS.

Despite this evidence, many issues remain to be elucidated. AMH physiology is still obscure, especially its exact role in ovarian folliculogenesis, significance of serum and follicular fluid concentrations and possible extraovarian actions. As far as PCOS is concerned, there is agreement that AMH concentrations are elevated in women with the syndrome as compared to controls. Nevertheless, it is still not known if this difference is the result of disrupted folliculogenesis, due to increased number of small antral follicles, or the cause of it, due AMH inhibition on folliculogenesis. Data on AMH pathophysiology in adolescent girls with PCOS are particularly scarce.

The answers to these questions will broaden the spectrum of AMH clinical applications. Adjustment of overall ART strategy and individualization of protocols according to AMH concentrations seems to constitute possibilities for the near future. More distant applications could include use of AMH in hormonal contraception, given its inhibitory action on follicular development, or even development of AMH-antagonists in the therapeutic approach of women with PCOS.

References

1. Cohen-Haguenauer O, Picard JY, Mattei MG, et al. Mapping of the gene for anti-Müllerian hormone to the short arm of human chromosome 19. Cytogenet Cell Genet. 1987;44(1):2–6.
2. Cate RL, Mattaliano RJ, Hession C, et al. Isolation of the bovine and human genes for Müllerian inhibiting substance and expression of the human gene in animal cells. Cell. 1986;45(5):685–98.
3. Massague J. The transforming growth factor-beta family. Annu Rev Cell Biol. 1990;6:597–641.
4. Massague J, Chen YG. Controlling TGF-beta signaling. Genes Dev. 2000;14(6):627–44.
5. Josso N, Cate RL, Picard JY, et al. Anti-müllerian hormone: the Jost factor. Recent Prog Horm Res. 1993;48:1–59.
6. Kretzschmar M, Massague J. SMADs: mediators and regulators of TGF-beta signaling. Curr Opin Genet Dev. 1998;8(1):103–11.
7. Teixeira J, Donahoe PK. Molecular biology of MIS and its receptors. J Androl. 1996;17(4):336–41.
8. Taguchi O, Cunha GR, Lawrence WD, Robboy SJ. Timing and irreversibility of Müllerian duct inhibition in the embryonic reproductive tract of the human male. Dev Biol. 1984;106(2):394–8.
9. Tran D, Josso N. Relationship between avian and mammalian anti-Mulllerian hormones. Biol Reprod. 1977;16(2):267–73.
10. Lee MM, Donahoe PK, Hasegawa T, et al. Müllerian inhibiting substance in humans: normal levels from infancy to adulthood. J Clin Endocrinol Metab. 1996; 81(2):571–6.
11. Schwindt B, Doyle LW, Hutson JM. Serum levels of müllerian inhibiting substance in preterm and term male neonates. J Urol. 1997;158(2):610–2.
12. Tran D, Meusy-Dessolle N, Josso N. Waning of anti-müllerian activity: an early sign of sertoli cell maturation in the developing pig. Biol Reprod. 1981;24(4): 923–31.
13. Vigier B, Tran D, du Mesnil du Buisson F, Heyman Y, Josso N. Use of monoclonal antibody techniques to study the ontogeny of bovine anti-Müllerian hormone. J Reprod Fertil. 1983;69(1):207–14.
14. Josso N, Legeai L, Forest MG, Chaussain JL, Brauner R. An enzyme linked immunoassay for anti-müllerian hormone: a new tool for the evaluation of testicular function in infants and children. J Clin Endocrinol Metab. 1990;70(1):23–7.
15. Kuroda T, Lee MM, Haqq CM, Powell DM, Manganaro TF, Donahoe PK. Müllerian inhibiting substance ontogeny and its modulation by follicle-stimulating hormone in the rat testes. Endocrinology. 1990;127(4):1825–32.
16. Hudson PL, Dougas I, Donahoe PK, et al. An immunoassay to detect human müllerian inhibiting substance in males and females during normal development. J Clin Endocrinol Metab. 1990;70(1): 16–22.

17. Munsterberg A, Lovell-Badge R. Expression of the mouse anti-müllerian hormone gene suggests a role in both male and female sexual differentiation. Development. 1991;113(2):613–24.
18. Rey R, al-Attar L, Louis F, et al. Testicular dysgenesis does not affect expression of anti-müllerian hormone by Sertoli cells in premeiotic seminiferous tubules. Am J Pathol. 1996;148(5):1689–98.
19. Rajpert-De Meyts E, Jorgensen N, Graem N, Muller J, Cate RL, Skakkebaek NE. Expression of anti-Müllerian hormone during normal and pathological gonadal development: association with differentiation of Sertoli and granulosa cells. J Clin Endocrinol Metab. 1999;84(10):3836–44.
20. Rota A, Ballarin C, Vigier B, Cozzi B, Rey R. Age dependent changes in plasma anti-Müllerian hormone concentrations in the bovine male, female, and freemartin from birth to puberty: relationship between testosterone production and influence on sex differentiation. Gen Comp Endocrinol. 2002;129(1):39–44.
21. Rey R, Lordereau-Richard I, Carel JC, et al. Anti-müllerian hormone and testosterone serum levels are inversely during normal and precocious pubertal development. J Clin Endocrinol Metab. 1993;77(5):1220–6.
22. Pasqualini T, Chemes H, Rivarla MA. Testicular testosterone levels during puberty in cryptorchidism. Clin Endocrinol. 1981;15(6):545–54.
23. Vigier B, Picard JY, Tran D, Legeai L, Josso N. Production of anti-Müllerian hormone: another homology between Sertoli and granulosa cells. Endocrinology. 1984;114(4):1315–20.
24. Bezard J, Vigier B, Tran D, Mauleon P, Josso N. Immunocytochemical study of anti-Müllerian hormone in sheep ovarian follicles during fetal and postnatal development. J Reprod Fertil. 1987;80(2):509–16.
25. Ueno S, Kuroda T, Maclaughlin DT, Ragin RC, Manganaro TF, Donahoe PK. Müllerian inhibiting substance in the adult rat ovary during various stages of the estrous cycle. Endocrinology. 1989;125(2):1060–6.
26. Rey RA, Lhomme C, Marcillac I, et al. Antimullerian hormone as a serum marker of granulosa cell tumors of the ovary: comparative study with serum alpha-inhibin and estradiol. Am J Obstet Gynecol. 1996;174(3):958–65.
27. Cook CL, Siow Y, Taylor S, Fallat ME. Serum müllerian-inhibiting substance levels during normal menstrual cycles. Fertil Steril. 2000;73(4):859–61.
28. de Vet A, Laven JS, de Jong FH, Themmen AP, Fauser BC. Antimullerian hormone serum levels: a putative marker for ovarian aging. Fertil Steril. 2002;77(2):357–62.
29. Hirobe S, He WW, Gustafson ML, MacLaughlin DT, Donahoe PK. Müllerian inhibiting substance gene expression in the cycling rat ovary correlates with recruited or graafian follicle selection. Biol Reprod. 1994;50(6):1238–43.
30. Baarends WM, Uilenbroek JT, Kramer P, et al. Anti-müllerian hormone and anti-müllerian hormone type II receptor messenger ribonucleic acid expression in rat ovaries during postnatal development, the estrous cycle, and gonadotropin-induced follicle growth. Endocrinology. 1995;136(11):4951–62.
31. Durlinger AL, Gruijters MJ, Kramer P, et al. Anti-Müllerian hormone inhibits initiation of primordial follicle growth in the mouse ovary. Endocrinology. 2002;143(3):1076–84.
32. Andersen CY, Schmidt KT, Kristensen SG, Rosendahl M, Byskov AG, Ernst E. Concentrations of AMH and inhibin-B in relation to follicular diameter in normal human small antral follicles. Hum Reprod. 2010;25(5):1282–7.
33. Hirobe S, He WW, Lee MM, Donahoe PK. Müllerian inhibiting substance messenger ribonucleic acid expression in granulosa and Sertoli cells coincides with their mitotic activity. Endocrinology. 1992;131(2):854–62.
34. Elvin JA, Clark AT, Wang P, Wolfman NM, Matzuk MM. Paracrine actions of growth differentiation factor-9 in the mammalian ovary. Mol Endocrinol. 1999;13(6):1035–48.
35. Gruijters MJ, Visser JA, Durlinger AL, Themmen AP. Anti-Müllerian hormone and its role in ovarian function. Mol Cell Endocrinol. 2003;211(1-2):85–90.
36. Durlinger AL, Gruijters MJ, Kramer P, et al. Anti-Müllerian hormone attenuates the effects of FSH on follicle development in the mouse ovary. Endocrinology. 2001;142(11):4891–9.
37. van Houten EL, Themmen AP, Visser JA. Anti-Müllerian hormone (AMH): regulator and marker of ovarian function. Ann Endocrinol (Paris). 2010;71(3):191–7.
38. Durlinger AL, Kramer P, Karels B, et al. Control of primordial follicle recruitment by anti-Müllerian hormone in the mouse ovary. Endocrinology. 1999;140(12):5789–96.
39. Visser JA, Durlinger AL, Peters IJ, et al. Increased oocyte degeneration and follicular atresia during the estrous cycle in anti-Müllerian hormone null mice. Endocrinology. 2007;148(5):2301–8.
40. Salmon NA, Handyside AH, Joyce IM. Oocyte regulation of anti-Müllerian hormone expression in granulosa cells during ovarian follicle development in mice. Dev Biol. 2004;266(1):201–8.
41. La Marca A, Volpe A. Anti-Müllerian hormone (AMH) in female reproduction: is measurement of circulating AMH a useful tool? Clin Endocrinol. 2006;64(6):603–10.
42. Pellatt L, Hanna L, Brincat M, et al. Granulosa cell production of anti-Müllerian hormone is increased in polycystic ovaries. J Clin Endocrinol Metab. 2007;92(1):240–5.
43. Andersen CY, Byskov AG. Estradiol and regulation of anti-Müllerian hormone, inhibin-A, and inhibin-B secretion: analysis of small antral and preovulatory human follicles' fluid. J Clin Endocrinol Metab. 2006;91(10):4064–9.
44. Teixeira J, Maheswaran S, Donahoe PK. Müllerian inhibiting substance: an instructive developmental

hormone with diagnostic and possible therapeutic applications. Endocr Rev. 2001;22(5):657–74.
45. Fanchin R, Taieb J, Lozano DH, Ducot B, Frydman R, Bouyer J. High reproducibility of serum anti-Müllerian hormone measurements suggests a multi-staged follicular secretion and strengthens its role in the assessment of ovarian follicular status. Hum Reprod. 2005;20(4):923–7.
46. Hehenkamp WJ, Looman CW, Themmen AP, De Jong FH, Te Velde ER, Broekmans FJ. Anti-Müllerian hormone levels in the spontaneous menstrual cycle do not show substantial fluctuation. J Clin Endocrinol Metab. 2006;91(10):4057–63.
47. La Marca A, Stabile G, Artenisio AC, Volpe A. Serum anti-Müllerian hormone throughout the human menstrual cycle. Hum Reprod. 2006;21(12):3103–7.
48. Tsepelidis S, Devreker F, Demeestere I, Flahaut A, Gervy C, Englert Y. table serum levels of anti-Müllerian hormone during the menstrual cycle: a prospective study in normo-ovulatory women. Hum Reprod. 2007; 22(7):1837–40.
49. Streuli I, Fraisse T, Pillet C, Ibecheole V, Bischof P, de Ziegler D. Serum antimullerian hormone levels remain stable throughout the menstrual cycle and after oral or vaginal administration of synthetic sex steroids. Fertil Steril. 2008;90(2):395–400.
50. Wunder DM, Guibourdenche J, Birkhauser MH, Bersinger NA. Anti-Müllerian hormone and inhibin B as predictors of pregnancy after treatment by in vitro fertilization/intracytoplasmic sperm injection. Fertil Steril. 2008;90(6):2203–10.
51. Streuli I, Fraisse T, Chapron C, Bijaoui G, Bischof P, de Ziegler D. Clinical uses of anti-Müllerian hormone assays: pitfalls and promises. Fertil Steril. 2009;91(1): 226–30.
52. La Marca A, Broekmans FJ, Volpe A, Fauser BC, Macklon NS. Anti-Müllerian hormone (AMH): what do we still need to know? Hum Reprod. 2009;24(9): 2264–75.
53. Gustafson ML, Donahoe PK. Male sex determination: current concepts of male sexual differentiation. Annu Rev Med. 1994;45:505–24.
54. Rey RA, Belville C, Nihoul-Fekete C, et al. Evaluation of gonadal function in 107 intersex patients by means of serum antimullerian hormone measurement. J Clin Endocrinol Metab. 1999;84(2):627–31.
55. Rey R, Mebarki F, Forest MG, et al. Anti-müllerian hormone in children with androgen insensitivity. J Clin Endocrinol Metab. 1994;79(4):960–4.
56. Lee MM, Donahoe PK, Silverman BL, et al. Measurements of serum müllerian inhibiting substance in the evaluation of children with nonpalpable gonads. N Engl J Med. 1997;336(21):1480–6.
57. Gustafson ML, Lee MM, Scully RE, et al. Müllerian inhibiting substance as a marker for ovarian sex-cord tumor. N Engl J Med. 1992;326(7):466–71.
58. Puls LE, Hamous J, Morrow MS, Schneyer A, MacLaughlin DT, Castracane VD. Recurrent ovarian sex cord tumor with annular tubules: tumor marker and chemotherapy experience. Gynecol Oncol. 1994; 54(3):396–401.
59. Rey R, Josso N. Regulation of testicular anti-Müllerian hormone secretion. Eur J Endocrinol. 1996;135(2): 144–52.
60. Rey R, Sabourin JC, Venara M, et al. Anti-Müllerian hormone is a specific marker of sertoli- and granulosa-cell origin in gonadal tumors. Hum Pathol. 2000;31(10): 1202–8.
61. Hughesdon PE. Morphology and morphogenesis of the Stein-Leventhal ovary and of so-called "hyperthecosis". Obstet Gynecol Surv. 1982;37(2):59–77.
62. Webber LJ, Stubbs S, Stark J, et al. Formation and early development of follicles in the polycystic ovary. Lancet. 2003;362(9389):1017–21.
63. Pache TD, Hop WC, de Jong FH, et al. 17 Beta-oestradiol, androstenedione and inhibin levels in fluid from individual follicles of normal and polycystic ovaries, and in ovaries from androgen treated female to male transsexuals. Clin Endocrinol. 1992;36(6):565–71.
64. van Santbrink EJ, Hop WC, Fauser BC. Classification of normogonadotropic infertility: polycystic ovaries diagnosed by ultrasound versus endocrine characteristics of polycystic ovary syndrome. Fertil Steril. 1997;67(3):452–8.
65. Fauser BC, Van Heusden AM. Manipulation of human ovarian function: physiological concepts and clinical consequences. Endocr Rev. 1997;18(1):71–106.
66. Piltonen T, MorinPapunen L, Koivunen R, Perheentupa A, Ruokonen A, Tapanainen JS. Serum anti-Müllerian hormone levels remain high until late reproductive age and decrease during metformin therapy in women with polycystic ovary syndrome. Hum Reprod. 2005;20(7):1820–6.
67. Jonard S, Pigny P, Jacquesson L, Demerle-Roux C, Robert Y, Dewailly D. The ovarian markers of the FSH insufficiency in functional hypothalamic amenorrhoea. Hum Reprod. 2005;20(1):101–7.
68. Jonard S, Robert Y, Cortet-Rudelli C, Pigny P, Decanter C, Dewailly D. Ultrasound examination of polycystic ovaries: is it worth counting the follicles? Hum Reprod. 2003;18(3):598–603.
69. Kevenaar ME, Themmen AP, van Kerkwijk AJ, et al. Variants in the ACVR1 gene are associated with AMH levels in women with polycystic ovary syndrome. Hum Reprod. 2009;24(1):241–9.
70. Fanchin R, Schonauer LM, Righini C, Frydman N, Frydman R, Taieb J. Serum anti-Müllerian hormone dynamics during controlled ovarian hyperstimulation. Hum Reprod. 2003;18(2):328–32.
71. Pigny P, Jonard S, Robert Y, Dewailly D. Serum anti-Müllerian hormone as a surrogate for antral follicle count for definition of the polycystic ovary syndrome. J Clin Endocrinol Metab. 2006;91(3):941–5.
72. Laven JS, Mulders AG, Visser JA, Themmen AP, De Jong FH, Fauser BC. Anti-Müllerian hormone serum concentrations in normoovulatory and anovulatory women of reproductive age. J Clin Endocrinol Metab. 2004;89(1):318–23.

73. Mulders AG, Laven JS, Eijkemans MJ, de Jong FH, Themmen AP, Fauser BC. Changes in anti-Müllerian hormone serum concentrations over time suggest delayed ovarian ageing in normogonadotrophic anovulatory infertility. Hum Reprod. 2004;19(9):2036–42.
74. Pigny P, Merlen E, Robert Y, et al. Elevated serum level of anti-müllerian hormone in patients with polycystic ovary syndrome: relationship to the ovarian follicle excess and to the follicular arrest. J Clin Endocrinol Metab. 2003;88(12):5957–62.
75. Eldar-Geva T, Margalioth EJ, Gal M, et al. Serum anti-Müllerian hormone levels during controlled ovarian hyperstimulation in women with polycystic ovaries with and without hyperandrogenism. Hum Reprod. 2005;20(7):1814–9.
76. Gilling-Smith C, Willis DS, Beard RW, Franks S. Hypersecretion of androstenedione by isolated thecal cells from polycystic ovaries. J Clin Endocrinol Metab. 1994;79(4):1158–65.
77. Gilling-Smith C, Mason H, Willis D, Franks S, Beard RW. In-vitro ovarian steroidogenesis in women with pelvic congestion. Hum Reprod. 2000;15(12):2570–6.
78. Carlsen SM. [Use of metformin in polycystic ovary syndrome]. Tidsskr Nor Laegeforen. 2009;129(16):1644–6.
79. Poretsky L. Commentary: polycystic ovary syndrome – increased or preserved ovarian sensitivity to insulin? J Clin Endocrinol Metab. 2006;91(8):2859–60.
80. Baillargeon JP, Nestler JE. Commentary: polycystic ovary syndrome: a syndrome of ovarian hypersensitivity to insulin? J Clin Endocrinol Metab. 2006;91(1):22–4.
81. Dunaif A, Segal KR, Futterweit W, Dobrjansky A. Profound peripheral insulin resistance, independent of obesity, in polycystic ovary syndrome. Diabetes. 1989;38(9):1165–74.
82. Dunaif A, Segal KR, Shelley DR, Green G, Dobrjansky A, Licholai T. Evidence for distinctive and intrinsic defects in insulin action in polycystic ovary syndrome. Diabetes. 1992;41(10):1257–66.
83. Conway GS, Jacobs HS. Clinical implications of hyperinsulinaemia in women. Clin Endocrinol. 1993;39(6):623–32.
84. Pache TD, de Jong FH, Hop WC, Fauser BC. Association between ovarian changes assessed by transvaginal sonography and clinical and endocrine signs of the polycystic ovary syndrome. Fertil Steril. 1993;59(3):544–9.
85. Carmina E, Orio F, Palomba S, Longo RA, Lombardi G, Lobo RA. Ovarian size and blood flow in women with polycystic ovary syndrome and their correlations with endocrine parameters. Fertil Steril. 2005;84(2):413–9.
86. Fulghesu AM, Villa P, Pavone V, et al. The impact of insulin secretion on the ovarian response to exogenous gonadotropins in polycystic ovary syndrome. J Clin Endocrinol Metab. 1997;82(2):644–8.
87. Barbieri RL, Makris A, Ryan KJ. Insulin stimulates androgen accumulation in incubations of human ovarian stroma and theca. Obstet Gynecol. 1984;64(3 Suppl):73S–80.
88. Nestler JE, Jakubowicz DJ, de Vargas AF, Brik C, Quintero N, Medina F. Insulin stimulates testosterone biosynthesis by human thecal cells from women with polycystic ovary syndrome by activating its own receptor and using inositolglycan mediators as the signal transduction system. J Clin Endocrinol Metab. 1998;83(6):2001–5.
89. La Marca A, Malmusi S, Giulini S, et al. Anti-Müllerian hormone plasma levels in spontaneous menstrual cycle and during treatment with FSH to induce ovulation. Hum Reprod. 2004;19(12):2738–41.
90. Crisosto N, Codner E, Maliqueo M, et al. Anti-Müllerian hormone levels in peripubertal daughters of women with polycystic ovary syndrome. J Clin Endocrinol Metab. 2007;92(7):2739–43.
91. Bayrak A, Terbell H, Urwitz-Lane R, Mor E, Stanczyk FZ, Paulson RJ. Acute effects of metformin therapy include improvement of insulin resistance and ovarian morphology. Fertil Steril. 2007;87(4):870–5.
92. Fleming R, Deshpande N, Traynor I, Yates RW. Dynamics of FSH-induced follicular growth in subfertile women: relationship with age, insulin resistance, oocyte yield and anti-Müllerian hormone. Hum Reprod. 2006;21(6):1436–41.
93. Fleming R, Harborne L, MacLaughlin DT, et al. Metformin reduces serum müllerian-inhibiting substance levels in women with polycystic ovary syndrome after protracted treatment. Fertil Steril. 2005;83(1):130–6.
94. Seifer DB, MacLaughlin DT, Christian BP, Feng B, Shelden RM. Early follicular serum müllerian-inhibiting substance levels are associated with ovarian response during assisted reproductive technology cycles. Fertil Steril. 2002;77(3):468–71.
95. van Rooij IA, Broekmans FJ, te Velde ER, et al. Serum anti-Müllerian hormone levels: a novel measure of ovarian reserve. Hum Reprod. 2002;17(12):3065–71.
96. Fallat ME, Siow Y, Marra M, Cook C, Carrillo A. Müllerian-inhibiting substance in follicular fluid and serum: a comparison of patients with tubal factor infertility, polycystic ovary syndrome, and endometriosis. Fertil Steril. 1997;67(5):962–5.
97. di Clemente N, Wilson C, Faure E, et al. Cloning, expression, and alternative splicing of the receptor for anti-Müllerian hormone. Mol Endocrinol. 1994;8(8):1006–20.
98. El-Halawaty S, Rizk A, Kamal M, et al. Clinical significance of serum concentration of anti-Müllerian hormone in obese women with polycystic ovary syndrome. Reprod Biomed Online. 2007;15(5):495–9.
99. Pellatt L, Rice S, Mason HD. Anti-Müllerian hormone and polycystic ovary syndrome: a mountain too high? Reproduction. 2010;139(5):825–33.

100. Catteau-Jonard S, Pigny P, Reyss AC, Decanter C, Poncelet E, Dewailly D. Changes in serum anti-müllerian hormone level during low-dose recombinant follicular-stimulating hormone therapy for anovulation in polycystic ovary syndrome. J Clin Endocrinol Metab. 2007;92(11):4138–43.
101. Toner JP. Ovarian reserve, female age and the chance for successful pregnancy. Minerva Ginecol. 2003; 55(5):399–406.
102. Abdalla H, Thum MY. An elevated basal FSH reflects a quantitative rather than qualitative decline of the ovarian reserve. Hum Reprod. 2004;19(4): 893–8.
103. Bezard J, Vigier B, Tran D, Mauleon P, Josso N. Anti-müllerian hormone in sheep follicles. Reprod Nutr Dev. 1988;28(4B):1105–12.
104. Fanchin R, Schonauer LM, Righini C, Guibourdenche J, Frydman R, Taieb J. Serum anti-Müllerian hormone is more strongly related to ovarian follicular status than serum inhibin B, estradiol, FSH and LH on day 3. Hum Reprod. 2003;18(2):323–7.
105. Muttukrishna S, McGarrigle H, Wakim R, Khadum I, Ranieri DM, Serhal P. Antral follicle count, anti-müllerian hormone and inhibin B: predictors of ovarian response in assisted reproductive technology? BJOG. 2005;112(10):1384–90.
106. Silberstein T, MacLaughlin DT, Shai I, et al. Müllerian inhibiting substance levels at the time of HCG administration in IVF cycles predict both ovarian reserve and embryo morphology. Hum Reprod. 2006;21(1):159–63.
107. La Marca A, Giulini S, Tirelli A, et al. Anti-Müllerian hormone measurement on any day of the menstrual cycle strongly predicts ovarian response in assisted reproductive technology. Hum Reprod. 2007;22(3): 766–71.
108. Feyereisen E, Mendez Lozano DH, Taieb J, Hesters L, Frydman R, Fanchin R. Anti-Müllerian hormone: clinical insights into a promising biomarker of ovarian follicular status. Reprod Biomed Online. 2006; 12(6):695–703.
109. Visser JA, de Jong FH, Laven JS, Themmen AP. Anti-Müllerian hormone: a new marker for ovarian function. Reproduction. 2006;131(1):1–9.
110. Hazout A, Bouchard P, Seifer DB, Aussage P, Junca AM, Cohen-Bacrie P. Serum antimüllerian hormone/müllerian-inhibiting substance appears to be a more discriminatory marker of assisted reproductive technology outcome than follicle-stimulating hormone, inhibin B, or estradiol. Fertil Steril. 2004;82(5): 1323–9.
111. Muttukrishna S, Suharjono H, McGarrigle H, Sathanandan M. Inhibin B and anti-Müllerian hormone: markers of ovarian response in IVF/ICSI patients? BJOG. 2004;111(11):1248–53.
112. Eldar-Geva T, Ben-Chetrit A, Spitz IM, et al. Dynamic assays of inhibin B, anti-Müllerian hormone and estradiol following FSH stimulation and ovarian ultrasonography as predictors of IVF outcome. Hum Reprod. 2005;20(11):3178–83.
113. Tremellen KP, Kolo M, Gilmore A, Lekamge DN. Anti-Müllerian hormone as a marker of ovarian reserve. Aust NZ J Obstet Gynaecol. 2005;45(1): 20–4.
114. Penarrubia J, Fabregues F, Manau D, et al. Basal and stimulation day 5 anti-Müllerian hormone serum concentrations as predictors of ovarian response and pregnancy in assisted reproductive technology cycles stimulated with gonadotropin-releasing hormone agonist – gonadotropin treatment. Hum Reprod. 2005;20(4):915–22.
115. Kwee J, Schats R, McDonnell J, Themmen A, de Jong F, Lambalk C. Evaluation of anti-Müllerian hormone as a test for the prediction of ovarian reserve. Fertil Steril. 2008;90(3):737–43.
116. Elgindy EA, El-Haieg DO, El-Sebaey A. Anti-Müllerian hormone: correlation of early follicular, ovulatory and midluteal levels with ovarian response and cycle outcome in intracytoplasmic sperm injection patients. Fertil Steril. 2008;89(6):1670–6.
117. McIlveen M, Skull JD, Ledger WL. Evaluation of the utility of multiple endocrine and ultrasound measures of ovarian reserve in the prediction of cycle cancellation in a high-risk IVF population. Hum Reprod. 2007;22(3):778–85.
118. Nelson SM, Yates RW, Fleming R. Serum anti-Müllerian hormone and FSH: prediction of live birth and extremes of response in stimulated cycles – implications for individualization of therapy. Hum Reprod. 2007;22(9):2414–21.
119. Gnoth C, Schuring AN, Friol K, Tigges J, Mallmann P, Godehardt E. Relevance of anti-Müllerian hormone measurement in a routine IVF program. Hum Reprod. 2008;23(6):1359–65.
120. Nardo LG, Gelbaya TA, Wilkinson H, et al. Circulating basal anti-Müllerian hormone levels as predictor of ovarian response in women undergoing ovarian stimulation for in vitro fertilization. Fertil Steril. 2009;92(5):1586–93.
121. Jayaprakasan K, Campbell B, Hopkisson J, Johnson I, Raine-Fenning N. A prospective, comparative analysis of anti-Müllerian hormone, inhibin-B, and three-dimensional ultrasound determinants of ovarian reserve in the prediction of poor response to controlled ovarian stimulation. Fertil Steril. 2010;93(3): 855–64.
122. Nelson SM, Yates RW, Lyall H, et al. Anti-Müllerian hormone-based approach to controlled ovarian stimulation for assisted conception. Hum Reprod. 2009;24(4):867–75.
123. La Marca A, Sighinolfi G, Radi D, et al. Anti-Müllerian hormone (AMH) as a predictive marker in assisted reproductive technology (ART). Hum Reprod Update. 2010;16(2):113–30.
124. Broer SL, Mol BW, Hendriks D, Broekmans FJ. The role of antimullerian hormone in prediction of outcome after IVF: comparison with the antral follicle count. Fertil Steril. 2009;91(3):705–14.
125. Ebner T, Sommergruber M, Moser M, Shebl O, Schreier-Lechner E, Tews G. Basal level of anti-Müllerian

hormone is associated with oocyte quality in stimulated cycles. Hum Reprod. 2006;21(8):2022–6.
126. Ficicioglu C, Kutlu T, Baglam E, Bakacak Z. Early follicular antimullerian hormone as an indicator of ovarian reserve. Fertil Steril. 2006;85(3):592–6.
127. Smeenk JM, Sweep FC, Zielhuis GA, Kremer JA, Thomas CM, Braat DD. Antimullerian hormone predicts ovarian responsiveness, but not embryo quality or pregnancy, after in vitro fertilization or intracyoplasmic sperm injection. Fertil Steril. 2007;87(1):223–6.
128. Gleicher N, Weghofer A, Barad DH. Anti-Müllerian hormone (AMH) defines, independent of age, low versus good live-birth chances in women with severely diminished ovarian reserve. Fertil Steril. 2010;94(7):2824–7.
129. Desforges-Bullet V, Gallo C, Lefebvre C, Pigny P, Dewailly D, Catteau-Jonard S. Increased anti-Müllerian hormone and decreased FSH levels in follicular fluid obtained in women with polycystic ovaries at the time of follicle puncture for in vitro fertilization. Fertil Steril. 2010;94(1):198–204.
130. Mashiach R, Amit A, Hasson J, et al. Follicular fluid levels of anti-Müllerian hormone as a predictor of oocyte maturation, fertilization rate, and embryonic development in patients with polycystic ovary syndrome. Fertil Steril. 2010;93(7):2299–302.
131. Nakhuda GS, Chu MC, Wang JG, Sauer MV, Lobo RA. Elevated serum Müllerian-inhibiting substance may be a marker for ovarian hyperstimulation syndrome in normal women undergoing in vitro fertilization. Fertil Steril. 2006;85(5):1541–3.
132. Lee TH, Liu CH, Huang CC, et al. Serum anti-Müllerian hormone and estradiol levels as predictors of ovarian hyperstimulation syndrome in assisted reproduction technology cycles. Hum Reprod. 2008;23(1):160–7.
133. Rey R. Anti-Müllerian hormone in disorders of sex determination and differentiation. Arq Bras Endocrinol Metabol. 2005;49:26–36.
134. Broekmans FJ, Visser JA, Laven JS, Broer SL, Themmen AP, Fauser BC. Anti-Müllerian hormone and ovarian dysfunction. Trends Endocrinol Metab. 2008;19(9):340–7.

The Role of Obesity in Reproduction

4

Barbara Luke

Abstract

Obesity has risen to epidemic proportions worldwide and affects more than two thirds of US adults. In both genders, obesity is associated with impaired fertility, primarily due to disorders of the reproductive hormonal profile. Across the reproductive spectrum, obesity is associated with greater risks for adverse health outcomes, including higher rates of infertility, subfertility, early pregnancy loss, fetal deaths and stillbirths, congenital anomalies, and pregnancy complications. The excess reproductive morbidity associated with obesity may increase with longer duration, making the current trends among children and young adults particularly critical in terms of their future reproductive potential. Clinical and epidemiologic studies strongly implicate prenatal growth restriction followed by early childhood catch-up growth with development of symptoms of polycystic ovary syndrome by early adolescence. Abnormal glycemic parameters, including high dietary glycemic load, fasting, and 2-h glucose levels, and fasting insulin have also been linked to adverse reproductive outcomes, further increased in the presence of obesity. A recent national study of ART reported reduced clinical pregnancy rate with increasing BMI with autologous but not donor oocytes and reduced live birth rate with increasing BMI regardless of oocyte source. These findings point to the need for dietary periconceptional and prenatal therapies targeted at improving the metabolic environment in obese women. Weight loss should be the first-line treatment for overweight men and women considering pregnancy. In addition to dietary modifications to facilitate weight loss, lifestyle factors such as regular physical exercise, elimination of tobacco use and alcohol consumption, behavior modification, and stress management may be of benefit.

B. Luke (✉)
Department of Obstetrics, Gynecology,
and Reproductive Biology, Michigan State University,
East Lansing, MI, USA
e-mail: lukeb@msu.edu

C. Racowsky et al. (eds.), *Biennial Review of Infertility: Volume 2*,
DOI 10.1007/978-1-4419-8456-2_4, © Springer Science+Business Media, LLC 2011

Keywords
Overweight • Obesity • Body mass index • Excess reproductive morbidity • Prenatal growth restriction • Abnormal glycemic parameters • Insulin resistance • Metabolic environment

4.1 Introduction

As the most common chronic disease in the United States, overweight or obesity affects more than two thirds of adults [1]. The prevalence of obesity has more than doubled since the 1970s and is a leading cause of morbidity and mortality, second only to tobacco use [2]. In both genders, obesity is associated with impaired fertility, primarily due to disorders of the reproductive hormonal profile. In obese men, this can result in hypotestosteronemia and even hypogonadotropic hypogonadism; in obese women, it can result in hyperandrogenism and the metabolic abnormalities which characterize the polycystic ovary syndrome (PCOS). The abdominal obesity phenotype amplifies these associations.

Obesity is associated with greater risks for adverse health outcomes across the reproductive spectrum, including higher rates of infertility [3–5], subfertility (increased time-to-pregnancy) [6–8], early pregnancy loss [9–15], fetal deaths, stillbirths and neonatal deaths [16–19], congenital anomalies [20], as well as pregnancy complications [21, 22]. The excess reproductive morbidity associated with obesity may increase with longer duration, making the current trends among children and young adults particularly critical in terms of their future reproductive potential. In the United States between 1971–1974 and 2005–2006, the proportion of young adults (ages 18–29 years) who were obese tripled (8–24%), compared to a doubling among most other adult age groups during the same time period [23]. Recent findings from the Study of Women's Health across the Nation indicate that adolescent obesity is associated with a threefold increased risk of lifetime nulliparity and a fourfold increased risk of lifetime nulligravidity [24].

4.2 Definitions

According to the World Health Organization [25], obesity is a disease defined as the condition of excess body fat to the extent that health is impaired. The most widely accepted measure is the body mass index (BMI, weight (kg)/height (m)^2), with cutpoints of 25 kg/m^2 (overweight) and 30 kg/m^2 (obese), respectively, recommended by the National Heart, Lung, and Blood Institute's and North American Association for the Study of Obesity expert committee [26] (see Table 4.1). In addition, this expert committee recommends using waist circumference cutpoints of 40 in. (102 cm) for men and 35 in. (88 cm) for women to define central obesity. This measure may be even more useful than BMI because of its greater predictive value for future health risks, as well as ease of measurement [26–28]. BMI is not the best measure to reflect body fat and does not account for racial and ethnic differences in body build [29]. Specifically, the proportion of Asians at high risk for type 2 diabetes and cardiovascular disease is considerable at lower cutoffs for overweight. The World Health Organization Expert Consultation recommended retaining the current BMI cutoffs, but adding additional cutoff points of 23, 27.5, 32.5, and 37.5 kg/m^2 for public health action (see Table 4.1).

4.3 Male Reproductive Health and Obesity

It has been suggested that semen quality has been declining during the second half of the last century [30–33], triggering debate regarding possible causes [34–37]. This trend corresponds with the international rise in obesity [1, 38]. Excess weight in adult men has been directly

Table 4.1 The World Health Organization's international classification of adult underweight, normal weight, overweight, and obesity according to BMI

Classification	Subclassification	BMI (kg/m²) Principal cutoff points	Additional cutoff points
Underweight		<18.5	
	Severe thinness	<16.0	
	Moderate thinness	16.00–16.99	
	Mild thinness	17.00–18.49	
Normal weight		18.50–24.99	18.50–22.99
			23.00–24.99
Overweight		≥25.00	25.00–27.49
	Preobese	25.00–29.99	27.50–29.99
Obese		≥30.0	
	Class I	30.00–34.99	30.00–32.49
			32.50–34.99
	Class II	35.00–39.99	35.00–37.49
			37.50–39.99
	Class III	≥40.0	

and indirectly related to biological changes that could reduce fertility [39]. Most, but not all studies, have reported an association between male infertility and elevated BMI.

Many studies have reported that adult BMI in males is dose-dependently associated with the levels of reproductive hormones, including: (1) lower concentrations of testosterone, sex hormone-binding globulin (SHBG), and inhibin B; and (2) higher concentrations of estradiol, but unaffected or only slightly lower concentrations of lutenizing hormone and follicle-stimulating hormone [40–47]. The results regarding semen quality are inconsistent, with some studies reporting a significant association between overweight and low semen quality [40, 41, 48–51], and other studies reporting no association [42, 43, 47, 52–54]. Several researchers have suggested that the adverse effect of male obesity on semen parameters is mediated by serum leptin, altering intracellular metabolism and peripheral tissue receptors in Leydig and germ cells [55–57]. Leptin inhibits testicular steroidogenesis, decreasing testosterone synthesis in Leydig cells and inhibiting sperm maturation, as well as suppressing Sertoli cell function [58, 59].

Although weight loss is the logical first-line therapy for obesity, there are few studies documenting its effect on fertility among obese men. Most published studies demonstrate an improvement in the reproductive hormonal profile, including an increase in SHBG, inhibin B, and total testosterone levels as well as a reduction in estradiol levels [60–63].

4.4 Female Reproductive Health and Obesity

In concert with the rise in obesity, there has been a long-term trend in delaying childbearing and an increased use of infertility treatments to achieve conception. Infertility affects an estimated 12% of women of reproductive age [64]. Research suggests that perinatal outcome may be worse for women with assisted vs. spontaneous conceptions, including greater risks for preterm birth (<32 and <37 weeks), low birth weight and very low birth weight, small-for-gestational age, cesarean delivery, NICU admission, and perinatal mortality [65, 66]. An important underlying mechanism may be a genetic predisposition to factors associated with infertility, including allelic variants in cytokine genes known to stimulate inflammation or those known to downregulate the anti-inflammatory response. Ness [67] suggests that although women with a robust inflammatory response may be more likely to survive to reproduce, their reproductive experiences may be less successful than women who are less responsive. Obesity has been shown to be a chronic inflammatory state with increased expression of proinflammatory factors and a reduction in anti-inflammatory factors [68, 69]. *In women with assisted conceptions, obesity may further potentiate this inflammatory response, increasing the known risks for adverse reproductive outcomes*, including fetal loss and stillbirths associated with higher body weight [16–18]. Inflammation and dyslipidemia early in pregnancy have been shown to be independently associated with preterm birth [70, 71]. In the presence of obesity, these factors are even greater and also include significant impairment of endothelial function [72, 73].

Among women, the reproductive axis is closely linked to nutritional status, with amenorrhea, anovulation, subfertility, and infertility occurring with higher body weights. Obese women are more likely to experience irregular menstrual cycles, anovulation, and signs of androgen excess, particularly when the excess weight occurred during adolescence [74, 75]. Obesity is strongly associated with PCOS, an abdominal phenotype of fat distribution, hyperandrogenism, and insulin resistance with compensatory hyperinsulinemia [76]. Obese women have a lower chance of pregnancy following in vitro fertilization, require higher dosage of gonadotropins, and have an increased miscarriage rate [9–15].

4.5 Prenatal Growth and PCOS

A growing body of research implicates prenatal growth to timing of puberty and subsequent symptoms of PCOS [77–85]. Even after achieving a normal body size by age two, children born small for their gestational age tend to become relatively adipose, hyperinsulinemic, and hypoadiponectinemic, with physiologic evidence of low-grade inflammation [83, 84]. By 6 years of age, these children are more likely to develop visceral adiposity, even with normal body weight. By 8 years of age, children born small for gestational age with catch-up growth develop high dehydroepiandrosterone sulfate (DHEAS) and low SHBG levels [85]. Precocious puberty (appearance of pubic hair before age eight) has also been demonstrated as part of this sequence, as well as anovulatory and hyperinsulinemic hyperandrogenism in late adolescence and adulthood [80–82]. Insulin resistance has been cited as a key mechanism linking prenatal growth restraint to early menarche [77], with insulin-sensitizing therapy improving ovulation rates [78, 79].

4.6 Diet, Obesity, and Adverse Reproductive Outcomes

Obesity is associated with alterations in carbohydrate and fat metabolism central to the development of insulin resistance. A diet with a high glycemic index has been associated with infertility, fetal loss, congenital anomalies, prematurity, as well as macrosomia. Greater carbohydrate intake and dietary glycemic load have been associated with an increased risk of infertility due to anovulation [86]. Jovanovic et al. [87] demonstrated a threefold increased risk of pregnancy losses at glycemic extremes in both normal and diabetic pregnancies, as measured by plasma glycated protein and fructosamine levels. A diet with a high glycemic load is associated with a twofold increased risk of neural tube defects [88, 89]; among women with BMIs greater than 29, this risk increases to more than fourfold [89]. Among normal-weight women treated with ART, Wei et al. [90] reported greater risk for preterm birth associated with abnormal preconception glycemic parameters, including higher fasting and 2-h glucose levels, fasting insulin, and homeostatic model assessment of insulin resistance.

4.7 Endometrial vs. Oocyte Factors

The endocrine and metabolic environment may influence oocyte quality, and therefore, embryo development and subsequent implantation and pregnancy outcome. One possible mechanism for the lower pregnancy rate associated with obesity may be altered receptivity of the uterus, due to disturbed endometrial function [10, 12]. Even studies limited to obese women using donor oocytes, eliminating the potential effect of older maternal age on lower quality of the embryos, have reported significantly reduced implantation and pregnancy rates and higher abortion rates [11, 12, 91, 92]. A recent national US study of ART reported reduced clinical pregnancy rate with increasing BMI with autologous but not donor oocytes and reduced live birth rate with increasing BMI regardless of oocyte source [91–93]. These findings are in accord with prior studies showing a progressive decline in pregnancy rates with rising obesity [4, 5, 10, 12]. The findings of an adverse effect of the maternal obese environment on a live birth outcome regardless of oocyte source point to the need for dietary periconceptional and prenatal therapies targeted at improving the metabolic environment.

4.8 Obesity and ART Therapy

Recent editorials have called for excluding women with high BMIs from receiving ART, suggesting a cutoff of 35 as the upper limit before initiation of treatment [94, 95], while others have advocated that weight loss be incorporated into the treatment for infertility, but prior to conception [96]. Weight loss should be the first-line treatment for overweight women considering pregnancy, particularly if they have a history of recurrent miscarriages [97]. In addition to dietary modifications to facilitate weight loss, lifestyle factors such as regular physical exercise, elimination of tobacco use and alcohol consumption, behavior modification, and stress management may be of benefit [98, 99].

4.9 Conclusions

Obesity is associated with greater risks for adverse health outcomes across the reproductive spectrum, including higher rates of infertility, subfertility (increased time-to-pregnancy), early pregnancy loss, fetal deaths, stillbirths and neonatal deaths, congenital anomalies, as well as pregnancy complications. Among males, obesity has been directly and indirectly related to biological changes that could reduce fertility. Obese women undergoing in vitro fertilization require higher dosages of gonadotropins, have a lower chance of pregnancy, and a greater miscarriage rate. Weight loss should be the primary therapy for overweight and obese men and women considering pregnancy, along with changes in lifestyle factors such as smoking, drinking, and stress management.

References

1. Flegal KM, Carroll MD, Ogden CL, Curtin LR. Prevalence and trends in obesity among US adults, 1999–2008. JAMA. 2010;303:235–41.
2. US Department of Health and Human Services. The surgeon general's call to action to prevent and decrease overweight and obesity. Rockville: Office of the Surgeon General; 2001 (www.surgeongeneral.gov/topics/obesity).
3. Law DCG, Maclehose RF, Longnecker MP. Obesity and time to pregnancy. Hum Reprod. 2007;22:414–20.
4. van der Steeg JW, Steures P, Eijkemans MJC, Habbema JDF, Hompes PGA, Burggraaff JM, et al. Obesity affects spontaneous pregnancy chances in subfertile, ovulatory women. Hum Reprod. 2008;23:324–8.
5. Awartani KA, Nahas S, Al Hassan SH, Al Deery MA, Coskun S. Infertility outcome in sub groups of obese population. Reprod Biol Endocrinol. 2009;7:52.
6. Nohr EA, Vaeth M, Rasmussen S, Ramlau-Hansen CH, Olsen J. Waiting time to pregnancy according to maternal birthweight and prepregnancy BMI. Hum Reprod. 2009;24:226–32.
7. Wise LA, Rothman KJ, Mikkelsen EM, Sørensen HT, Riis A, Hatch EE. An internet-based prospective study of body size and time-to-pregnancy. Hum Reprod. 2010;25:253–64.
8. Bolúmar F, Olsen J, Rebagliato M, Sáez-Lloret I, Bisanti L, European Study Group on Infertility and Subfecundity. Body mass index and delayed conception: a European multicenter study on infertility and subfecundity. Am J Epidemiol. 2000;151:1072–9.
9. Fedorcsák P, Storeng R, Dale PO, Tanbo T, Åbyholm T. Obesity is a risk factor for early pregnancy loss after IVF or ICSI. Acta Obstet Gynecol Scand. 2000;79:43–8.
10. Wang JX, Davies M, Norman RJ. Body mass index and probability of pregnancy during assisted reproduction treatment: retrospective study. BMJ. 2000;321:1320–1.
11. Bellver J, Rossal LP, Bosch E, Zúñiga A, Corona JT, Meléndez F, et al. Obesity and the risk of spontaneous abortion after oocyte donation. Fertil Steril. 2003;79:1136–40.

12. Bellver J, Melo MAB, Bosch E, Serra V, Remohí J, Pellicer A. Obesity and poor reproductive outcome: the potential role of the endometrium. Fertil Steril. 2007;88:446–51.
13. Bellver J, Ayllón Y, Ferrando M, Melo M, Goyri E, Pellicer A, et al. Female obesity impairs in vitro fertilization outcome without affecting embryo quality. Fertil Steril. 2010;93:447–54.
14. Lashen H, Fear K, Sturdee DW. Obesity is associated with increased risk of first trimester and recurrent miscarriage: matched case-control study. Hum Reprod. 2004;19:1644–6.
15. Veleva Z, Tiitinen A, Vilska S, Hydén-Granskog C, Tomás C, Martikainen H, et al. High and low BMI increase the risk of miscarriage after IVF/ICSI and FET. Hum Reprod. 2008;23:878–84.
16. Cnattingius S, Bergström R, Lipworth L, Kramer MS. Prepregnancy weight and the risk of adverse pregnancy outcomes. N Engl J Med. 1998;338:147–52.
17. Nohr EA, Bech BH, Davies MJ, Frydenberg M, Henriksen TB, Olsen J. Prepregnancy obesity and fetal death: a study within the Danish National Birth Cohort. Obstet Gynecol. 2005;106:250–9.
18. Kristensen J, Vestergaard M, Wisborg K, Kesmodel U, Secher NJ. Pre-pregnancy weight and the risk of stillbirth and neonatal death. BJOG. 2005;112: 403–8.
19. Chen A, Feresu SA, Fernandez C, Rogan WJ. Maternal obesity and the risk of infant death in the United States. Epidemiology. 2009;20:74–81.
20. Stothard KJ, Tennant PW, Bell R, Rankin J. Maternal overweight and obesity and the risk of congenital anomalies: a systematic review and meta-analysis. JAMA. 2009;301:636–50.
21. Cedergren MI. Maternal morbid obesity and the risk of adverse pregnancy outcome. Obstet Gynecol. 2004;103:219–24.
22. Dokras A, Baredziak L, Blaine J, Syrop C, VanVoorhis BJ, Sparks A. Obstetric outcomes after in vitro fertilization in obese and morbidly obese women. Obstet Gynecol. 2006;108:61–9.
23. National Center for Health Statistics. Health, United States 2008. Hyattsville, Md. 2009.
24. Polotsky AJ, Hailpern SM, Skurnick JH, Lo JC, Sternfeld B, Santoro N. Association of adolescent obesity and lifetime nulliparity – The Study of Women's Health Across the Nation (SWAN). Fertil Steril. 2010;93:2004–11.
25. World Health Organization (WHO). Obesity: preventing and managing the global epidemic: report of a WHO consultation. Geneva: World Health Organization; 2000. (Technical report series no. 894).
26. National Institutes of Health (NIH) National Heart, Lung, and Blood Institute's (NHLBI) North American Association for the Study of Obesity (NAASO). The practical guide: identification, evaluation, and treatment of overweight and obesity in adults. Rockville: National Institutes of Health. 2000. (Publication no. 00-4084).
27. Zhu S, Heymsfield SB, Toyoshima H, et al. Race-ethnicity-specific waist circumference cutoffs for identifying cardiovascular disease risk factors. Am J Clin Nutr. 2005;81:409–15.
28. Wang Y, Rimm EB, Stampfer MJ, et al. Comparison of abdominal adiposity and overall obesity in predicting risk of type 2 diabetes among men. Am J Clin Nutr. 2005;81:555–63.
29. WHO Expert Consultation. Appropriate body-mass index for Asian populations and its implications for policy and intervention strategies. Lancet. 2004;363:157–63.
30. Carlsen E, Giwercman A, Keiding N, Skakkebæk NE. Evidence for decreasing quality of semen during past 50 years. BMJ. 1992;305:609–13.
31. Vermeulen A. Environment, human reproduction, menopause, and andropause. Environ Health Perspect Suppl. 1993;101 Suppl 2:91–100.
32. Bonde JP, Ernst E, Jensen TK, Hjollund NH, Kolstad H, Henriksen TB. Relation between semen quality and fertility: a population-based study of 430 first-pregnancy planners. Lancet. 1998;352:1172–7.
33. Skakkebæk NE, Jørgensen N, Main KM, Rajpert-De Meyts E, Leffers H, Andersson A-M, et al. Is human fecundity declining? Int J Androl. 2006;29:2–11.
34. Irvine DS. Male reproductive health: cause for concern? Andrologia. 2000;32:195–208.
35. Storgaard L, Bonde JP, Ernst E, Spanô M, Andersen CY, Frydenberg M, et al. Does smoking during pregnancy affect sons' sperm counts? Epidemiology. 2003;14:278–86.
36. Fisch H. Declining worldwide sperm counts: disproving a myth. Urol Clin North Am. 2008;35:137–46.
37. Velde E, Burdorf A, Nieschlag E, Eijkemans R, Kremer JAM, Roeleveld N, et al. Is human fecundity declining in Western countries? Hum Reprod. 2010;25:1348–53.
38. The International Obesity Task Force. http://www.iotf.org. Accessed 20 July 2010.
39. Nguyen R, Wilcox A, Skjærven R, Baird DD. Men's body mass index and infertility. Hum Reprod. 2007; 22:2488–93.
40. Jensen TK, Andersson A-M, Jørgensen N, Andersen A-G, Carlsen E, Petersen JH, et al. Body mass index in relation to semen quality and reproductive hormones among 1,558 Danish men. Fertil Steril. 2004; 82:863–70.
41. Fejes I, Koloszar S, Zavaczki Z, Daru J, Szollosi J, Pal A. Effect of body weight on testosterone/estradiol ratio in oligoospermic patients. Arch Androl. 2006; 52:97–102.
42. Aggerholm AS, Thulstrup AM, Toft G, Ramlau-Hansen CH, Bonde JP. Is overweight a risk factor for reduced semen quality and altered serum sex hormone profile? Fertil Steril. 2008;90:619–26.
43. Pauli EM, Legro RS, Demers LM, Kunselman AR, Dodson WC, Lee PA. Diminished paternity and gonadal function with increasing obesity in men. Fertil Steril. 2008;90:346–51.

44. Vermeulen A. Decreased androgen levels and obesity in men. Ann Med. 1996;28:13–5.
45. Winters SJ, Wang C, Abdelrahaman E, Hadeed V, Dyky MA, Brufsky A. Inhibin-B levels in healthy young adult men and prepubertal boys: is obesity the cause for the contemporary decline in sperm count because of fewer Sertoli cells? J Androl. 2006;27:560–4.
46. Pasquali R. Obesity and androgens: facts and perspectives. Fertil Steril. 2006;85:1319–40.
47. Ramlau-Hansen CH, Hansen M, Jensen CR, Olsen J, Bonde JP, Thulstrup AM. Semen quality and reproductive hormones according to birthweight and body mass index in childhood and adult life: two decades of follow-up. Fertil Steril. 2010;94:610–8.
48. Magnusdottir EV, Thorsteinsson T, Thorsteindottir S, Heimisdottir M, Olafsdottir K. Persistent organochlorines, sedentary occupation, obesity and human male subfertility. Hum Reprod. 2005;20:208–15.
49. Fejes I, Koloszar S, Szollosi J, Zavaczki Z, Pal A. Is semen quality affected by male body fat distribution? Andrologia. 2005;37:155–9.
50. Kort HI, Massey JB, Elsner CW, Mitchell-Leef D, Shapiro DB, Witt MA. Impact of body mass index values on sperm quantity and quality. J Androl. 2006; 27:450–2.
51. Hammoud AO, Wilde N, Gibson M, Parks A, Carrell DT, Meikle AW. Male obesity and alteration in sperm parameters. Fertil Steril. 2008;90:897–904.
52. Qin DD, Yuan W, Zhou WJ, Cui YQ, Wu JQ, Gao ES. Do reproductive hormones explain the association between body mass index and semen quality? Asian J Androl. 2007;9:827–34.
53. Martini AC, Tissera A, Estofán D, Molina RI, Mangeaud A, Fiol de Cuneo M, et al. Overweight and seminal quality: a study of 794 patients. Fertil Steril. 2010;94:1739–43.
54. Duits FH, van Wely M, van der Veen F, Gianotten J. Healthy overweight male partners of subfertile couples should not worry about their semen quality. Fertil Steril. 2010;94:1356–9.
55. Hofny ERM, Ali ME, Abdel-Hafez HZ, El-Dien Kamal E, Mohamed EE, El-Azeem HGA, et al. Semen parameters and hormonal profile in obese fertile and infertile males. Fertil Steril. 2010;94:581–4.
56. Tena-Sempere M, Pinilla L, Gonzalez LC, Dieguez C, Cazanueva FF, Aguilar E. Leptin inhibits secretion from adult rat testis in vitro. J Endocrinol. 1999;161:211–8.
57. Soyupek S, Armağan A, Serel TA, Hoğcan MB, Perk H, Karaöz E. Leptin expression in the testicular tissue of fertile and infertile men. Arch Androl. 2005;51: 239–46.
58. Tena-Sempere M, Barreiro ML. Leptin in male reproduction: the testis paradigm. Mol Cell Endocrinol. 2002;188:9–13.
59. Margetic S, Gazzola C, Pegg GG, Hill RA. Leptin: a review of its peripheral actions and interactions. Int J Obes Relat Metab Disord. 2002;26:1407–33.
60. Globerman H, Shen-Orr Z, Karnieli E, Aloni Y, Charuzi I. Inhibin B in men with severe obesity and after weight reduction following gastroplasty. Endocr Res. 2005;31:17–26.
61. Kaukua J, Pekkarinen T, Sane T, Mustajoki P. Sex hormones and sexual function in obese men losing weight. Obes Res. 2003;11:689–94.
62. Niskanen L, Laaksonen DE, Punnonen K, Mustajoki P, Kaukua J, Rissanen A. Changes in sex hormone binding globulin and testosterone during weight loss and weight maintenance in abdominally obese men with the metabolic syndrome. Diabetes Obes Metab. 2004;6:208–15.
63. Bastounis EA, Karayiannakis AJ, Syrigos K, Zbar A, Makri GG, Alexious D. Sex hormone changes in morbidly obese patients after vertical banded gastroplasty. Eur Surg Res. 1998;30:43–7.
64. Chandra A, Martinez GM, Mosher WD, Abma JC, Jones J. Fertility, family planning, and reproductive health of US women: data from the 2002 National Survey of Family Growth. National Center for Health Statistics. Vital Health Stat. 2005;23(25):1–160.
65. Helmerhorst FM, Perquin DAM, Donker D, Keirse MJNC. Perinatal outcome of singletons and twins after assisted conception: a systematic review of controlled studies. BMJ. 2004. doi: 10.1136/bmj.37957.560278.EE.
66. Shevell T, Malone FD, Vidaver J, Porter TF, Luthy DA, Comstock CH, et al. Assisted reproductive technology and pregnancy outcome. Obstet Gynecol. 2005; 106:1039–45.
67. Ness RB. The consequences for human reproduction of a robust inflammatory response. Q Rev Biol. 2004; 79:383–93.
68. Hotamisligil GS, Shargill NS, Spiegelman BM. Adipose expression of tumor necrosis factor-alpha: direct role in obesity-linked insulin resistance. Science. 1993;259:87–91.
69. Cancello R, Clément K. Is obesity an inflammatory illness? Role of low-grade inflammation and macrophage infiltration in human white adipose tissue. Br J Obstet Gynaecol. 2006;113:1141–7.
70. Catov JM, Bodnar LM, Ness RB, Barron SJ, Roberts JM. Inflammation and dyslipidemia related to risk of spontaneous preterm birth. Am J Epidemiol. 2007; 166:1312–9.
71. Catov JM, Bodnar LM, Kip KE, Hubel C, Ness RB, Harger G, et al. Early pregnancy lipid concentrations and spontaneous preterm birth. Am J Obstet Gynecol. 2007;197:610.e1–7.
72. Stewart FM, Freeman DJ, Ramsay JE, Greer IA, Caslake M, Ferrell WR. Longitudinal assessment of maternal endothelial function and markers of inflammation and placental function throughout pregnancy in lean and obese mothers. J Clin Endocrinol Metab. 2007;92:969–75.
73. Ramsay JE, Ferrell WR, Crawford L, Wallace AM, Greer IA, Sattar N. Maternal obesity is associated with dysregulation of metabolic, vascular, and inflammatory pathways. J Clin Endocrinol Metab. 2002;87: 4231–7.

74. Grodstein F, Goldman MB, Cramer DW. Body mass index and ovulatory infertility. Epidemiology. 1994; 5:247–50.
75. Pelusi C, Pasquali R. Polycystic ovary syndrome in adolescents: pathophysiology and treatment implications. Treat Endocrinol. 2003;2:215–30.
76. The Rotterdam ESHRE/ASRM-Sponsored PCOS Consensus Workshop Group. Revised 2003 consensus on diagnostic criteria and long-term health risks related to polycystic ovary syndrome (PCOS). Hum Reprod. 2004;19:41–7.
77. Ibáñez L, de Zegher F. Puberty and prenatal growth. Mol Cell Endocrinol. 2006;254–255:22–5.
78. Ibáñez L, López-Bermejo A, Diaz M, Marcos MV, de Zegher F. Pubertal metformin therapy to reduce total, visceral, and hepatic adiposity. J Pediatr. 2010;156: 98–102.
79. Ibáñez L, López-Bermejo A, Diaz M, Marcos MV, de Zegher F. Metformin treatment for four years to reduce total and visceral fat in low birth weight girls with precocious pubarche. J Clin Endocrinol Metab. 2008;93:1841–5.
80. Ibáñez L, Potau N, Zampolli M, Street ME, Carrascosa A. Girls diagnosed with premature pubarche show an exaggerated ovarian androgen synthesis from the early stages of puberty: evidence from gonadotropin-releasing hormone agonist testing. Fertil Steril. 1997;67:849–55.
81. Zegher F, Ibáñez L. Prenatal growth restraint followed by catch-up of weight: a hyperinsulinemic pathway to polycystic ovary syndrome. Fertil Steril. 2006;86 Suppl 1:S4–5.
82. Ibáñez L, Jaramillo A, Enríquez G, Miró E, López-Bermejo A, Dunger D, et al. Polycystic ovaries after precocious pubarche: relation to prenatal growth. Hum Reprod. 2007;22:395–400.
83. Ibáñez L, Suárez L, López-Bermejo A, Diaz M, Valls C, de Zegher F. Early development of visceral fat excess after spontaneous catch-up growth in children with low birth weight. J Clin Endocrinol Metab. 2008;93:925–8.
84. Ibáñez L, López-Bermejo A, Suárez L, Marcos MV, Diaz M, de Zegher F. Visceral adiposity without overweight in children born small for gestational age. J Clin Endocrinol Metab. 2008;93:2079–83.
85. Ibáñez L, López-Bermejo A, Diaz M, Suárez L, de Zegher F. Low-birth weight children develop lower sex hormone binding globulin and higher dehydroepiandrosterone sulfate levels and aggravate their visceral adiposity and hypoadiponectinemia between six and eight years of age. J Clin Endocrinol Metab. 2009; 94:3696–9.
86. Chavarro JE, Rich-Edwards JW, Rosner BA, Willett WC. A prospective study of dietary carbohydrate quantity and quality in relation to risk of ovulatory infertility. Eur J Clin Nutr. 2009;63:78–86.
87. Jovanovic L, Knopp RH, Kim H, Cefalu WT, Zhu X-D, Lee YJ, et al. Elevated pregnancy losses at high and low extremes of maternal glucose in early normal and diabetic pregnancy. Diabetes Care. 2005;28: 1113–7.
88. Yazdy MM, Liu S, Mitchell AA, Werler MM. Maternal dietary glycemic intake and the risk of neural tube defects. Am J Epidemiol. 2009;171:407–14.
89. Shaw GM, Quach T, Nelson V, Carmichael SL, Schaffer DM, Selvin S, et al. Neural tube defects associated with maternal periconceptional dietary intake of simple sugars and glycemic index. Am J Clin Nutr. 2003;78:972–8.
90. Wei H-J, Young R, Kuo I-L, Liaw C-M, Chiang H-S, Yeh C-Y. Abnormal preconception oral glucose tolerance test predicts an unfavorable pregnancy outcome after an in vitro fertilization cycle. Fertil Steril. 2008;90:613–8.
91. Luke B, Brown MB, Stern JE, Missmer SA, Fujimoto VY, Leach R. Maternal obesity adversely affects assisted reproductive technology (ART) pregnancy rates and obstetric outcomes. Fertil Steril. 2009;92 Suppl 1:S1.
92. Luke B, Brown MB, Stern JE, Missmer SA, Fujimoto VY, Leach R. Effect of maternal body mass index (BMI) on assisted reproductive technology (ART) pregnancy rates and obstetric outcomes. Fertil Steril. 2009;92 Suppl 1:S79.
93. Luke B, Brown MB, Stern JE, Missmer SA, Leach R, Fujimoto VY. The effect of maternal body mass index (BMI) and oocyte source on assisted reproductive technology (ART) pregnancy rates and obstetric outcomes. Fertil Steril. 2009;92 Suppl 1:S52.
94. Jauniaux E, Farquharson RG, Christiansen OB, Exalto N. Evidence-based guidelines for investigation and medical management of recurrent miscarriage. Hum Reprod. 2006;21:2216–22.
95. Balen AH, Dresner M, Scott EM, Drife JO. Should obese women with polycystic ovary syndrome receive treatment for infertility? (Editorial). BMJ. 2006;332: 434–5.
96. Farquhar CM, Gillett WR. Prioritizing for fertility treatments – should a high BMI exclude treatment? (Commentary). BJOG. 2006;113:1107–9.
97. Nelson SM, Fleming RF. The preconceptual contraception paradigm: obesity and infertility. Hum Reprod. 2007;22:912–5.
98. Moran LJ, Pasquali R, Tede HJ, Hoeger KM, Norman RJ. Treatment of obesity in polycystic ovary syndrome: a position statement of the androgen excess and Polycystic Ovary Syndrome Society. Fertil Steril. 2009;92:1966–82.
99. ESHRE Task Force on Ethics and Law. Lifestyle-related factors and access to medically assisted reproduction. Hum Reprod. 2010;25:578–83.

Endometrial Receptivity in Natural and Controlled Ovarian-Stimulated Cycles

5

José A. Horcajadas, José A. Martínez-Conejero, and Carlos Simón

Abstract

The development of endometrial receptivity is a prerequisite for successful embryonic implantation in mammals. The receptive status is reached only during a short period of time in the midluteal phase, this being maximal 7 days after the endogenous peak of LH (LH+7), named as the window of implantation (WOI). At this time, the endometrial epithelium acquires the functional ability to support blastocyst adhesion. In ART, controlled ovarian stimulation (COS) induces lower implantation rates per embryo transferred than natural or ovum donation cycles, suggesting suboptimal endometrial development due to the abnormal endocrine/paracrine milieu. Researchers have investigated the functional genomics of endometrial receptivity in natural cycles and the impact of COS on the gene expression pattern of the endometrium, even with the use of different drugs such as gonadotrophin-releasing hormone (GnRH) agonists or antagonists. This paper reviews results obtained in different studies to elucidate the changes induced by the different clinical protocols with the objective to introduce a new molecular objective tool to analyze the endometrial receptivity status in natural cycles and to understand the impact of COS in the human endometrium.

Keywords

Endometrial receptivity • Gene expression • Controlled ovarian stimulation • Microarray

C. Simón (✉)
Fundación IVI-Instituto Universitario IVI-University of Valencia, Valencia 46015, Spain
and
Valencia Stem Cell Bank, Centro de Investigaciones Príncipe Felipe, Valencia 46012, Spain
e-mail: csimon@ivi.es

C. Racowsky et al. (eds.), *Biennial Review of Infertility: Volume 2*,
DOI 10.1007/978-1-4419-8456-2_5,

5.1 Introduction

Human endometrium is a dynamic tissue that undergoes well-defined cycles of proliferation, differentiation, and shedding (menstruation) in response to the prevailing endocrine and paracrine environment, the main objective being to reach the receptive status. In the natural cycle, the ovary releases one oocyte in a standard ovulation, approximately 14 days before the next menstruation. If the oocyte is fertilized, the resulting embryo will arrive at the endometrium at the morula stage (days 4–5). At this time, receptiveness of the endometrium will occur, in a synchronized manner with the development of the embryo.

In assisted reproduction technologies (ART), the main goal of ovarian stimulation is to trigger oocyte maturation of an appropriate number of follicles to obtain 6–8 mature oocytes. However, lower implantation rates per transferred embryo than those in natural cycles remain a major problem that is compensated by increasing the number of transferred embryos [1] at the cost of increased numbers of multiple pregnancies. Furthermore, implantation rates obtained in ovum donation programs are higher than in patients under controlled ovarian stimulation (COS), suggesting that the low rates observed when the ovaries are stimulated are related to a detrimental effect on the endometrium. This issue remains more evident in high responders patients where supraphysiological concentrations of estradiol on the day of human chorionic gonadotrophin (hCG) administration are deleterious to embryonic implantation [2–5]. Furthermore, it has been demonstrated in animal models that while low doses of estradiol maintain the uterus in a receptive state, high doses cause it to become refractory [6]. Uterine receptivity is diminished during ovarian stimulation compared with natural cycles [7]. A substantial number of endometrial alterations inducing have been documented in COS cycles using morphological methods. An advancement in the early luteal phase using histology [8–11] and scanning electron microscopy [12, 13] has been previously demonstrated. Others researchers have elucidated biochemical changes in the endometrium induced by ovarian stimulation. In this context, down-regulation of the endometrial estrogen and progesterone receptors [14] and biochemical changes in the endometrial fluid [15] have been described. As has been mentioned before, this is not surprising, considering that the aim of COS is to recruit a sufficient number of oocytes, having as a side-effect supraphysiological concentrations of steroid hormones and paracrine mediators that might target the endometrium. The impact of some specific molecules on the development of endometrial receptivity has been reported from different perspectives, encompassing the impact of progesterone on endometrial stromal cell development in vitro [16] such as interleukin (IL)-1β [17] or IL-11 [18]. More recently, the in vitro effects of steroids on freshly isolated endometrial endothelial cells have also been reported [19].

However, the most attractive strategy to investigate the genomic profile of the endometrium and the impact of COS protocols on endometrial receptivity has been the use of microarray technology, which allows studying of the entire transcriptome of a given tissue in a single experiment.

5.2 The Endometrium as a Tissue

The lining of the human uterus is a complex mucosa composed of a basal layer (basalis), which persists from cycle to cycle, and a transient superficial layer (functionalis). The function of the latter is to accommodate the implanting blastocyst and provide the maternal component that will interact with the placenta. The tissue components of the endometrium are a luminal and glandular epithelium with a connective stroma in which is embedded an elaborate vascular tree. Endometrial components features change along the menstrual cycle [20]. Cyclic changes of the endometrium have been well described at the light microscopy level [21]. Although some authors prefer to simplify the menstrual cycle and divide it into two main phases, proliferative and secretory, others prefer to consider three different phases: the proliferative phase (days 5–14), the secretory phase [14–28], and menses (days 1–4) if no implantation occurs.

For more than 50 years, histological evaluation of the endometrium has been the gold standard for clinical diagnosis set on the basis of the morphological observations of Noyes et al. [22, 23]. These authors described "specific" morphological features of the different endometrial compartments throughout the menstrual cycle. The early proliferative phase (days 5–7) is characterized by straight, fairly undifferentiated glands with circular cross-section lined by a columnar epithelium with basally located nuclei. Their luminal diameter (below 50 mm) changes little in the proliferative and the height of the cells remains fairly constant (around 21 mm). Few mitotic figures can be seen. By the midproliferative phase (days 8–10), the endometrial glands are longer with slight tortuosity. Mitotic figures are prominent and cells appear pseudostratified. In the late proliferative phase [11–14], the glands appear with a marked tortuosity and wider lumena. Pseudostratification increases and stromal edema starts to be evident. During secretory phase (LH+2/3), there is still a moderate degree of glandular and stromal mitosis. The cells appear taller and less pseudostratified than before. At LH+4, only occasional mitoses can be seen. Sub- and supranuclear vacuoles within the gland cells are maximal on this day. Gland cell size is also maximal on this day. At LH+5, mitosis activity has ceased absolutely in glands although can be visualized in stroma. Around 25% of the endometrium is occupied by glands in this phase. At LH+7, the gland cells contain little secretor material and have acquired a low columnar to cuboidal appearance. This is the point of maximal receptivity for clinical researchers. The amounts of secretory product within the glands and stromal edema are both maximal by day LH+8. In the last week of the secretory phase are few changes and they mainly occur in stroma and blood vessels. The late secretory phase is characterized by regression and glandular involution. At day LH+10, stromal edema has decreased, and at LH+11, the stromal predecidual reaction is mainly confined to the perivascular regions, but may also extend to adjacent glands and there is lymphocytic infiltration. By day LH+12, the predecidual reaction extends beneath the luminal epithelium. There is an increase in the lymphocyte number. The predecidual reaction is extensive on days LH+13/14, with a sheet-like formation in the stroma. Stroma disintegration and extravasation of erythrocytes are evident. If no implantation occurs, shedding of the functionalis layer of the endometrium ensues [20].

5.3 Hormonal Regulation of The Endometrium

The human endometrium undergoes cyclical variation in each menstrual cycle during the reproductive life. Endometrial changes are driven by the ovarian steroid hormones. Estradiol peaks at the end of the proliferative phase and progesterone increases at the beginning of the secretory phase, reaching the maximum 7 days later (Fig. 5.1). Esteroid hormones elicit their actions by binding to specific high-affinity nuclear receptors, which modulate the transcription of a large variety of genes. Global gene expression analyses performed along the menstrual cycle have revealed the relationship between molecular profiling and hormonal regulation.

Both estrogen receptor a (ERa) and b (ERb) are expressed in the endometrium, being ERa dominant. This receptor is present in both epithelial glands and stroma of the functionalis, being its expression maximal during the proliferative phase and declining during the secretory phase. Epithelial ERb also decreases during the secretory phase, but it is not detected in stroma. Progesterone receptor A and B are coexpressed in endometrium and are stimulated by estrogen during the proliferative phase and downregulated by progesterone in the secretory phase.

The coordinated action of steroids, through their nuclear receptors in the endometrial cells, promotes the gene regulation of hundreds of genes, inducing the formation of a receptive phenotype. Endometrial cells undergo specific

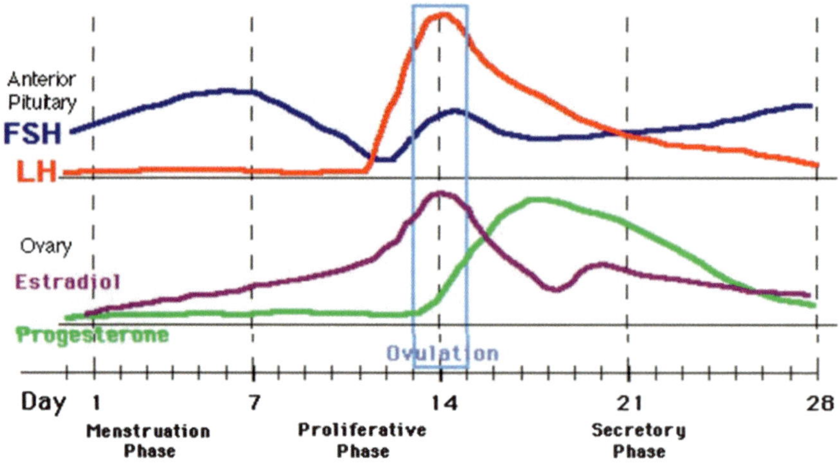

Fig. 5.1 Profile of expression of the hormones during the menstrual cycle

structural and functional changes that allow adhesiveness for the trophoectoderm. Detailed analyses, phase by phase, by using microarray technology are published by Ponnampalam et al. [24] and Talbi et al. [25].

5.4 Functional Genomics Studies of the Human Endometrium in Natural Cycles

Following completion of the human genome sequence, the main goal of researchers has been to identify the genes involved in the physiological and pathological processes of their particular fields of expertise. Parallelly, the development of new technologies and the bioinformatics have made possible to take the best from the information coming from the Human Genome. The success of this project has generated a burst of the "-omics" sciences: genomics is the study of genomes and the complete collection of genes that they contain; functional genomics, also known as transcriptomics, attempts to analyze patterns of gene expression and to relate this to function; metabolomics is a large-scale approach to monitoring as many as possible of the compounds involved in cellular processes in a single assay to derive metabolic profiles; proteomic approaches examine the collection of proteins to determine how, when, and where they are expressed; and bioinformatics, although not graced with the -omics suffix, remains a key element in collection, management, and analysis of large-scale data sets that are generated by the approaches described here. These technologies allow the analysis of thousands of molecules in a single experiment that ultimately makes possible a global view of the molecular profile of a biological sample. One of these newly developed tools is microarray technology, initially described in 1995 [26]. In the field of human reproduction, most of the studies performed have been functional genomics analyses, directed mainly to deepen the molecular knowledge of human endometrial physiology. Studies with human endometrial cells include cDNA and oligonucleotide analyses of endometrial stromal cell decidualization stimulated by cAMP ± progesterone [27–29], compared with nondecidualized endometrial stromal cells. Some of these were time-courses and have resulted in important insights into biochemical pathways participating in the process of endometrial stromal decidualization, with new players being involved.

Much information has been gained, in a whole functional genomics context, by employing endometrial biopsies. Some authors have analyzed the gene expression profile of the endometrium throughout the menstrual cycle [24, 25]. One of them concluded that it is possible to classify endometria precisely according to their transcriptional profile, regardless of the morphological appearance. More importantly, they established the existence of clusters of genes characteristic of the different phases of the cycle, highlighting the potential of gene expression profiling for the development of molecular tools in the evaluation of endometrial status [24]. This study has been confirmed and extended by the work of Linda Giudice and her group, who have dissected the molecular phenotyping of human endometrium throughout the menstrual cycle phases underlying its biological processes in normo-ovulatory women [25].

Other studies have focused on the receptive endometrium and have defined the gene expression profile of this tissue during the WOI [30–34]. Although only one gene, osteopontin, was consistently upregulated in all five studies, there are several important molecules that have been highlighted by their presence in four of the five papers. Some of them are proteins previously identified in the endometrium, with or without a described function. Genes are involved in lipid metabolism (apolipoprotein D), immune response (decay accelerating factor for complement, serine or cysteine proteinase, interleukin [IL]-15), regulation of cell cycle (growth arrest and DNA-damage inducible, alpha), ion binding (annexin IV), or enzymes with different functions in different tissues (monoamine oxidase A). More detailed reviews of these studies can be found in Giudice [13] and Horcajadas et al. [35].

The results obtained by these laboratories, taken together, have demonstrated that endometrial receptivity is an equilibrated, complex, and active process involving hundreds of up- and downregulated genes. These results also indicate that a key molecule with the capacity to regulate endometrial receptiveness by itself does not exist. Rather, an endometrial gene signature composed of 25 genes is prevalent in the development of receptiveness in natural cycles and dysregulated in nonoptimal conditions [36].

One of the main drawbacks of the previous studies is the inability to differentiate among the different cell types present in the endometrium. Therefore, the findings described above obtained by microarray technology have to be added to other findings obtained by other methods. Some authors have assigned separately essential candidates to the different phases of embryonic implantation. MUC1 (also with a role in first attachment), MUC4, MUC6, and MUC16 which form the epithelial glycocalyx are necessary for epithelial polarity, a key characteristic of the epithelial surface. A brief review of the relevance of candidate adhesion systems for the second phase attachment, such as basigin (CD147), CD44, osteopontin, several integrin subfamilies, trophinin, and CD9, is given by Aplin [37].

The race for finding is still continuing, every year many papers are published with the discovery of new biomarkers of endometrial receptivity. In any case, the role of these genes should be tested by functional analysis in animal or in in vitro models in the near future.

5.5 Functional Genomics Studies of the Human Endometrium in Stimulated Cycles

Following the studies performed in natural cycles, efforts were concentrated on the genomic impact of COS on the human endometrium during ART treatments. The aim of the first study was to investigate the impact of ovarian stimulation using urinary gonadotrophins in a long protocol with gonadotrophin-releasing hormone (GnRH) agonists without progesterone supplementation (similar to the natural cycle) on endometrial gene expression profiles during the WOI by comparing the endometrial transcriptomic profiles at hCG+7 of COS cycles vs. LH+7 of a previous natural cycle in the same women. For this purpose, microarray technology by Affymetrix (GeneChip HG_U133A, USA) was used, which contained more than 22,000 genes to be tested simultaneously [38]. Results were validated by semiquantitative polymerase chain reaction (PCR) and quantitative PCR experiments. It was found that more than 558 genes showed a differential expression of more than twofold when ovarian stimulation and normal cycles were compared at hCG+7 vs. LH+7.

Analyzing this list of genes, a surprisingly high number of genes involved in endometrial receptivity (WOI genes) were found to be aberrantly expressed in endometria following ovarian stimulation (342 genes), showing the expression levels to be more similar to those in a nonreceptive endometrium. It clearly showed that endometrial development is hampered and delayed under these conditions, as other authors previously had suggested [38]. This study simultaneously reanalyzed the LH+2 vs. LH+7 endometrial gene expression profiles in previous natural cycles in the same subject using a specific GeneChip, and the results obtained were consistent with previously published results [33].

5.6 Functional Genomics Studies of the Human Endometrium in Ovarian Stimulation Cycles: Agonists vs. Antagonists

In 2004, Mirkin et al. compared the gene expression profile in the peri-implantation endometrium in natural vs. gonadotrophin-stimulated cycles using recombinant FSH (rFSH), with either GnRH agonist or GnRH antagonist, with or without progesterone supplementation of the luteal phase [39]. Endometrial biopsies were collected in the previous natural cycle LH+8 and 9 days after hCG administration (hCG+9) in the next ovarian stimulation cycle. Analysis was performed with high-density oligonucleotide microarrays (GeneChip HG_U95Av2 Array; Affymetrix), containing more than 12,000 gene targets. Other structural and functional features of the endometrium were also investigated. The observations made corroborated the morphological changes previously described by other authors. However, those changes were associated with significant, albeit small, variations in gene expression (18 genes per expressed sequence tag, with a fold change ranging between 1.55 and 3.40). Mirkin et al. concluded that although ovarian stimulation causes structural and functional changes compared with natural cycles, small changes were found when gene expression patterns were compared, and that ovarian stimulation may therefore not have a major impact on endometrial receptivity. They also concluded that significant changes were found when comparing cycles using GnRH agonist vs. GnRH antagonist (13 genes significantly different) [39]. In our laboratory, a second study was performed to evaluate the impact of standard and high doses of a GnRH antagonist (ganirelix) in stimulated cycles compared with GnRH agonist (buserelin); both protocols were supplemented with progesterone. All the groups were initiated with a fixed dose of rFSH, and endometrial biopsies were collected at hCG+2 and hCG+7 in ovarian stimulation cycles. Endometrial collection at LH+2 and LH+7 from the previous natural cycle was included as a control. At day hCG+2, endometrial dating, estrogen and progesterone receptors, and pinopode appearance were comparable in all the groups, including the natural cycle. At hCG+7, endometrial dating, steroid receptors, and the presence of pinopodes were comparable in both GnRH antagonist groups and the natural cycles. In the protocol employing a GnRH agonist, however, endometrial dating and pinopode expression suggested an arrested endometrial development compared with the other regimens. Gene expression profiles of the treatment cycles were largely comparable with that of the natural cycle at LH+2 [40].

For WOI genes, expression patterns were closer to those in the natural cycle following standard (50 genes dysregulated) or high-dose ganirelix (23 dysregulated) administration compared with buserelin administration (85 dysregulated) [40]. To reflect clinical practice, progesterone supplementation was given in the luteal phase in all three arms of the study. Under this homogenous condition, in each of the treatment groups, expression of about 100 genes was different compared to the natural cycle. This suggests that endometrial gene dysregulation under COS is affected in a global manner, and as a result, a different endometrial profile arises. The endometrial genomic profile after daily treatment with standard or high-dose GnRH antagonist in women undergoing ovarian stimulation mimics more closely the natural cycle as compared with GnRH agonist.

Table 5.1 Different studies of the gene expression profile of the endometrium performed at the time of implantation comparing natural and stimulated cycles in human using wide functional genomics analysis [45] (with permission)

Study	# Samples	Day in natural cycle	Day in stimulated cycle	Paired analysis	FC	# Genes Up	# Genes Down
Mirkin et al. [39]	13	LH+8 (n=5)	hCG+9 (n=5) Atg	Partially	>1.19	6	6
		LH+8 (n=5)	hCG+9 (n=5) Ag		>1.2	5	1
Horcajadas et al. [38]	19	LH+7 (n=14)	hCG+7 (n=5)	No	>3	281	277
Simón et al. [40]	28	LH+7 (n=14)	hCG+7 (n=4) Atg standard dose	No		22	69
		LH+7 (n=14)	hCG+7 (n=5) Atg high dose		>2	88	24
		LH+7 (n=14)	hCG+7 (n=5) Ag			22	100
Horcajadas et al. [45]	49	LH+1 (n=5)	hCG+1 (n=5)	No		0	0
		LH+2 (n=5)	hCG+2 (n=5)			0	0
		LH+3 (n=5)	hCG+3 (n=5)			0	0
		LH+5 (n=5)	hCG+5 (n=4)			0	0
		LH+7 (n=5)	hCG+7 (n=5)			69	0
		LH+9 (n=5)	hCG+9 (n=5)		–	0	73
Liu et al. [42]	13	LH+7 (n=5)	hCG+7 (n=4) high-serum E2 levels	No	>2	244	159
		LH+7 (n=5)	hCG+7 (n=4) low serum E2 levels			5	2
Haouzi et al. [43]	84	LH+2 (n=21)	hCG+2 (n=21)	Yes		321	4
		LH+7 (n=21)	hCG+5 (n=21)		>2	657	0

FC: fold change

Many groups have continued the investigations about the impact of the ovarian stimulation protocols in the gene expression profile of the endometrium. Some of them analyzed the expression of molecules of interest such as angiopoitins or vascular factors by using classical techniques of immunohistochemistry, quantitative PCR, or western blot [41] to conclude that there is an advanced endometrial angiogenesis after gonadotrophin stimulation. But the most interesting for us are those that have continued analyzing the endometrium in a global manner using microarray technology. Liu et al. presented in 2008 a work where they analyzed the effect of high-serum estradiol levels in gonadotrophin-stimulated cycles at hCG+7 comparing the results to natural cycle at LH+7 [42]. They found 441 genes differentially expressed among the three different groups (natural cycle, moderate-responder, and high-responder). In 2009, the group of Dr. Hamamah has published information analyzing the impact of different stimulation cycles compared to natural cycles in the same patients [43, 44]. These works, with similar approach to ours in 2005 [38], showed similar results emphasizing the concept that GnRH antagonist protocol is more similar to the natural cycle receptivity than under the GnRH agonist protocol [44]. A brief summary of the results is represented in Table 5.1.

5.7 Endometrial Receptivity as a Global Process

The significant histological, biological, and physiological features that occur in the endometrium throughout the menstrual cycle are ultimately the result of changes at the gene transcription level, together with the posttranscriptional modifications and epigenetic changes. Most of the laboratories have their favorite protein or molecule and have tried to elaborate its function in endometrial receptivity. But, at the moment, functional studies have not demonstrated the existence of a magic bullet for human endometrial receptivity as we have mentioned previously. Probably, we will never be able to understand this complex process with the narrow focus of one gene, because it is the result of an equilibrated expression of many genes involved in specific pathways. For this reason, our laboratory analyzed the transcriptomics of the early and midsecretory phase day by day and compared natural vs. COH cycles [45]. Data obtained from the microarray analyses of 50 endometrial biopsies were analyzed using different methods such as sample and gene clustering, biological processes, or selection of differentially expressed genes, as implemented in several microarray data analysis platforms [45]. The first conclusion that could be drawn from that work was that the development of the human endometrium in natural cycle follows a genetic program with a well-defined molecular transition from the prereceptive (unable to accept the adhesion of the human blastocysts) to the receptive endometrium (LH+7), which is comparable among the different subjects investigated (Fig. 5.2). In stimulated cycles, the endometrial gene expression pattern was very similar to natural cycles during the WOI in the prereceptive phase from hCG-1 to hCG-5 (Fig. 5.2). This observation was confirmed using hierarchical clustering. However, the gene expression profile of the receptive endometrium in the COS cycle at hCG-7 showed significant statistical differences compared with the natural cycle at LH-7 (Fig. 5.2).

In order to understand how cellular functionalities are activated and deactivated along the WOI in natural and stimulated cycles, we analyzed their corresponding temporal functional profiles. For that end, we used the first day as reference and we compared each subsequent day to this reference time by a gene set enrichment analysis,

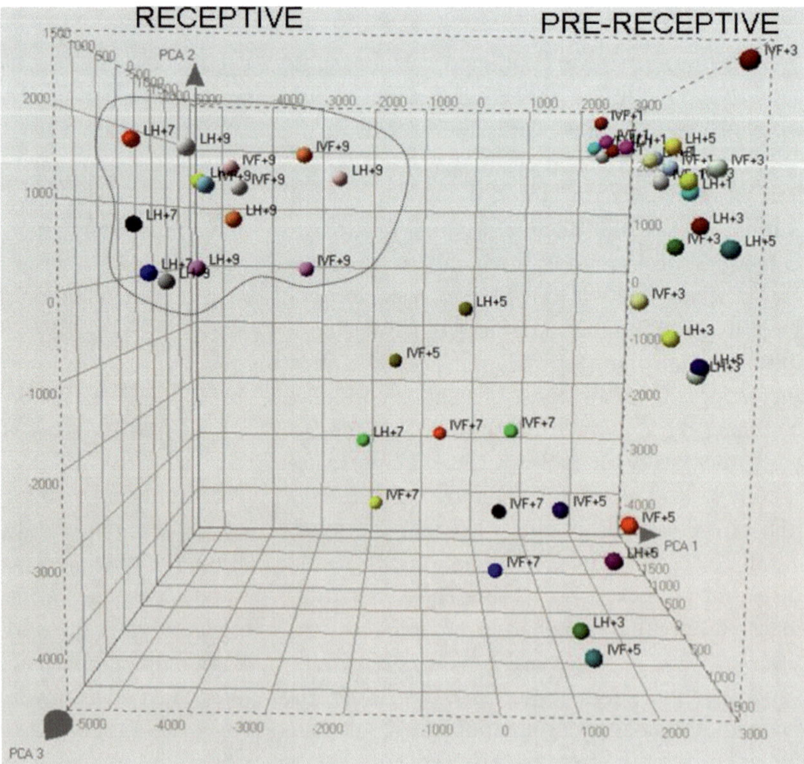

Fig. 5.2 Principal Component Analysis (PCA) of human endometrium throughout the development of the secretory phase (after the endogenous peak of LH) in natural cycle and after hCG injection in stimulated cycle [45] (with permission)

as implemented in the FatiScan tool of Babelomics [46]. Many overrepresented biological terms were shared in both natural and COS categories, particularly on days +3 and +5, suggesting a similar development on the first days of the WOI. On day +7, however, the natural cycle showed a higher number of overrepresented biological terms, such as localization, response to external stimulus, locomotion, response to biotic stimulus, and others [45]. Interestingly, most of these Gene Ontology (GO) terms are not present in the transition from day hCG+5 to hCG+7 in COS cycles. Only two GO terms are conserved in the transition from the prereceptive to receptive state in natural and COS cycles; these terms are the response to the stress and cellular physiological process.

We also found similarities in the biological terms underrepresented in the prereceptive endometrium, except on day LH+7 when more differences were observed. On this specific day (LH+7), no common biological term was identified in natural and COS cycles. Furthermore, some terms appeared to be underrepresented in hCG+7 of COS cycles, such as response to external stimulus or organismal physiological process, which are overrepresented in LH+7 of natural cycles [45]. These results show us that we can consider a function or a dysfunction taking into account a gene, a couple of genes, or a short number of genes. Endometrial receptivity is a complex process in which every regulated gene contributes to the global process in a particular manner.

5.8 New Methods for Endometrial Receptivity Studies

The most widely used techniques to study the receptive endometrium included microscopy [47], quantitative PCR, in situ hybridization and gene expression microarrays [36], and proteomics and metabolomics of endometrial flushings or secretions [48]. It is evident that evaluation of endometrial function cannot be aside of new technologies. The histological studies suggest that new technologies should be added for objective identification of biological samples and the study of endometrial development in health and disease [49, 50].

During the last decade, several groups have attempted to create an objective and modern tool for endometrial evaluation. However, at the present, commercially available kits have demonstrated not to be strong enough for clinical use. This year, our laboratory has presented the *E*ndometrial *R*eceptivity *A*rray (ERA) [51]. During the last 5 years, we have analyzed the differential gene expression profile of endometria at LH+1, LH+3, LH+5 (prereceptive phase) vs. LH+7 (receptive phase) by a T-test. A list of 569 probes representing 238 genes was selected to create our ERA according to very strict criteria. This molecular tool can be classified as receptive or nonreceptive endometrial biopsies from different phases of the menstrual cycle (Fig. 5.3). The functional sense of these genes was assessed by FATIGO-GEPAS [46]. A significant number of these genes are implicated in the response to stress, defense response, and cell adhesion. This molecular method that contents a gene selection for endometrial receptivity offers a new objective tool for endometrial diagnosis. We are now in the functional validation of this array using endometrial samples with specific pathologies such as implantation failure, endometriosis, and others. In addition to this method, the future of endometrial evaluation has to be directed to noninvasive methods such as endometrial fluids or serum markers. Researchers are now working in these two lines of investigation to provide noninvasive diagnostic tools.

An alternative approach to study endometrial receptivity and also embryonic implantation has been culture models. We can divide these models in: explants, monolayer cultures, coculture, and three-dimensional (3D) cultures. Organ explants would appear to provide perfect models for mimicking the in vivo environment, as the 3D structure and integrity of the endometrium are preserved and all layers of the endometrium are included. Landgren et al. [52] developed a model using endometrial biopsies taken 4, 5, and 6 days after the LH peak from healthy women with normal regular menstrual cycles. It was used for placing embryos on the lining epithelium of the explant

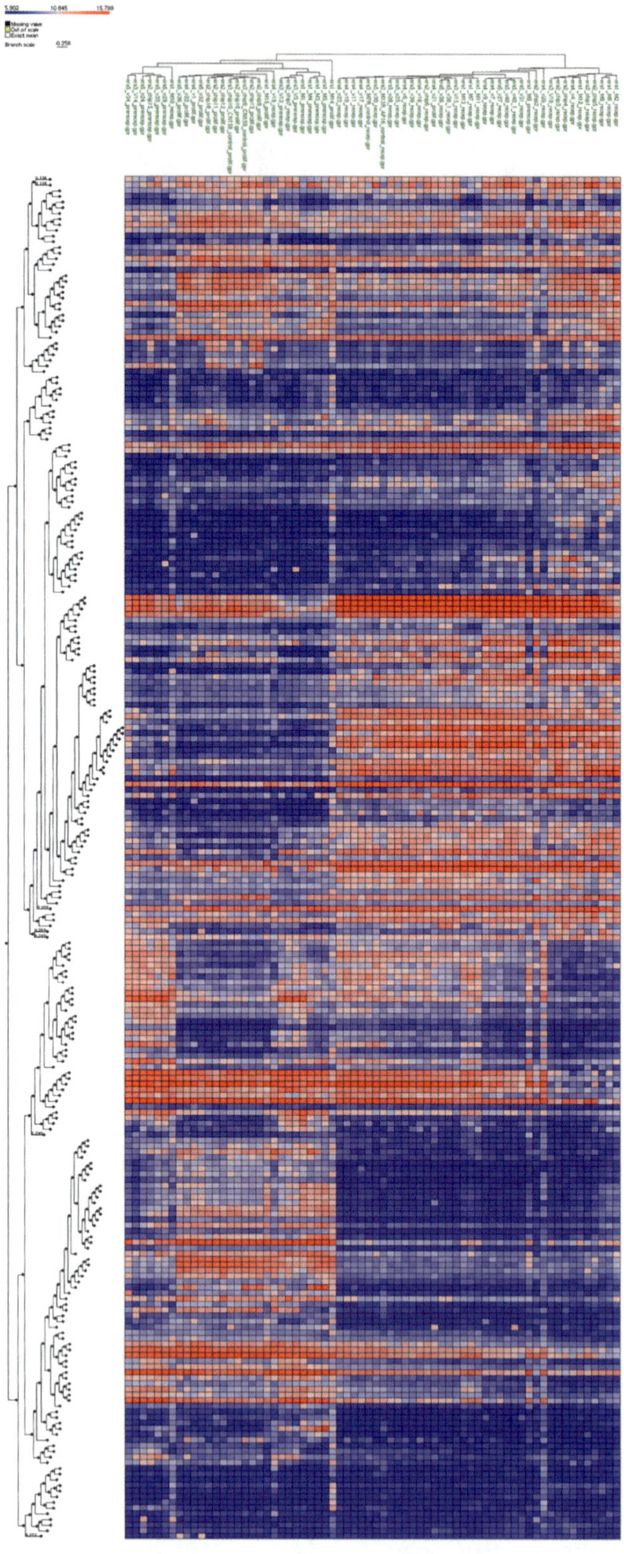

Fig. 5.3 Hierarchical clustering of the 68 samples of menstrual cycle. Samples are represented in vertical and values of gene expression in horizontal. *Color* indicates gene expression value intensities (*blue* low; *red* high)

within 3h of the biopsy being taken. Monolayer culture consists in single cultures of endometrial epithelial cells in flasks and wells. These cultures can be performed using primary cell culture coming from endometrial biopsies or established endometrial epithelial cell lines. These cultures have been used mainly for studying the response to drugs and for embryo adhesion assays [53]. Coculture consists in a separated but communicated culture of epithelial and stromal endometrial cells. This has been used to get high rates of blastocyst formation in clinic, especially as a salvage treatment option in couples with repeated implantation failures [54, 55]. The ultimate in vitro model to study the endometrial receptivity and the embryonic implantation therefore would contain all the cell types of the endometrium (epithelium, stroma, endothelial, and immune cells) so that the complex interactions between the maternal tissue and the blastocyst could be characterized. However, mimicking the physiological 3D architecture of the endometrium is clearly a challenge. Several approaches have been reported, consisting of layers of epithelial and stromal cells grown in and below tissue culture well inserts (reviewed in [56]). One arrangement consists of endometrial stromal cells seeded into a collagen type1 gel in culture well inserts, on top of which there is a thin layer of matrigel, and upon which endometrial epithelial cells are seeded. In a second model, stromal cells are seeded into a culture well below the insert, and epithelial cells are plated on the surface of matrigel in the insert described. A third configuration consists of stromal cells seeded into a mixture of collagen type I and matrigel, and epithelial cell clumps placed on the surface. However, human studies using the 3D models in conjunction with blastocysts are still very limited, but constitute part of the future in endometrial receptivity investigation.

5.9 Conclusions

The molecular basis of endometrial receptivity and the interactions that occur between the blastocyst and the endometrium are still poorly understood [57, 58]. Researchers have found many molecules whose expressions are directly related with the receptive status and are altered during COS cycles [59]. Gene-by-gene analyses and microarray technology have produced huge amount of data. However, it has been demonstrated that endometrial receptivity does not depend on a single molecule. All the functional genomics studies have shown that endometrial receptivity is a very complex process, in which an uncountable number of genes are involved. Now it is the time to learn about what the genomic era can add to our understanding of human endometrial receptivity. In this sense, the use of specific customized microarray such as the ERA [51] could help to evaluate the endometrium in an objective manner. Future directions in endometrial receptivity studies will also require complementarily with proteomics and functionomics.

References

1. American Society for Reproductive Medicine. Assisted reproductive technology in the United States and Canada: 1999 results generated from the American Society for Reproductive Medicine/Assisted Reproductive Technology Registry. Fertil Steril. 2002;78:5.
2. Simón C, Cano F, Valbuena D, et al. Clinical evidence for a detrimental effect on uterine receptivity of high serum estradiol levels in high and normal responder patients. Hum Reprod. 1995;10:2432–4.
3. Simón C, García-Velasco J, Valbuena D, et al. Increasing uterine receptivity by decreasing estradiol levels during the preimplantation period in high responders with the use of a follicle-stimulating hormone step-down regimen. Fertil Steril. 1998;70: 234–9.
4. Simón C, Domínguez F, Valbuena D, et al. The role of estrogen in uterine receptivity and blastocyst implantation. Trends Endocrinol Metabol. 2003;14:197–9.
5. Pellicer A, Valbuena D, Cano F, et al. Lower implantation rates in high responders: evidence for an altered endocrine milieu during the preimplantation period. Fertil Steril. 1996;65:1190–5.
6. Ma WG, Song H, Das SK, et al. Estrogen is a critical determinant that specifies the duration of the window of uterine receptivity for implantation. Proc Natl Acad Sci U S A. 2003;100:2963–8.
7. Paulson RJ, Sauer MV, Lobo RA. Embryo implantation after human in vitro fertilization: importance of endometrial receptivity. Fertil Steril. 1990;53:870–4.
8. Seif MW, Pearson JM, Ibrahim ZH, et al. Endometrium in in-vitro fertilization cycles: morphological and

functional differentiation in the implantation phase. Hum Reprod. 1992;7:6–11.
9. Psychoyos A. The implantation window; basic and clinical aspects. In: Mori T, Aono T, Tominaga T, Hiroi M, editors. Perspectives on assisted reproduction. Ares-Serono symposium, vol. 4. Roma; 1994. p. 57–63.
10. Kolb BA, Paulson RJ. The luteal phase of cycles utilizing controlled ovarian hyperstimulation and the possible impact of this hyperstimulation on embryo implantation. Am J Obstet Gynecol. 1997;176:1262–7.
11. Kolibianakis EM, Bourgain C, Platteau P, et al. Abnormal endometrial development occurs during the luteal phase of nonsupplemented donor cycles treated with recombinant follicle stimulating hormone and gonadotropin-releasing hormone antagonists. Fertil Steril. 2003;80:464–6.
12. Nikas G, Develioglu OH, Toner JP, et al. Endometrial pinopodes indicate a shift in the window of receptivity in IVF cycles. Hum Reprod. 1999;14:787–92.
13. Giudice LC. Elucidating endometrial function in the postgenomic era. Hum Reprod Update. 2003;9: 223–35.
14. Develioglu OH, Hsiu JG, Nikas G, et al. Endometrial estrogen and progesterone receptor and pinopode expression in stimulated cycles of oocyte donors. Fertil Steril. 1999;71:1040–7.
15. Simón C, Mercader A, Francés A, et al. Hormonal regulation of serum and endometrial IL-1α, IL-1β and IL-1Ra: IL-1 endometrial microenvironment of the human embryo at the apposition phase under physiological and supraphysiological steroid level conditions. J Reprod Immunol. 1996;31:165–84.
16. Okada H, Nakajima T, Yoshimura T, et al. Microarray analysis of genes controlled by progesterone in human endometrial stromal cells in vitro. Gynecol Endocrinol. 2003;17:271–80.
17. Rossi M, Sharkey AM, Vigano P, et al. Identification of genes regulated by interleukin-1beta in human endometrial stromal cells. Reproduction. 2005;130: 721–9.
18. White CA, Dimitriadis E, Sharkey AM, Salamonsen LA. Interleukin-11 inhibits expression of insulin-like growth factor binding protein-5 mRNA in decidualizing human endometrial stromal cells. Mol Hum Reprod. 2005;11:649–58.
19. Krikun G, Schatz F, Taylor R, et al. Endometrial endothelial cell steroid receptor expression and steroid effects on gene expression. J Clin Endocrinol Metabol. 2005;90:1812–8.
20. Dockery B, Burke MJ. The fine structure of mature human endometrium. In: Aplin JD, Fazleabas AT, Glasser SR, Giudice LC, editors. The endometrium: molecular, cellular and clinical perspectives. 2nd ed. London: Informa Healthcare; 2008. p. 46–65.
21. Wynn RM. The human endometrium: cyclic and gestational changes. In: Wynn RM, Jollie WP, editors. Biology of the uterus. 2nd ed. New York: Plenum; 1989. p. 289–332.
22. Noyes RW, Hertig AT, Rock J. Dating the endometrial biopsy. Fertil Steril. 1950;1:3–17.
23. Noyes RW, Hertig AT, Rock J. Dating the endometrial biopsy. Am J Obstet Gynecol. 1975;122:262–3.
24. Ponnampalam AP, Weston GC, Trajstman AC, et al. Molecular classification of human endometrial cycle stages by transcriptional profiling. Mol Hum Reprod. 2004;10:879–93.
25. Talbi S, Hamilton AE, Vo KC, et al. Molecular phenotyping of human endometrium distinguishes menstrual cycle phases and underlying biological processes in normo-ovulatory women. Endocrinology. 2006;147:1097–121.
26. Schena M, Shalon D, Davis RW, Brown PO. Quantitative monitoring of gene expression patterns with a complementary DNA microarray. Science. 1995;270:467–70.
27. Popovici RM, Kao LC, Giudice LC. Discovery of new inducible genes in in vitro decidualized human endometrial stromal cells using microarray technology. Endocrinology. 2000;141:3510–3.
28. Brar AK, Handwerger S, Kessler CA, Aronow BJ. Gene induction and categorical reprogramming during in vitro human endometrial fibroblast decidualization. Physiol Genomics. 2001;7:135–48.
29. Tierney EP, Tulac S, Huang STJ, Giudice LC. Sequential induction of gene expression during human endometrial stromal cell decidualization using microarray expression profile analysis. In: Proceedings of the 84th annual meeting of the endocrine society, vol. 537. San Francisco; 2002, p. P3–192.
30. Carson DD, Lagow E, Thathiah A, et al. Changes in gene expression during the early to mid-luteal (receptive phase) transition in human endometrium detected by high-density microarray screening. Mol Hum Reprod. 2002;8:871–9.
31. Kao LC, Tulac S, Lobo S, et al. Global gene profiling in human endometrium during the window of implantation. Endocrinology. 2002;143:2119–38.
32. Borthwick JM, Charnock-Jones DS, Tom BD, et al. Determination of the transcript profile of human endometrium. Mol Hum Reprod. 2003;9:19–33.
33. Riesewijk A, Martin J, van Os R, et al. Gene expression profiling of human endometrial receptivity on days LH+2 versus LH+7 by microarray technology. Mol Hum Reprod. 2003;9:253–64.
34. Mirkin S, Arslan M, Churikov D, et al. In search of candidate genes critically expressed in the human endometrium during the window of implantation. Hum Reprod. 2005;20:2104–17.
35. Horcajadas JA, Riesewijk A, Martin J, et al. Global gene expression profiling of human endometrial receptivity. J Reprod Immunol. 2004;63:41–9.
36. Horcajadas JA, Pellicer A, Simon C. Wide genomic analysis of human endometrial receptivity: new times, new opportunities. Hum Reprod Update. 2007;13: 77–86.
37. Aplin J. Embryo implantation: the molecular mechanisms remain elusive. RBM Online. 2006;13:833–9.

38. Horcajadas JA, Riesewijk A, Polman J, et al. Effect of controlled ovarian hyperstimulation in IVF on endometrial gene expression profiles. Mol Hum Reprod. 2005;11:195–205.
39. Mirkin S, Nikas G, Hsiu JG, et al. Gene expression profiles and structural/functional features of the peri-implantation endometrium in natural and gonadotropin-stimulated cycles. J Clin Endocrinol Metab. 2004;89:5742–52.
40. Simón C, Bellver J, Vidal C, et al. Similar endometrial development in oocyte donors treated with high- or low-dose GnRH-antagonist compared to GnRH-agonist treatment and natural cycles. Hum Reprod. 2005;12:3318–27.
41. Lee Y-L, Liu Y, Ng P-Y, et al. Aberrant expression of angiopoietins-1 and -2 and vascular growth factor-A in peri-implantation endometrium after gonadotrophin stimulation. Hum Reprod. 2008;23:894–903.
42. Liu Y, Lee K-F, Ng E H-Y, et al. Gene expression profiling of human peri-implantation endometria between natural and stimulated cycles. Fertil Steril. 2008; 90:2152–64.
43. Haouzi D, Assou S, Mahmoud K, et al. Gene expression profile of human endometrial receptivity: comparison between natural and stimulated cycles for the same patients. Hum Reprod. 2009;24:1436–45.
44. Haouzi D, Assou S, Dechanet C, et al. Controlled ovarian hyperstimulation for in vitro fertilization alters endometrial receptivity in humans: protocol effects. Biol Reprod. 2010;82:679–86.
45. Horcajadas JA, Mínguez P, Dopazo J, et al. Controlled ovarian stimulation induces a functional genomic delay of the endometrium with potential clinical implications. J Clin Endocrinol Metab. 2008;93:4500–10.
46. Al-Shahrour F, Diaz-Uriarte R, Dopazo J. FatiGO: a web tool for finding significant associations of gene ontology terms with groups of genes. Bioinformatics. 2004;20:578–80.
47. Bourgain C, Devroey P. Histologic and functional aspects of the endometrium in the implantatory phase. Gynecol Obstet Invest. 2007;64:131–3.
48. Boomsma CM, Kavelaars A, Eijkemans MJ, et al. Cytokine profiling in endometrial secretions: a non-invasive window on endometrial receptivity. Reprod Biomed Online. 2009;18:85–94.
49. Murray MJ, Meyer WR, Zaino RJ, et al. A critical analysis of the accuracy, reproducibility, and clinical utility of histologic endometrial dating in fertile women. Fertil Steril. 2004;81:1333–43.
50. Coutifaris C, Myers ER, Guzick DS, et al. Histological dating of timed endometrial biopsy tissue is not related to fertility status. Fertil Steril. 2004;82: 1264–72.
51. Díaz-Gimeno P, Horcajadas JA, Martínez-Conejero JA, et al. A genomic diagnostic tool for human endometrial receptivity based on the transcriptomic signature. Fertil Steril. 2011;95:50–60.
52. Landgren BM, Johannisson E, Stavreus-Evers A, et al. A new method to study the process of implantation of a human blastocyst in vitro. Fertil Steril. 1996;65:1067–70.
53. Martin JC, Jasper D, Valbuena D, et al. Increased adhesiveness in cultured endometrial-derived cells is related to the absence of moesin expression. Biol Reprod. 2000;63:1370–6.
54. Simón C, Mercader A, Garcia-Velasco J, et al. Coculture of human embryos with autologous human endometrial epithelial cells in patients with implantation failure. J Clin Endocrinol Metab. 1999;84: 2638–46.
55. Barmat LI, Liu HC, Spandorfer SD, et al. Autologous endometrial co-culture in patients with repeated failures of implantation after in vitro fertilization-embryo transfer. J Assist Reprod Genet. 1999;16:121–7.
56. Mardon H, Grewal S, Mills K. Experimental models for investigating implantation of the human embryo. Semin Reprod Med. 2007;25:410–7.
57. Dey SK, Lim H, Das SK, et al. Molecular cues to implantation. Endocr Rev. 2004;25:341–73.
58. Yoshinaga K. Review of factors essential for blastocyst implantation for their modulating effects on the maternal immune system. Semin Cell Dev Biol. 2008;19:161–9.
59. Martínez-Conejero JA, Simón C, Pellicer A, Horcajadas JA. Is ovarian stimulation detrimental to the endometrium? RBM Online. 2007;15:45–50.

Current Understanding of Mullerian-Inhibiting Substance

6

Antonio La Marca, Giovanna Sighinolfi, and Annibale Volpe

Abstract

In the ovary, Mullerian-Inhibiting Substance (MIS) is produced by the granulosa cells of early developing follicles and inhibits the transition from the primordial to the primary follicular stage. MIS levels can be measured in serum and have been shown to be proportional to the number of small antral follicles. In women, serum MIS levels decrease with age and are undetectable in the postmenopausal period. In patients with premature ovarian failure, MIS is undetectable or greatly reduced depending on the number of antral follicles in the ovaries. In contrast, MIS levels have been shown to be increased in women with PCOS. MIS levels appear to represent the quantity of the ovarian follicle pool and may become a useful marker of ovarian reserve. In IVF, MIS may permit the identification of both the extremes of ovarian stimulation; a possible role for its measurement may be in the individualization of treatment strategies in order to reduce the clinical risk of ART along with optimized treatment burden.

While MIS has the potential to increase our understanding of ovarian pathophysiology, and to guide clinical management in a broad range of conditions, a number of important questions relating to both the basic physiology of MIS and its clinical implications need to be answered.

Keywords

MIS • Folliculogenesis • POI • PCOS • Ovarian reserve • Ovarian ageing • IVF • Poor response • OHSS

A. La Marca (✉)
Mother-Infant Department, Section of Obstetrics and Gynecology, University of Modena and Reggio Emilia, Modena, Italy
e-mail: antlamarca@libero.it

C. Racowsky et al. (eds.), *Biennial Review of Infertility: Volume 2*,
DOI 10.1007/978-1-4419-8456-2_6,

6.1 The Mullerian-Inhibiting Substance (MIS) and MIS Receptors

MIS (also called anti-Mullerian hormone, AMH) is a member of the transforming growth factor-beta (TGF-beta) superfamily [1]. MIS is a homodimeric disulfide-linked glycoprotein with a molecular weight of 140 kD. The gene is located on the short arm of chromosome 19 in humans, band 19p 13.3 [2]. The MIS gene is 2,750 bp long, and it is divided into five exons. The 3′ part of the fifth exon codes for the bioactive part of the molecule and is extremely GC rich. MIS is strongly expressed in Sertoli cell from testicular differentiation up to puberty and to a much lesser degree in granulosa cells from birth up to menopause [3, 4]

MIS seems to act only in the reproductive organs [4]. The most striking effect of MIS is its capacity to induce regression of the Müllerian ducts, the anlage of the female internal reproductive organs. In the absence of MIS, Müllerian ducts of both sexes develop into uterus, Fallopian tubes and the upper part of the vagina [5, 6]. MIS is expressed also in the ovarian granulosa cells. MIS expression in the ovaries has been observed as early as 36-week gestation in humans [7].

MIS employs a heteromeric receptor system consisting of single membrane spanning serine threonine kinase receptors called types I and II. The type II receptor imparts ligand-binding specificity and the type I receptor mediates downstream signalling when activated by the type II receptor.

The human gene for MIS type II receptor was isolated in 1995 [8]. It is located on chromosome 12 and constituted by 11 exons spread over more than 8 kbp. The MISRII messenger is expressed by MIS target organs, namely the Müllerian ducts, and the gonads. MIS type II receptor is localized to the mesenchyme around the Müllerian duct in the urogenital ridge of both the male and female rat and mouse. It is interesting to note that loss of function mutations in the type II receptor as well as the MIS ligand itself are causes of Persistent Müllerian Duct Syndrome in humans [9]. In the ovary of rats, MIS type II receptor is expressed both in granulosa and theca cells [10].

The identity of MIS type I receptor(s) is not yet clear, particularly in gonads. At least three type I receptors have been extensively studied [11]. It has been hypothesized that MIS could share a type I receptor with another member of the TGF-family. The first identified MIS type I receptor [12], Alk6, was singled out from the six type I receptors of the TGF-β family because of its ability to interact in a ligand-dependent manner with MISRII in CHO cells, permanently expressing human MISRII (CHO-3W) [18]. Alk 2 and Alk 3 have been successively proposed as alternative possible MIS type I receptor [11]. Alk6 and Alk 2 [13, 14] may mediate MIS action in other target cells, whereas Alk 3 is the only one to have been clearly shown to mediate MIS action upon Müllerian ducts [15].

6.2 The Role of MIS in Ovarian Folliculogenesis

In primordial follicles, MIS expression seems to be absent. MIS immunostaining can first be observed in granulosa cells of follicles at the primary stage of development. In one study, approximately 75% of secondary follicles were positive for MIS immunostaining. The strongest staining was observed in preantral and small antral follicles [16].

MIS continues to be expressed in the growing follicles in the ovary until they have reached the size and differentiation state at which they may be selected for dominance. In the mouse, this occurs at the early antral stage in small growing follicles, whereas in the human it is evident in antral follicles 4–6 mm in diameter [16]. Thus, MIS is expressed in follicles that have undergone recruitment from the primordial follicle pool, but have not been selected for dominance. MIS is not expressed in atretic follicles or theca cells [17–19]

It has recently been demonstrated that oocytes from early preantral, late preantral and preovulatory follicles up-regulate MIS mRNA levels in granulosa cells, in a fashion that is dependent upon the developmental stage of the oocyte. These findings therefore suggest that oocyte regulation of granulosa cell gene expression occurs during extended periods of follicle development and that oocyte regulation of MIS expression may play a role in intra- and inter-follicular coordination of follicle development [20]

The main physiological role of MIS in the mouse ovary seems to be limited to the inhibition of the early stages of follicular development [21, 22], since both in vivo and in vitro experiments have indicated that the transition from primordial into growing follicles becomes enhanced in the absence of MIS, leading to early exhaustion of the primordial follicle pool [23] (Fig. 6.1).

In one study, the ovaries of 4-month-old MIS knockout mice contained 3 times as many small non-atretic growing follicles and a reduced number of primordial follicles compared to their wild-type littermates [25]. The increased rate of recruitment from the primordial pool observed in the MIS null-mice was already evident before the initiation of the oestrous cycle. These studies confirmed the concept that in the absence of MIS, primordial follicles are recruited at a faster rate, resulting in premature exhaustion of the primordial follicle pool [25]. Since MIS null-mice have low levels of FSH, with increased numbers of growing follicles, it has been hypothesized that follicles are more sensitive to FSH in absence of MIS. The possible inhibitory effect of MIS on follicular sensitivity to FSH could play a role in the process of follicular selection [25]. Diminished expression of MIS within the follicles would reduce the threshold level for FSH, allowing follicles to continue growing and to ovulate in the next estrous cycle [23, 26].

Very recently, ovaries from rats placed in organ culture and incubated in the absence and presence of MIS permitted to show that MIS

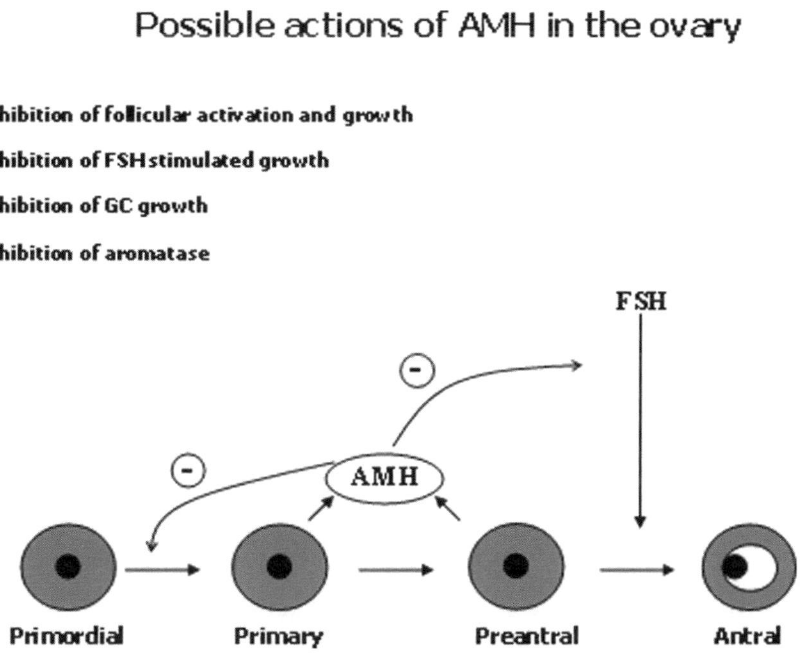

Fig. 6.1 In women, MIS expression can first be observed in primary follicles, and is strongest in preantral and small antral follicles. MIS may play an inhibiting role in initial recruitment and in the selection of the dominant follicle (from ref [24] with permission)

alters the expression of several hundred genes [27]. The overall effects of MIS exposure were to decrease the expression of stimulatory factors, increase the expression of inhibitory factors and regulate cellular pathways that result in the inhibition of primordial follicle development [27]. At present, however, these views remain largely speculative as few in vitro or in vivo studies have been conducted which address physiological role of MIS in the human ovary.

Current theories also suggest a role for MIS as a co-regulator of steroidogenesis in granulosa cells, as MIS levels appear to be related to oestradiol levels in follicular fluid (FF) from small antral follicles [28]. This was confirmed by a recent study which showed that polymorphisms in the gene for MIS or MIS receptor type II seem to be related to follicular phase oestradiol levels, suggesting a role for MIS in the FSH-induced steroidogenesis in the human ovary [29].

Although MIS has been shown to have mainly autocrine and paracrine actions in follicle development, the protein is also measurable in serum. Antral follicles are considered the primary source of circulating MIS as they contain a large number of granulosa cells. A body of clinical data suggests that MIS is preferentially and constantly secreted by small rather than large antral follicles. The amount and the rate of MIS production by a single antral follicle should be investigated and in

Granulosa cells secrete MIS into both the bloodstream and FF, although concentrations are very much higher in the latter. However, the exact role of MIS in this compartment has not been elucidated.

6.3 Circulating MIS in Women

6.3.1 Current Assays

Until recently, MIS assays were only available in a few laboratories around the world. The lack of access to a single reliable and standardized commercial assay has hindered the development of MIS as a clinical marker of ovarian reserve. A sensitive ELISA assay capable of detecting levels as low as 2 ng/mL was developed 9 years ago [30]. However, recently new commercial ultrasensitive sandwich ELISA assays have been developed capable of detecting concentrations less than 0.1 ng/mL. The increased sensitivity and availability of different assays have highlighted the urgent need to agree on the standard preparations used, in order to avoid confusion in reported levels and interpretation.

At present, there are two highly sensitive sandwich ELISA assays available: the diagnostic systems laboratories (DSL) and the Immunotech-Beckman assay. The sensitivity of the DSL is reported to be 0.025 ng/mL compared with 0.07 ng/mL for the Immunotech-Beckman assay, although this difference was not confirmed in a recent clinical study [31]. The intra- and inter-assay variations of the two assays are similar (<7 and <5%, respectively). The DSL assay is not species-specific, a feature which can be advantageous for research laboratories using rodent models.

Initial studies comparing the two assays have shown that MIS levels appear to be four to five-fold lower with the DSL assay compared to the Immunotech-Beckman assay [32, 33]. In their report, Bersinger and coll. [33] alluded to problems inherent to MIS measurements which stem from residual matrix effects and instabilities of certain antigenic determinants. However, although developed independently, these assays are now both produced by a single company (Beckman-Coulter), and cross-referencing has shown that the correlation between the two assays is >0.9 (personal communication from Beckman-Coulter representative). While a uniform conversion factor has never been published, the manufacturers suggest that 1.5 may be a good figure for this purpose (personal communication).

Both kits are likely to remain in production over the next few years as approximately half of researchers are using the DSL assay and the other half the Immunotech-Beckman product. However, it is anticipated that within 2 years, an automated system for MIS measurement will probably become available, and industry sources indicate that it is likely that this will be calibrated to the Immunotech-Beckman kit (personal communication).

6.3.2 Factors Modulating Serum MIS Levels

In women, MIS levels are almost undetectable at birth. After a slight increase in the weeks after birth, MIS levels reach the highest values during late puberty [34] and then show a progressive decline along reproductive life as the follicular reserve becomes depleted [34, 35], becoming undetectable after menopause [36, 37]. Further evidence that circulating MIS appears to be solely of ovarian origin comes from a study in which MIS was undetectable 3–5 days following bilateral ovariectomy [37]. As MIS levels essentially reflect the follicular ovarian pool, reduction in the number of small growing follicles may be followed by a reduction in circulating MIS. The reduction in ovarian reserve is a physiological process occurring in the late reproductive period and consistently associated to a decrease in MIS levels [38, 39]. The strong correlation existing between MIS levels and the resting pool of follicles has recently been highlighted by some papers showing that MIS measurement may be used to predict the occurrence of menopause [40, 41].

MIS may constitute a unique endocrine parameter for the investigation of ovarian function, since several studies have demonstrated that, in contrast to sex steroids, gonadotropins and peptides such as inhibin Band MIS serum levels do not significantly change throughout the menstrual cycle [42–45]. However, others have reported significant cyclical fluctuations in MIS levels with a rapid decrease in MIS levels in the early luteal phase [46, 47]. Excursions from mean levels of +3% and to −19% have been reported [46, 47]. These variations are similar to reported intercycle fluctuations for MIS [45]. In the clinical setting, the inter- and intra-cycle variability in serum MIS levels may be considered to be low enough to permit random timing of MIS measurements during the menstrual cycle. Of course, further studies on a large sample of patients, based on daily blood samples, are needed to clarify whether MIS levels vary significantly during the menstrual cycle. Up to now, reported fluctuations appear to be of small amplitude, and therefore, probably of minor significance when interpreting data for clinical purposes.

Furthermore, MIS levels appear to be unmodified in conditions under which endogenous gonadotrophin release is substantially diminished, such as during pregnancy [48], under GnRH agonist pituitary downregulation [49] and oral contraceptive administration [45, 50, 51]. This indicates that non-cyclic FSH-independent ovarian activity persists even when pituitary FSH secretion is suppressed. These findings are consistent with the concept that MIS levels reflect the continuous FSH-independent non cyclic growth of small follicles in the ovary (Fig. 6.2)

Obesity has been associated to reduced fertility even in the presence of ovulatory menstrual cycles and to increased probability of miscarriage than normal weight women [52, 53]. Non-PCOS obese women show reduced levels of inhibin B and MIS [54, 55], suggesting that obesity may be associated to impaired ovarian reserve. However, a recent study [56] examined the correlation of obesity with hormonal and ultrasound-derived markers of ovarian reserve and found that serum MIS levels are lower in obese women compared with age-matched women of normal weight, despite similar antral follicular count. This suggests that MIS levels in obese women may be lower for physiological reasons related to obesity itself and may not be necessarily indicative of impaired ovarian reserve [56]. Other factors related to reduced MIS levels are smoking [57], alcohol use [58] and race or ethnicity [59].

6.4 The Role of MIS in Investigating Ovarian Dysfunction

The observed relationship between the follicular ovarian pool and serum MIS levels indicates that serum levels could provide additional information (linked to the follicle dynamics) during the diagnostic evaluation of hypogonadism. MIS serum levels have been found to be normal in women with hypogonadotropic amenorrhea, indicating that initial follicle recruitment is not abolished in hypogonadotropic hypogonadism [60].

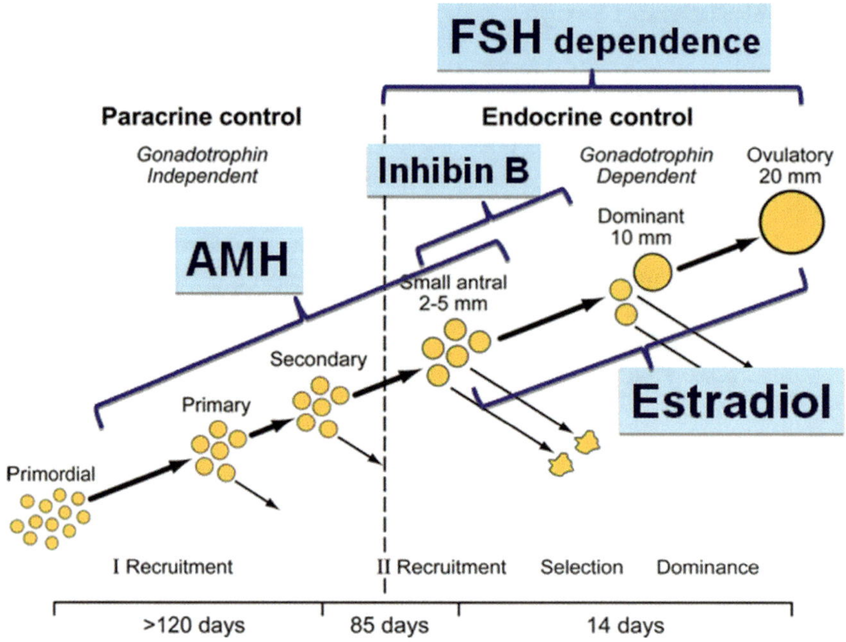

Fig. 6.2 In contrast to the other known ovarian reserve markers, AMH may not only reflect the number of early and developing antral follicles, but also earlier stages of follicle development. The FSH, estradiol, and inhibin secretions are mutually connected by a negative feedback. Therefore, their circulating levels are only an indirect reflection of the number of antral follicles. The E2 levels are less a reflection of the number of antral follicles, but rather of their growth activity during the follicular phase. On the basis of this reason, highest biological plausibility as marker of ovarian reserve is to be attributed to AMH, followed by inhibin B, FSH, and E2 (from ref [24] with permission)

This finding has been recently confirmed in young women with anorexia nervosa-related amenorrhea [61]. In contrast, in women with hypergonadotropic amenorrhea (premature ovarian insufficiency, POI), serum MIS levels are very low or undetectable. In a recent study in POI patients, the number of MIS immunopositive follicles present in ovarian biopsy material was closely correlated with serum MIS levels [62], suggesting a diagnostic role for MIS in the evaluation of hypogonadism.

In a recent study, we measured serum concentrations of MIS in 26 women with POI due to steroidogenic cell autoimmunity (SCA-POI) and 66 with non-autoimmune idiopathic POI (iPOI) [63] and found significantly higher MIS levels in women with SCA-POI than in women with iPOI. MIS was detected in 11/26 (42%) women with SCA-POI and in 7/66 (11%) with iPOI. Serum concentrations above the fifth percentile of the normal range were detected in 9/26 (35%) women with SCA-POI and in 4/66 (6%) with iPOI. Eight of 12 (67%) women with SCA-POI with less than 5 years and 1/14 (7%) with longer disease duration had MIS concentrations within the normal range. These findings indicate that women with SCA-POI, differently from those with iPOI, present a preserved ovarian follicle pool for several years after diagnosis of ovarian insufficiency. The results of our study on women with SCA-POI may be of high relevance for future clinical studies aimed at modulating the autoimmune process and at preserving the residual functional tissue and/or delay the progression of the destructive autoimmune process [63] (Figs. 6.3 and 6.4).

Serum MIS measurement may also have a role in identifying incipient ovarian failure in young eumenorrheic women with moderate hypergonadotropism. Incipient ovarian failure [64] may precede the onset of cycle irregularity (transitional ovarian failure) and hence the menopausal transition by 3–10 years .In a recent study, serum levels

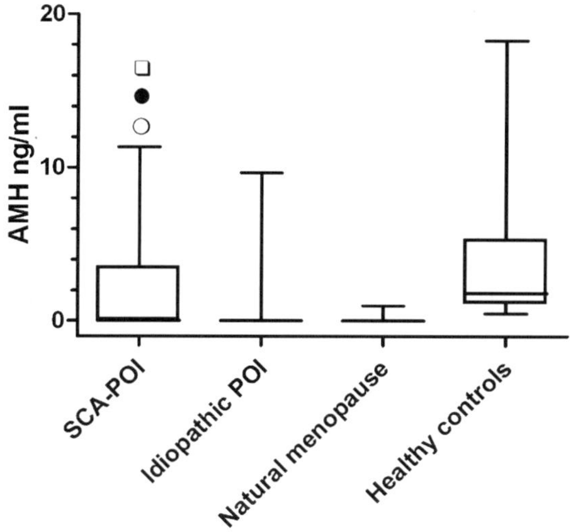

Fig. 6.3 *Box*-and-*whisker* plot of AMH serum concentrations in patients with POI due to steroidogenic cell autoimmunity (SCA-POI), in patients with idiopathic POI, in post-menopausal women and in healthy control women. *Boxes* represent median (*thick line* in the *middle* of the *boxes*) and interquartile ranges (25th and 75th percentile; *thick lines* at the *bottom* and the *top* of *boxes*). *Error bars* represent 10th and 90th percentiles. Open square, $p=0.03$ SCA-POI vs. idiopathic POI; *closed circle*, $p=0.018$ SCA-POI vs. natural menopause; open circle, $p<0.0001$ SCA-POI vs. healthy controls (Bonferroni's corrected p values) (from ref [63], with permission)

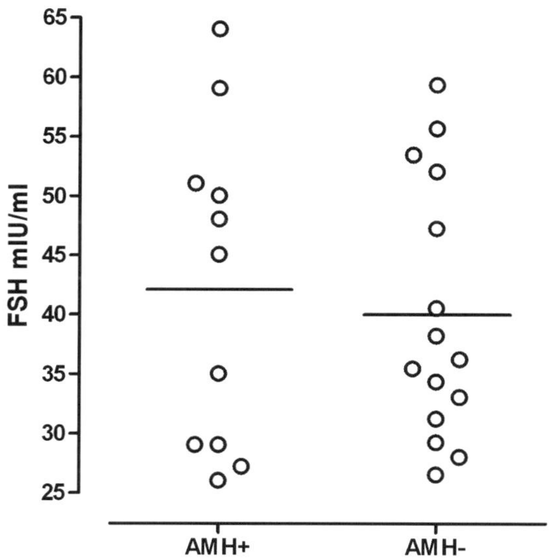

Fig. 6.4 Distribution of FSH serum concentration in women with SCA-POI, according to AMH serum concentration ($n=11$ women with detectable (+) AMH and $n=15$ women with undetectable (–) AMH). Bars represent mean values (from ref [63], with permission)

of MIS were able to discriminate between incipient and transitional ovarian failure, defined as elevated follicular phase FSH levels along with a regular menstrual cycle or cycle disturbances, respectively. In women with incipient failure, levels were below the fifth percentile of normo-ovulatory women in 25% and undetectable in 7%, compared with 66 and 52% in women with transitional ovarian failure [65]. This finding indicates that MIS provides an accurate assessment of ovarian follicle pool in young hypergonadotropic patients especially in the clinically challenging subgroups of patients with elevated FSH who do not fulfil the strict definition of POF [65].

Moreover, young sisters or daughters of women affected by POF, patients undergoing ovarian surgery, and patients affected by Turner syndrome may all benefit from the information which MIS levels might provide in this context. This is illustrated in a recent report on the fertility preservation in girls with Turner Syndrome [66]. Forty-seven young girls with Turner Syndrome underwent laparoscopy for ovarian tissue cryopreservation and 15 of them had follicles in the tissue piece analysed. When investigating which factors had the highest predictive value for finding follicles, the most powerful were the presence of 46XX/XO chromosomal mosaicism, serum FSH levels below 11 IU/L and serum MIS levels greater than 0.28 ng/mL [66]. MIS may therefore have a role in the diagnostic work-up and fertility counselling of patients with Turner Syndrome.

A particularly promising field for further research is assessing the value of MIS as a potential marker of ovarian function in women who underwent chemotherapy or radiotherapy for malignant disease. Longitudinal studies have demonstrated that MIS measurement can be used as a reliable and early marker of ovarian damage, and that a decrease in MIS precedes alterations in other markers [67–71]. The ability to predict the impact of these treatments on ovarian follicular pool (including future fertility) in individual cases may be of considerable value in guiding clinicians and patients when considering whether or not fertility preservation strategies should be employed, and if so, which strategy is most appropriate. At present, care is guided largely by the nature of the intervention and the age of the woman.

A number of studies have shown serum MIS levels to be increased in women with PCOS compared to controls [72–77]. This is thought to be the result of increased granulosa cells synthesis and secretion of MIS in the polycystic ovaries [78]. Indeed, levels of MIS are on average 75 times higher in granulosa cells from polycystic ovaries, compared with levels in normal ovaries [79]. In addition, increased MIS levels in PCOS may be due to the disruption in folliculogenesis leading to an excess accumulation of preantral and small antral follicles [80].

Increased MIS levels have also been found in prepubertal [81] and peripubertal [82] daughters of PCOS women as well as in adolescent PCOS girls with normal menstrual cycles [83], suggesting that altered follicle development is already present during infancy and early adulthood before the clinical phenotype of ovarian dysfunction is present.

MIS levels appear to be related to the severity of the syndrome since levels have been observed to be higher in insulin-resistant PCOS women than in patients with normal insulin sensitivity [84]. Similarly, MIS is higher in amenorrheic compared to oligomenorrheic women with PCOS [75], which could indicate a role for MIS in the pathogenesis of PCOS-related anovulation. Alternatively, high MIS values could reflect more impaired disruption in folliculogenesis and granulosa cell function in the ovary of amenorrheic compared to oligomenorrheic PCOS women [75].

In a recent longitudinal study, serum MIS levels were measured in 98 women with PCOS and 41 controls at 2 time points (interval between the visits: 0.3–9 years). Although serum MIS levels declined over time in both groups, the reduction observed in PCOS patients was less than that in controls. The authors of this study postulated that this may indicate a longer reproductive life span in PCOS patients [78]. On histological examination, polycystic ovaries exhibit the same number of primordial follicles, whereas the number of developing follicles is doubled compared with normal ovaries [85]. Hence, it may be proposed that the process of ovarian ageing is delayed in women with PCOS since high MIS levels may inhibit the primordial follicle pool depletion [78].

MIS measurement has been found to offer a relatively high specificity and sensitivity (92 and 67%, respectively) as a diagnostic marker for PCOS [86]. On this basis, it has been proposed that in situations where accurate ultrasound data are not available, MIS could be used instead of the follicle count as a diagnostic criterion for PCOS [86].

Other than for diagnostic evaluation, MIS measurement may also be useful in the therapeutic approach of PCOS patients. Indeed, overweight women with PCOS who respond to weight loss with menstrual improvements have significantly reduced preweight-loss MIS levels, indicating that baseline MIS may provide a potential clinical predictor of menstrual improvements with weight loss in PCOS [87]. Similarly, basal MIS levels evaluation may be useful in the prediction of ovarian response to clomiphene citrate [88]. Finally, it has been shown that metformin administration in women affected by PCOS is associated with a reduction in both MIS serum levels and antral follicles, suggesting that the measurement of MIS could be used to evaluate the treatment efficacy with insulin sensitizers [89].

6.5 MIS as a Marker for Ovarian Ageing

The age-related decline in female reproductive function due to the reduction of the ovarian follicle pool and the quality of oocytes has been well established. A reliable marker for the age at which subfertility will occur would have great potential value as a predictor of future reproductive lifespan. The ideal marker would show a significant change in levels from adolescence to the late reproductive period. Increased basal levels of FSH and a decrease in inhibin B and in the antral follicle count (AFC) on ultrasound examination are widely taken to indicate a reduced ovarian reserve.

Recent studies have indicated that MIS may constitute an important novel measure of ovarian reserve. Evidence for this come from studies demonstrating that serum MIS levels fall throughout reproductive life [90], with levels becoming undetectable after spontaneous menopause [34, 36] (Figs. 6.5 and 6.6).

Serum levels on day 3 of the menstrual cycle show a progressive decrease with age and appear to correlate well with AFCs age and FSH [90]. In an interesting prospective study, a group of women was followed longitudinally, with an interval between the two visits ranging from 1.1 to 7.3 years. Although the number of antral follicles and the levels of FSH and inhibin B did not change, a reduction in mean MIS levels of about 38% was observed [90].

The same group prospectively studied 81 women for 4 years (mean age 39.6 and 43.6 at the beginning and at the end of the study, respectively). Although the AFCs did not change over this time period, MIS, FSH and inhibin B all demonstrated significant changes. However, MIS was the only marker of ovarian reserve showing a mean longitudinal decline over time both in younger women (<35 years) and in women over 40 years [36].

Recently, MIS levels were measured in 144 fertile normal volunteers and used to determine an estimate of mean MIS as a function of age [41]. There was good conformity between the observed distribution of age at menopause and that predicted from declining MIS levels, further supporting the hypothesis that MIS levels may predict the age of onset of menopause. Other studies have recently confirmed that a single MIS measurement may be a good predictor for the onset of menopause in ageing women [40, 92].

In conclusion, compared to other known markers, MIS seems to better reflect the continuous decline of the oocyte / follicle pool with age [36]. The decrease in MIS with advancing age may be present before changes in currently known ageing-related variables, suggesting that serum MIS levels may be the best marker of ovarian ageing and menopausal transition.

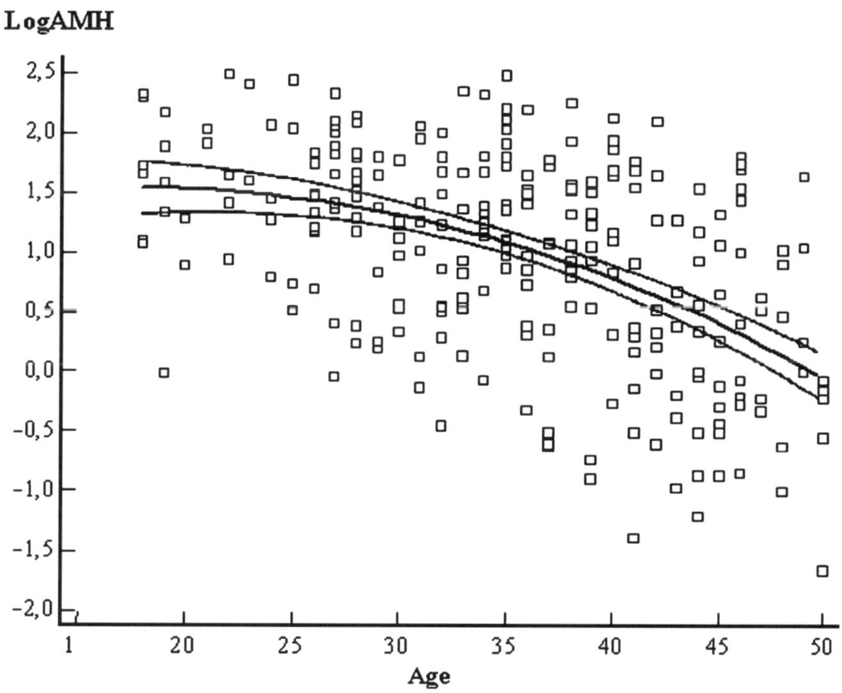

Fig. 6.5 Correlation between logAMH and age of women. Regression analysis revealed that age-related changes were bestfittedbyapolynomialfunction(logAMH = 1.0547 + 0.0546 age–0.0015 age^2). Ninety five percent confidence interval is shown ($R2=0.24$; $P<0.001$). *X* axis: age (years); *Y* axis: logAMH (from ref [91] with permission)

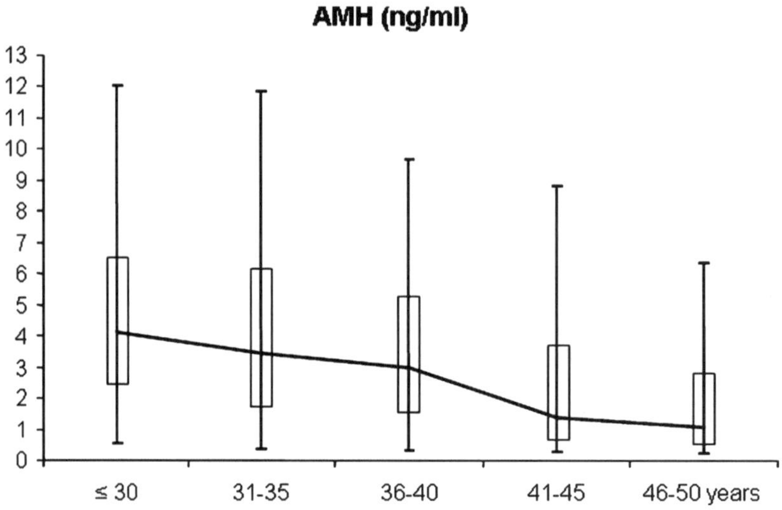

Fig. 6.6 AMH levels throughout the reproductive period. Median, lower (2.5th centile) and upper (97.5th centile) limits are reported. *Box* indicates 25th and 75th centiles (from ref [91] with permission)

6.6 MIS as Predictive Marker in IVF

Recently, Anti-Mullerian Hormone (MIS) has been evaluated by several groups as a potential novel clinical marker of ovarian reserve and response to gonadotropins (see ref [93] for review). In particular, in the last few years several large prospective studies have been published reporting extremely interesting new data on the possible clinical application of MIS measurement in the prediction of quantitative and qualitative ovarian response in ART.

6.6.1 Prediction of Quantitative Ovarian Response

Much data show a strong and positive correlation between basal MIS serum levels and the number of retrieved oocytes in women undergoing ovarian stimulation. In the evaluation of MIS as a marker of ovarian response to FSH, the first paper reporting an association between circulating MIS and ovarian response to gonadotropin was by Seifer and colleagues, 7 years ago [94]. The author observed that higher day 3 MIS was associated with a greater number of retrieved oocytes. In particular, MIS levels were 2.5-fold higher in patients with at least 11 oocytes compared with those with 6 oocytes or fewer retrieved. Results from this study were successively confirmed by several retrospective and prospective studies by different independent groups.

In Table 6.1, all retrospective and prospective studies that have found a correlation between the number of retrieved oocytes and MIS levels have been summarized. The majority of authors have compared MIS with age and other hormonal markers (FSH, estradiol and Inhibin B) and only few of them also with ultrasound markers of ovarian reserve. The balance of the published studies seems to indicate that MIS is a better marker in predicting ovarian response to COS than age of the patient, day 3 FSH, oestradiol and inhibin B.

With high probability, AFC and MIS perform with similar power in the prediction of the number of retrieved oocytes. This is confirmed by a recent meta-analysis in which the value of serum MIS levels as a test to predict ovarian response in IVF in comparison to the performance of the AFC has been assessed [115]. A total of thirteen studies were analysed reporting on MIS and seventeen on AFC. The ROC curves for the prediction of

Table 6.1 Studies on AMH as marker of ovarian response to COH

		R with	AMH better than					
References	*n*	oocytes	AFC	Ov. Vol	d3 FSH	d3 E2	d3 inhB	Age
Seifer et al. [94]	107	0.48			√	√		
Van Rooij et al. [95]	130	0.57	=		√	√	√	√
Fanchin et al. [96]	93	0.43						
Muttukrishna et al. [97]	69	0.69			√		√	
Hazout et al. [98]	109	0.38			√	√	√	√
Muttukrishna et al. [99]	108	0.5	=		√			
Elder Geva et al. [100]	56	0.64	X		√		√	
Silberstein et al. [101]	257	0.33			√			
Ficicioglu et al. [102]	50	0.56	√		√	√		√
Lekamge et al. [103]	126	0.34	=					
La Marca et al. [104]	48	0.7						
Kwee et al. [105]	110	0.63	X	√	√			√
Nakhuda et al. [106]	77	0.63			√			
McIlveen et al. [107]	84	0.78	√	√	√		=	√
Nelson et al. [108]	340	0.71			√			√
Elgindy et al. [109]	33	0.88	=	√	√			
Lie Fong et al. [110]	125	0.47						
Jee et al. [111]	59	0.53					X	
Jayaprakasan et al. [112]	135	0.47	=	√	√	√		√
Wunder et al. [113]	276	0.35			√		X	
Nelson et al. [114]	538	0.64						

Comparison with other predictors (from ref [93])

ovarian response indicated no significant difference between the performances of MIS and AFC. Hence, it may be concluded that at present MIS appears to offer at least the same level of accuracy and clinical value for the prediction of ovarian response as AFC [115].

6.6.1.1 Prediction of Poor Response and Cycle Cancellation

A proportion of women (2–30%) undergoing COS experience poor response [116] for which there is no universally accepted definition. Numerous criteria have been used to characterize poor response. The number of developed follicles and the number of retrieved oocytes are two of the most important criteria for defining poor response. The proposed number varies among different authors and ranges from less than three to less than five dominant follicles on the day of hCG and from less than three to less than five retrieved oocytes (reviewed in ref [117]). More logically, poor response is generally considered to have occurred if the cycle is cancelled due to an inadequate ovarian response to stimulation. Whatever definition is used, poor responders have definitely lower pregnancy rates compared to normal responders of similar age [117].

In the clinical setting, it may be useful to correctly predict the occurrence of poor response as this may lead to avoiding treatment for women destined not to respond to COS thus contributing to reducing the cycle cancellation rate, the treatment costs and psychological stress for the couple. Finally, an improved counselling for the prediction of poor response may ameliorate disappointment and distress.

A large number of clinical parameters have been shown to predict the poor ovarian response to stimulation with exogenous gonadotropins and have been introduced in the clinical practice. These include age, basal serum FSH and inhibin

B levels, AFC, ovarian volume, a number of dynamic tests and more recently MIS.

Several authors investigated the utility of MIS in the prediction of poor response to FSH. Reported sensitivity and specificity ranged between 44–97 and 41–100%, respectively (Table 6.2). It is clear that not all studies found for MIS an optimal sensitivity (>0.75) and specificity (>0.85). However, if MIS is measured with the aim of refraining bad prognosis couples from IVF, then in order to have a low number of false positive results, specificity more than sensitivity should be taken into consideration. On this basis, it should be highlighted that half of the studies on MIS have reported a specificity higher than 0.85.

One of the main advantages of MIS with respect to the other hormonal markers of ovarian reserve is the possibility to be used as a menstrual

Table 6.2 Sensitivity and specificity of AMH for the prediction of poor response to gonadotropin stimulation (from ref [93])

References	*n*	Study design	CUT-OFF value	Sens (%)	Spec (%)	Definition of poor response	AMH assay
Van Rooij et al. [95]	119	Prosp	0.3 μg/L	60	89	<4 oocytes	Immunotech-Beckman-Coulter
Muttukrishna et al. [97]	69	Prosp	0.1 ng/mL	87.5[a]	72.2[a]	<4 oocytes or cancellation	Immunotech-Beckman-Coulter
Muttukrishna et al. [99]	108	Retro	0.2 ng/mL	87	64	≤4 oocytes	Immunotech-Beckman-Coulter
Tremellen et al. [118]	75	Prosp	8.1 pmol/L	80	85	≤4 oocytes	Immunotech-Beckman-Coulter
Panarrubia et al. [119]	80	Prosp	4.9 pmol/L	53[a]	96[a]	Cancellation	Immunotech-Beckman-Coulter
Ebner et al. [120]	141	Prosp	1.66 ng/mL	69	86	<4 oocytes	Immunotech-Beckman-Coulter
Ficicioglu et al. [102]	50	Prosp	0.25 pg/mL	90.9	90.9	<5 oocytes	Diagnostic system laboratories
La Marca et al. [104]	48	Prosp	0.75 ng/mL	80	93	<4 oocytes or cancellation	Immunotech-Beckman-Coulter
Freour et al. [121]	69	Prosp	1.3 μg/L	44	100	<6 oocytes	Immunotech-Beckman-Coulter
Smeenk et al. [122]	80	Prosp	1.4 μg/L	62	73	≤4 oocytes	Immunotech-Beckman-Coulter
McIlveen et al. [107]	84	Prosp	1.25 ng/mL	58	75	≤4 oocytes	Immunotech-Beckman-Coulter
Kwee et al. [105]	110	Prosp	1.4 μg/L	76	86	<6 oocytes	Diagnostic system laboratories
Nakhuda et al. [106]	77	Prosp	0.35 ng/mL	90.1[a]	81.8[a]	Cancellation	Diagnostic system laboratories
Lekamge et al. [103]	126	Retro	14 pmol/L	73	73	≤4 oocytes	Immunotech-Beckman-Coulter
Nelson et al. [108]	340	Prosp	5 pmol/L	75[b]		≤2 oocytes	Diagnostic system laboratories
Gnoth et al. [123]	132	Prosp	1.26 ng/mL	97	41	≤4 oocytes	Diagnostic system laboratories
Nardo et al. [124]	165	Prosp	1.0 ng/mL	87	67	≤4 follicles on day 8 of COH	Diagnostic system laboratories
Jayaprakasan et al. [112]	135	Prosp	0.99 ng/mL	100	73	<4 oocytes or cancellation	Diagnostic system laboratories

Retro retrospective study; *Prosp* prospective study
[a]For cycle cancellation identification
[b]Percentage of correctly classified poor responder patients

cycle-independent marker since MIS seems to be stable and to have very low inter- and intra-cycle variability. In the first published study based on a single random measurement of MIS, a sensitivity of 80% and specificity of 93% has been calculated for the prediction of poor response [104].

Variable predictive performance for MIS was reported in the various studies and this has been considered by some authors to be partly due to the use of different variants of MIS assay.

Most importantly, the performance of any test of ovarian reserve, including MIS, is strictly dependent on the prevalence of the disease (poor response) we want to identify. Throughout the published studies, the prevalence of poor response may vary on the basis of the percentage of older (high incidence of poor response) and younger (low incidence of poor response) patients included in the study and of course on the basis of the adopted definition for poor response. As a consequence, the same test, measured at the same laboratory, will have different predictive performance if the proportion of older patient and the definition of poor response will change.

In conclusion, the balance of all the clinical studies on MIS seems to suggest that MIS measurement prior to gonadotropin secretion may be useful in the prediction of women at risk for poor response or no response to gonadotropins. Moreover, the absence of modifications in serum MIS levels throughout the menstrual cycle permits clinicians to have a reliable serum marker of ovarian reserve that can be measured independently of the day of the cycle.

6.6.1.2 Prediction of Hyper-Response and OHSS

Ovarian hyper-response is the opposite side of the spectrum of ovarian reserve and might lead to a potentially life-threatening condition, the ovarian hyperstimulation syndrome (OHSS).

OHSS refers to an exaggerated ovarian response to gonadotropin treatment. The syndrome has a broad spectrum of clinical manifestations, from mild illness needing only careful observation to severe illness requiring hospitalization and intensive care being a potentially life-threatening condition. Mild and moderate forms of OHSS may occur in 15–20% of all ovarian stimulation cycles; however, the severe form of the syndrome has been reported as frequently as 1–3% [125].

The specific risk factors for OHSS include young age, low BMI, signs of PCOS, previous history of OHSS and high estradiol on the day of hCG [125]. The key to preventing OHSS is the recognition of risk factors for OHSS leading to an individualization of gonadotropin starting dose which should be the minimum dose necessary to achieve the therapeutical goal. However, the accurate prediction of OHSS in an individual IVF cycle remains a difficult task. Indeed, PCOS (the main risk factor used in the prediction of OHSS) is present only in 20% of women undergoing COH and in less than 20% of patients developing symptoms of impending OHSS [126].

The recognition of a dose-response relationship between MIS and ovarian response to FSH leads to the hypothesis that hyper-response to ovulation induction might result from high MIS. In this context, high basal MIS may be associated with an increased risk of developing OHSS.

At present, few studies have been published reporting on this issue (Table 6.3). However, it seems that hyper-response and OHSS may be associated to significantly higher mean basal MIS levels. In the last years, four prospective studies performed on large number of subjects have been published reporting relevant value for MIS for the prediction of hyper-response and OHSS (Table 6.4).

Particularly, the studies by Lee et al. [128] and Nardo et al. [124] have independently calculated a similar performance of MIS for the prediction of hyper-response and OHSS. The reported cut-off value is of about 3.5 ng/mL, above which hyper-response/OHSS may be anticipated. In the study by Lee et al. [128], a cohort of 262 IVF cycles was investigated, in order to evaluate the predictive value for OHSS by means of age, BMI, estradiol and MIS levels. Authors found that the ROC of the basal MIS was larger than age and BMI and works as well as the number of follicles and estradiol levels on the day of hCG. Basal MIS levels predicted OHSS with a sensitivity of

Table 6.3 Basal AMH levels in women with normal and hyper-response to COH and OHSS (from ref [93])

			Mean AMH levels (ng/mL)		
References	Design	*n*	Normal response	Excessive response (>20 oocytes)	OHSS
Tremellen et al. [118]	Prosp	75	2.1		2.95
Eldar Geva et al. [100]	Prosp	56	2	5.3	
Nakhuda et al. [127]	Retro	30	0.63		3.6
Nelson et al. [108]	Prosp	340	1.4	3.9	
Nardo et al. [124]	Prosp	165	3.04	5.56	

Retro retrospective study; *Prosp* prospective study

Table 6.4 AMH cut-off values for the prediction of hyper-response to COS and OHSS (from ref [93])

References	*n*	Study design	CUT-OFF value	Sens (%)	Spec (%)	Prediction of hyper-response	Prediction of OHSS
Kwee et al. [105]	110	Prosp	5 μg/L	53	91	√[a]	
Nelson et al. [108]	340	Prosp	25 pmol/L	60	94.9	√[b]	
Lee et al. [128]	262	Prosp	3.36 ng/mL	90.5	81.3		√
Nardo et al. [124]	165	Prosp	3.5 ng/mL	88	70	√[a]	

Prosp prospective study
[a]Excessive response if >20 oocytes retrieved
[b]Excessive response if ≥21 oocytes retrieved

90.5% and specificity of 81.3%. Interestingly, the cut-off value calculated (3.36 ng/mL) corresponded to the highest quartile of the MIS values in their population, suggesting that hyper-response and OHSS may be caused by gonadotropin administration to women with “enhanced ovarian reserve” [128]. This was also evident in a previous study by our group [104] in which all cases with ovarian hyper-response to COS were in the group of patients with basal MIS levels in the highest MIS quartile. Considering that PCOS has been associated to high MIS levels, it is logical to conclude that the prevalence of PCOS patients among women with MIS levels in the highest MIS quartile may be increased thus in part explaining the observed high rate of OHSS in this group of women.

In conclusion, according to published papers, MIS measurement prior to gonadotropin stimulation could provide useful information to direct the application of mild patient friendly stimulation protocols in order to avoid OHSS.

6.6.2 Prediction of Qualitative Ovarian Response

It is extensively recognized that pregnancy in ART is mostly related to the qualitative than quantitative aspects of IVF. As the status of the ovarian reserve includes both the quantity and quality of ovarian follicle pool, MIS may reflect not only quantitative but also qualitative ovarian responsiveness. Indeed, several authors have found a significant positive correlation between MIS levels, oocyte quality [98, 101, 103, 120, 129, 130] and embryo morphology [101]. However, this relationship has not been confirmed by others [110, 122]. In order to clarify the complex relationship between MIS and oocyte quality, embryo quality and implantation and pregnancy rate, we should separately comment studies on MIS in the FF and in serum.

In an elegant study, MIS was measured in the FF obtained from both small and large follicles on the day of oocyte retrieval [131]. MIS levels in FF were found to be roughly 3 times higher in small than in large follicles confirming the hypothesis that MIS production by granulosa cells probably declines during final follicular maturation. Moreover, in both small and large follicles, FF MIS levels correlated positively with the number of early antral follicles on cycle day 3 before COS, growing follicles on the day of hCG administration and oocytes retrieved. This interesting finding may indicate that peripheral MIS levels are not exclusively dependent on the number of follicles; they are also modulated by individual follicular ability to produce MIS. Hence, elevated peripheral MIS levels indicate not only that the number of antral follicles is increased, but also that each follicle probably produces more MIS individually. This offers us a new understanding of the reported association between peripheral MIS levels and the ovarian fertility potential and leads the author to speculate that serum MIS measurement could reflect not only quantitative but also qualitative ovarian responsiveness to COS [131].

In a successive study by the same group [130], 118 monodominant follicle cycles were prospectively studied. MIS was measured in the FF and the fate of oocytes and embryos generated was observed. It was found that embryo implantation, clinical pregnancy and ongoing pregnancy rate increase dramatically from the low to the high FF MIS groups. The embryo morphology was similar within the groups so indicating that MIS in FF may be an additional factor in the selection of the oocyte [130]. This is particularly relevant in countries with restrictive law limiting the number of oocytes that may be inseminated. A recent study on a large number of subjects ($n = 276$) confirmed the previous finding that levels of MIS in FF were significantly increased in women who became pregnant in the respective IVF/ICSI treatment cycle [113].

While studies on FF seem to indicate that MIS may be useful in the prediction of oocyte and embryo quality and finally pregnancy, the same could not be said for circulating MIS. At present, only few studies concluded that serum MIS measurement may be able to give relevant information on gametes and embryo quality and on the outcome of the treatment cycle.

Silberstein and coll [101] found that serum MIS measured on the day of hCG correlated with the quality of embryos obtained permitting to discriminate between embryos with high and low implantation potential. Consequently, implantation rate but not pregnancy rate was higher in the group with high basal MIS levels [101]. However, the lack of a consistent correlation between serum MIS and embryo morphology and embryo aneuploidy rate, which is not in favour of a direct relationship between oocyte quantity and embryo quality, has been clearly demonstrated [110]. Hence, serum MIS seems not to be an adequate marker for embryo quality.

The vast majority of the studies investigating the performance of serum MIS in the prediction of pregnancy occurrence following IVF reported that MIS measurement is not useful in the prediction of success. Until present, only one study has been published relating serum MIS levels to the live birth rate following IVF [108]. In this large prospective study of 340 patients, it was demonstrated that the live birth rate dramatically increased with increasing basal MIS values. However, this was valid only for women with basal levels less than 7.8 pmol/L. Above this value, there was no discrimination for the live birth. Basal MIS seems not able to predict pregnancy or non-pregnancy, but simply enables patients to be identified as being at a low or high probability of pregnancy after IVF. As concluded by the same author, this finding may at least in part be explained by the very good correlation existing between basal MIS and the number of retrieved oocytes [108].

In conclusion, the possible prediction of qualitative aspects of ART programs by serum MIS measurement remains largely controversial. Evidence suggests that this relationship may only be indirect and related to the strong correlation existing between serum MIS and the quantitative ovarian response to COS.

6.7 Conclusions

In summary, the currently available data indicate that MIS is produced by growing preantral and early antral follicles. It has been demonstrated in mice that MIS inhibits initial follicle recruitment from the resting primordial stage. In addition, MIS may affect FSH-dependent growth of more mature follicles. However, the precise nature of the function of MIS within the human, ovary, and in particular the paracrine role of MIS on ovarian folliculogenesis and steroidogenesis in the human remains largely speculative.

As MIS is related to the ovarian follicular status, circulating MIS measurement may provide useful information in women with ovarian dysfunction. Circulating MIS levels are increased in women with PCOS and its use as a clinical diagnostic marker for the syndrome has been proposed. It is still unclear whether MIS levels may reflect the severity of ovarian function disruption or have a role in predicting the outcome of individual treatment regimens.

MIS could be a valuable marker of ovarian reserve in the general population, which may facilitate reproductive life planning for women. However, longitudinal data on MIS values during the reproductive life span are not available, and it remains unknown whether MIS levels may enable age-independent prediction of an individuals reproductive lifespan and spontaneous pregnancy in the general population. At present, the application of the MIS measurement for fertility assessment in the general population outwit the context of research studies, which is inappropriate.

For women who desire to become pregnant by means of ART, it is important to offer counselling about the optimal balance between benefit and risk. Since these outcomes are highly dependent on ovarian reserve, much effort has been put into identifying good clinical markers of ovarian reserve regarding individual prognosis for success and to design appropriate stimulation protocols.

Although MIS measurement is of course more expensive than age evaluation as a single marker of ovarian reserve, it clearly performs better in the prediction of both poor and hyper-response to COS (Table 6.5). Furthermore, MIS ease of measurement confers a relevant advantage to FSH which is cycle-dependent and less powerful. MIS may be informative on ovarian reserve also in women during GnRH agonist treatment or hormonal contraception that consequently exhibits suppressed FSH levels. Finally, it seems that poor response may be predicted by MIS with a performance which is similar to the AFC. Conversely, MIS seems superior to AFC in the prediction of hyper-response [124]. While AFC is a very common and useful measurement, it may be sometimes technically challenging and operator-dependent. Considering all these peculiar characteristics, it may be concluded that MIS is a candidate to be proposed as the ideal test for the ovarian reserve evaluation [132] (Table 6.5).

One new interesting field of application for MIS measurement, may be its use in the individualization of ovarian stimulation regimens. In many centres, the starting FSH dose for the first IVF is often selected on the basis of age and possibly also BMI of the patient. Some authors have recently proposed adjusting the treatment strategy on the basis of MIS levels [108, 114, 123].

As low and high MIS values are predictive of poor- and high-response to gonadotropins, respectively, it has been proposed to administer the FSH daily dose according to the pre-IVF MIS levels and independently of the age and BMI of the patient [108, 114, 123].

In summary, published studies indicate a relevant role for MIS measurement in the identification of both the extremes of ovarian response to stimulation and probably in the consequent individualization of treatment strategies in order to possibly reduce the incidence of cycle cancellation and OHSS. It still remains to clarify the cost/benefit of its use as a single assay before beginning an IVF cycle and whether the MIS-determined strategy of COS for assisted conception may be associated to improved live birth rate.

Table 6.5 Comparison of characteristics of the most widely used markers of ovarian reserve (from ref [93])

Characteristics for a good marker	Age	AMH	FSH	AFC
Prediction of poor response	+	+++	++	+++
Prediction of hyper-response	+	+++	–	+++
Low inter-cycle variability	+++	++	–	+
Low intra-cycle variability	+++	++	–	+
Blinded to the operator	+++	+++	+++	–
Applicable to all patients[a]	+++	+++	+	++
Cheapness	+++	–	–	–

[a]FSH and AFC are not informative in patients on hormonal contraception or GnRH agonist treatment. Moreover, the count of antral follicles may be difficult in women with ovarian cysts or with previous pelvic surgery

References

1. Cate RL, Mattaliano RJ, Hession C, Tizard R, Farber NM, Cheung A, et al. Isolation of the bovine and human genes for Mullerian inhibiting substance and expression of the human gene in animal cells. Cell. 1986;45:685–98.
2. Cohen-Haguenauer O, Picard JY, Mattei MG, Serero S, Nguyen VC, de Tand MF, et al. Mapping of the gene for anti-mullerian hormone to the short arm of human chromosome 19. Cytogenet Cell Genet. 1987;44:2–6.
3. Rey R, Lukas-Croisier C, Lasala C, Bedecarras P. AMH/MIS: what we know already about the gene, the protein and its regulation. Mol Cell Endocrinol. 2003;15:21–31.
4. Teixeira J, Maheswaran S, Donahoe PK. Mullerian inhibiting substance: an instructive developmental hormone with diagnostic and possible therapeutic applications. Endocr Rev. 2001;22:657–74.
5. Knebelmann B, Boussin L, Guerrier D, Legeai L, Kahn A, Josso N, et al. Anti-Mullerian hormone Bruxelles: a nonsense mutation associated with the persistent Mullerian duct syndrome. Proc Natl Acad Sci USA. 1991;88:3767–71.
6. Behringer RR, Finegold MJ, Cate RL. Mullerian-inhibiting substance function during mammalian sexual development. Cell. 1994;79:415–25.
7. Rajpert-De Meyts E, Jorgensen N, Graem N, Muller J, Cate RL, Skakkebaek NE. Expression of anti-Mullerian hormone during normal and pathological gonadal development: association with differentiation of Sertoli and granulosa cells. J Clin Endocrinol Metab. 1999;84:3836–44.
8. Imbeaud S, Faure E, Lamarre I, Mattei MG, di Clemente N, Tizard R, et al. Insensitivity to anti-Müllerian hormone due to a spontaneous mutation in the human anti-Müllerian hormone receptor. Nat Genet. 1995;11:382–8.
9. Imbeaud S, Carre-Eusebe D, Rey R, Belville C, Josso N, Picard JY. Molecular genetics of the persistent mullerian duct syndrome: a study of 19 families. Hum Mol Genet. 1994;3:125–31.
10. Ingraham HA, Hirokawa Y, Roberts LM, Mellon SH, McGee E, Nachtigal MW, et al. Autocrine and paracrine Mullerian inhibiting substance hormone signaling in reproduction. Recent Prog Horm Res. 2000;55:53–67.
11. di Clemente N, Josso N, Gouedard L, Belville C. Components of the anti-Mullerian hormone signaling pathway in gonads. Mol Cell Endocrinol. 2003;211:9–14.
12. Gouédard L, Chen YG, Thevenet L, Racine C, Borie S, Lamarre I, et al. Engagement of bone morphogenetic protein type IB receptor and Smad1 signaling by anti-Müllerian hormone and its type II receptor. J Biol Chem. 2000;275:27973–8.
13. Clarke TR, Hoshiya Y, Yi SE, Liu X, Lyons KM, Donahoe PK. Mullerian inhibiting substance signaling uses a bone morphogenetic protein (BMP)-like pathway mediated by ALK2 and induces SMAD6 expression. Mol Endocrinol. 2001;15:946–59.
14. Visser JA, Olaso R, Verhoef-Post M, Kramer P, Themmen AP, Ingraham HA. The serine/threonine transmembrane receptor ALK2 mediates Mullerian inhibiting substance signaling. Mol Endocrinol. 2001;15:936–45.
15. Jamin SP, Arango NA, Mishina Y, Hanks MC, Behringer RR. Requirement of Bmpr1a for Mullerian duct regression during male sexual development. Nat Genet. 2002;32:408–10.
16. Weenen C, Laven JS, Von Bergh AR, Cranfield M, Groome NP, Visser JA, et al. Anti-Mullerian hormone expression pattern in the human ovary: potential implications for initial and cyclic follicle recruitment. Mol Hum Reprod. 2004;10:77–83.
17. Munsterberg A, Lovell-Badge R. Expression of the mouse anti-mullerian hormone gene suggests a role in both male and female sexual differentiation. Development. 1991;113:613–24.
18. Ueno S, Kuroda T, Maclaughlin DT, Ragin RC, Manganaro TF, Donahoe PK. Mullerian inhibiting substance in the adult rat ovary during various stages of the estrous cycle. Endocrinology. 1989;125:1060–6.

19. Hirobe S, He WW, Gustafson ML, MacLaughlin DT, Donahoe PK. Mullerian inhibiting substance gene expression in the cycling rat ovary correlates with recruited or graafian follicle selection. Biol Reprod. 1994;50:1238–43.
20. Salmon NA, Handyside AH, Joyce IM. Oocyte regulation of anti-Müllerian hormone expression in granulosa cells during ovarian follicle development in mice. Dev Biol. 2004;266:201–8.
21. Visser JA, Themmen AP. Anti-Müllerian hormone and folliculogenesis. Mol Cell Endocrinol. 2005; 234:81–6.
22. Themmen AP. Anti-Müllerian hormone: its role in follicular growth initiation and survival and as an ovarian reserve marker. J Natl Cancer Inst Monogr. 2005;34:18–21.
23. Durlinger AL, Gruijters MJ, Kramer P, Karels B, Kuman TR, Matzuk MM, et al. Anti-Müllerian hormone attenuates the effects of FSH on follicle development in the mouse ovary. Endocrinology. 2001;142:4891–9.
24. La Marca A, Broekmans FJ, Volpe A, Fauser BC. ESHRE special interest group for reproductive endocrinology – AMH Round Table. Anti-Mullerian hormone (AMH): what do we still need to know? Hum Reprod. 2009;24(9):2264–75.
25. Durlinger AL, Kramer P, Karels B, de Jong FH, Uilenbroek JT, Grootegoed JA, et al. Control of primordial follicle recruitment by anti-Müllerian hormone in the mouse ovary. Endocrinology. 1999; 140:5789–96.
26. Visser JA, de Jong FH, Laven JS, Themmen AP. Anti-Müllerian hormone: a new marker for ovarian function. Reproduction. 2006;131:1–9.
27. Nilsson E, Rogers N, Skinner MK. Actions of anti-Mullerian hormone on the ovarian transcriptome to inhibit primordial to primary follicle transition. Reproduction. 2007;134:209–21.
28. Andersen CY, Byskov AG. Estradiol and regulation of anti-Müllerian hormone, inhibin-A, and inhibin-B secretion: analysis of small antral and preovulatory human follicles' fluid. J Clin Endocrinol Metab. 2006;91:4064–9.
29. Kevenaar ME, Themmen AP, Laven JS, Sonntag B, Fong SL, Uitterlinden AG, et al. Anti-Müllerian hormone and anti-Müllerian hormone type II receptor polymorphisms are associated with follicular phase estradiol levels in normo-ovulatory women. Hum Reprod. 2007;22:1547–54.
30. Long WQ, Ranchin V, Pautier P, Belville C, Denizot P, Cailla H, et al. Detection of minimal levels of serum anti-Mullerian hormone during follow-up of patients with ovarian granulosa cell tumor by means of a highly sensitive enzyme-linked immunosorbent assay. J Clin Endocrinol Metab. 2000;85: 540–4.
31. Taieb J, Belville C, Coussieu J, Guibourdenche J, Picard JY, di Clemente N. Deux dosages de l'hormone antimüllérienne: performances analytiques et cliniques. Ann Biol Clin. 2008;66:537–47.
32. Fréour T, Miralllié S, Bach-Ngohou K, Denis M, Barrière P, Masson D. Measurement of serum anti-Müllerian hormone by Beckman Coulter ELISA and DSL ELISA: comparison and relevance in assisted reproduction technology (ART). Clin Chim Acta. 2007;375:162–4.
33. Bersinger NA, Wunder D, Birkhäuser MH, Guibourdenche J. Measurement of anti-mullerian hormone by Beckman Coulter ELISA and DSL ELISA in assisted reproduction: differences between serum and follicular fluid. Clin Chim Acta. 2007;384:174–5.
34. Lee MM, Donahoe PK, Hasegawa T, Silverman B, Crist GB, Best S, et al. Mullerian inhibiting substance in humans: normal levels from infancy to adulthood. J Clin Endocrinol Metab. 1996;81:571–6.
35. Guibourdenche J, Lucidarme N, Chevenne D, Rigal O, Nicolas M, Luton D, et al. Anti-Müllerian hormone levels in serum from human foetuses and children: pattern and clinical interest. Mol Cell Endocrinol. 2003;211:55–63.
36. Van Rooij IA, Tonkelaar I, Broekmans FJ, Looman CW, Scheffer GJ, de Jong FH, et al. Anti-mullerian hormone is a promising predictor for the occurrence of the menopausal transition. Menopause. 2004;11:601–6.
37. La Marca A, De Leo V, Giulini S, Orvieto R, Malmusi S, Giannella L, et al. Anti-Mullerian hormone in premenopausal women and after spontaneous or surgically induced menopause. J Soc Gynecol Investig. 2005;12:545–8.
38. van Rooij IA, Broekmans FJ, Scheffer GJ, Looman CW, Habbema JD, de Jong FH, et al. Serum anti-mullerian hormone levels best reflect the reproductive decline with age in normal women with proven fertility: a longitudinal study. Fertil Steril. 2005;83: 979–87.
39. Robertson DM, Hale GE, Fraser IS, Hughes CL, Burger HG. A proposed classification system for menstrual cycles in the menopause transition based on changes in serum hormone profiles. Menopause. 2008;15:1139–44.
40. Sowers MR, Eyvazzadeh AD, McConnell D, Yosef M, Jannausch ML, Zhang D, et al. Anti-mullerian hormone and inhibin B in the definition of ovarian aging and the menopause transition. J Clin Endocrinol Metab. 2008;93:3478–83.
41. Van Disseldorp J, Faddy MJ, Themmen AP, de Jong FH, Peeters PH, van der Schouw YT, et al. Relationship of serum antimullerian hormone concentration to age at menopause. J Clin Endocrinol Metab. 2008;93: 2129–34.
42. La Marca A, Stabile G, Artenisio AC, Volpe A. Serum anti-Mullerian hormone throughout the human menstrual cycle. Hum Reprod. 2006;21:3103–7.
43. Hehenkamp WJ, Looman CW, Themmen AP, de Jong FH, Te Velde ER, Broekmans FJ. Anti-Müllerian hormone levels in the spontaneous menstrual cycle do not show substantial fluctuation. J Clin Endocrinol Metab. 2006;91:4057–63.

44. Tsepelidis S, Devreker F, Demeestere I, Flahaut A, Gervy Ch, Englert Y. Stable serum levels of anti-Müllerian hormone during the menstrual cycle: a prospective study in normo-ovulatory women. Hum Reprod. 2007;22:1837–40.
45. Streuli I, Fraisse T, Pillet C, Ibecheole V, Bischof P, de Ziegler D. Serum antimüllerian hormone levels remain stable throughout the menstrual cycle and after oral or vaginal administration of synthetic sex steroids. Fertil Steril. 2008;90:395–400.
46. Streuli I, Fraisse T, Chapron C, Bijaoui G, Bischof P, de Ziegler D. Clinical uses of anti-Müllerian hormone assays: pitfalls and promises. Fertil Steril. 2009;91: 226–30.
47. Wunder DM, Bersinger NA, Yared M, Kretschmer R, Birkhäuser MH. Statistically significant changes of antimüllerian hormone and inhibin levels during the physiologic menstrual cycle in reproductive age women. Fertil Steril. 2008;89:927–33.
48. La Marca A, Giulini S, Orvieto R, De Leo V, Volpe A. Anti-Müllerian hormone concentrations in maternal serum during pregnancy. Hum Reprod. 2005;20: 1569–72.
49. Mohamed KA, Davies WA, Lashen H. Antimüllerian hormone and pituitary gland activity after prolonged down-regulation with goserelin acetate. Fertil Steril. 2006;86:1515–7.
50. Arbo E, Vetori DV, Jimenez MF, Freitas FM, Lemos N, Cunha-Filho JS. Serum anti-mullerian hormone levels and follicular cohort characteristics after pituitary suppression in the late luteal phase with oral contraceptive pills. Hum Reprod. 2007;22:3192–6.
51. Somunkiran A, Yavuz T, Yucel O, Ozdemir I. Anti-Mullerian hormone levels during hormonal contraception in women with polycystic ovary syndrome. Eur J Obstet Gynecol Reprod Biol. 2007;134:196–201.
52. Rich-Edwards JW, Spiegelman D, Garland M, Hertzmark E, Hunter DJ, Colditz GA, et al. Physical activity, body mass index, and ovulatory disorder infertility. Epidemiology. 2002;13:184–90.
53. Fedorcsák P, Dale PO, Storeng R, Ertzeid G, Bjercke S, Oldereid N, et al. Impact of overweight and underweight on assisted reproduction treatment. Hum Reprod. 2004;19:2523–8.
54. Gracia CR, Freeman EW, Sammel MD, Lin H, Nelson DB. The relationship between obesity and race on inhibin B during the menopause transition. Menopause. 2005;12:559–66.
55. Freeman EW, Gracia CR, Sammel MD, Lin H, Lim LC, Strauss 3rd JF. Association of anti-mullerian hormone levels with obesity in late reproductive-age women. Fertil Steril. 2007;87:101–6.
56. Su HI, Sammel MD, Freeman EW, Lin H, DeBlasis T, Gracia CR. Body size affects measures of ovarian reserve in late reproductive age women. Menopause. 2008;15:857–61.
57. Freour T, Masson D, Mirallie S, Jean M, Bach K, Dejoie T, et al. Active smoking compromises IVF outcome and affects ovarian reserve. Reprod Biomed Online. 2008;16:96–102.
58. Nardo LG, Christodoulou D, Gould D, Roberts SA, Fitzgerald CT, Laing I. Anti-Müllerian hormone levels and antral follicle count in women enrolled in in vitro fertilization cycles: relationship to lifestyle factors, chronological age and reproductive history. Gynecol Endocrinol. 2007;24:1–8.
59. Seifer DB, Golub ET, Lambert-Messerlian G, Benning L, Anastos K, Watts DH, et al. Variations in serum müllerian inhibiting substance between white, black, and Hispanic women. Fertil Steril. 2009;92: 1674–8.
60. La Marca A, Pati M, Orvieto R, Stabile G, Carducci Artenisio A, Volpe A. Serum anti-Mullerian hormone levels in women with secondary amenorrhea. Fertil Steril. 2006;85:1547–9.
61. Van Elburg AA, Eijkemans MJ, Kas MJ, Themmen AP, de Jong FH, van Engeland H, et al. Predictors of recovery of ovarian function during weight gain in anorexia nervosa. Fertil Steril. 2007;87:902–8.
62. Méduri G, Massin N, Guibourdenche J, Bachelot A, Fiori O, Kuttenn F, et al. Serum anti-Müllerian hormone expression in women with premature ovarian failure. Hum Reprod. 2007;22:117–23.
63. La Marca A, Marzotti S, Brozzetti A, Stabile G, Artenisio AC, Bini V, et al. Italian Addison Network. Primary ovarian insufficiency due to steroidogenic cell autoimmunity is associated with apreserved pool of functioning follicles. J Clin Endocrinol Metab. 2009;94:3816–23.
64. Soules MR, Sherman S, Parrott E, Rebar R, Santoro N, Utian W, et al. Executive summary: stages of reproductive aging workshop (STRAW). Fertil Steril. 2001;76:874–8.
65. Knauff EA, Eijkemans MJ, Lambalk CB, Ten Kate-Booij MJ, Hoek A, Beerendonk CC, Laven JS, Goverde AJ, Broekmans FJ, Themmen AP, de Jong FH, Fauser BC. Anti Mullerian hormone, inhibin B, and antral follicle count in young women with varying degrees of hypergonadotropic ovarian failure. J Clin Endocrinol Metab. 2008; [Epub ahead of print].
66. Borgström B, Hreinsson J, Rasmussen C, Sheikhi M, Fried G, Keros V, et al. Fertility preservation in girls with Turner Syndrome – prognostic signs of the presence of ovarian follicle. J Clin Endocrinol Metab. 2009;94(1):74–80.
67. Anderson RA, Themmen AP, Al-Qahtani A, Groome NP, Cameron DA. The effects of chemotherapy and long-term gonadotrophin suppression on the ovarian reserve in premenopausal women with breast cancer. Hum Reprod. 2006;21:2583–92.
68. Loverro G, Guarini A, Di Naro E, Giacomantonio L, Lavopa C, Liso V. Ovarian function after cancer treatment in young women affected by Hodgkin disease (HD). Hematology. 2007;12:141–7.
69. Van Beek RD, van den Heuvel-Eibrink MM, Laven JS, de Jong FH, Themmen AP, Hakvoort-Cammel FG, et al. Anti-Mullerian hormone is a sensitive serum marker for gonadal function in women treated for Hodgkin's lymphoma during childhood. J Clin Endocrinol Metab. 2007;92:3869–74.

70. Lutchman Singh K, Muttukrishna S, Stein RC, McGarrigle HH, Patel A, Parikh B, et al. Predictors of ovarian reserve in young women with breast cancer. Br J Cancer. 2007;96:1808–16.
71. Lie Fong S, Lugtenburg PJ, Schipper I, Themmen AP, de Jong FH, Sonneveld P, et al. Anti-müllerian hormone as a marker of ovarian function in women after chemotherapy and radiotherapy for haematological malignancies. Hum Reprod. 2008;23:674–8.
72. Fallat ME, Siow Y, Marra M, Cook C, Carrillo A. Mullerian-inhibiting substance in follicular fluid and serum: a comparison of patients with tubal factor infertility, polycystic ovary syndrome, and endometriosis. Fertil Steril. 1997;67:962–5.
73. Cook CL, Siow Y, Brenner AG, Fallat ME. Relationship between serum mullerian-inhibiting substance and other reproductive hormones in untreated women with polycystic ovary syndrome and normal women. Fertil Steril. 2002;77:141–6.
74. Pigny P, Merlen E, Robert Y, Cortet-Rudelli C, Decanter C, Jonard S, et al. Elevated serum level of anti-mullerian hormone in patients with polycystic ovary syndrome: relationship to the ovarian follicle excess and to the follicular arrest. J Clin Endocrinol Metab. 2003;88:5957–62.
75. La Marca A, Orvieto R, Giulini S, Jasonni VM, Volpe A, De Leo V. Mullerian-inhibiting substance in women with polycystic ovary syndrome: relationship with hormonal and metabolic characteristics. Fertil Steril. 2004;82:970–2.
76. Laven JS, Mulders AG, Visser JA, Themmen AP, De Jong FH, Fauser BC. Anti-Mullerian hormone serum concentrations in normoovulatory and anovulatory women of reproductive age. J Clin Endocrinol Metab. 2004;89:318–23.
77. Wachs DS, Coffler MS, Malcom PJ, Chang RJ. Serum anti-mullerian hormone concentrations are not altered by acute administration of follicle stimulating hormone in polycystic ovary syndrome and normal women. J Clin Endocrinol Metab. 2007;92:1871–4.
78. Mulders AG, Laven JS, Eijkemans MJ, de Jong FH, Themmen AP, Fauser BC. Changes in anti-Mullerian hormone serum concentrations over time suggest delayed ovarian ageing in normogonadotrophic anovulatory infertility. Hum Reprod. 2004;19:2036–42.
79. Pellatt L, Hanna L, Brincat M, Galea R, Brain H, Whitehead S, et al. Granulosa cell production of anti-Müllerian hormone is increased in polycystic ovaries. J Clin Endocrinol Metab. 2007;92:240–5.
80. Wang JG, Nakhuda GS, Guarnaccia MM, Sauer MV, Lobo RA. Müllerian inhibiting substance and disrupted folliculogenesis in polycystic ovary syndrome. Am J Obstet Gynecol. 2007;196:77e1–5.
81. Sir-Petermann T, Maliqueo M, Codner E, Echiburú B, Crisosto N, Pérez V, et al. Early metabolic derangements in daughters of women with polycystic ovary syndrome. J Clin Endocrinol Metab. 2007;92:4637–42.
82. Crisosto N, Codner E, Maliqueo M, Echiburú B, Sánchez F, Cassorla F, et al. Anti-Müllerian hormone levels in peripubertal daughters of women with polycystic ovary syndrome. J Clin Endocrinol Metab. 2007;92:2739–43.
83. Siow Y, Kives S, Hertweck P, Perlman S, Fallat ME. Serum Müllerian-inhibiting substance levels in adolescent girls with normal menstrual cycles or with polycystic ovary syndrome. Fertil Steril. 2005;84:938–44.
84. Fleming R, Deshpande N, Traynor I, Yates RW. Dynamics of FSH-induced follicular growth in subfertile women: relationship with age, insulin resistance, oocyte yield and anti-Mullerian hormone. Hum Reprod. 2006;21:1436–41.
85. Webber LJ, Stubbs S, Stark J, Trew GH, Margara R, Hardy K, et al. Formation and early development of follicles in the polycystic ovary. Lancet. 2003;362:1017–21.
86. Pigny P, Jonard S, Robert Y, Dewailly D. Serum anti-Mullerian hormone as a surrogate for antral follicle count for definition of the polycystic ovary syndrome. J Clin Endocrinol Metab. 2006;91:941–5.
87. Moran LJ, Noakes M, Clifton PM, Norman RJ. The use of anti-mullerian hormone in predicting menstrual response after weight loss in overweight women with polycystic ovary syndrome. J Clin Endocrinol Metab. 2007;92:3796–802.
88. El-Halawaty S, Rizk A, Kamal M, Aboulhassan M, Al-Sawah H, Noah O, et al. Clinical significance of serum concentration of anti-Müllerian hormone in obese women with polycystic ovary syndrome. Reprod Biomed Online. 2007;15:495–9.
89. Piltonen T, Morin-Papunen L, Koivunen R, Perheentupa A, Ruokonen A, Tapanainen JS. Serum anti-Mullerian hormone levels remain high until late reproductive age and decrease during metformin therapy in women with polycystic ovary syndrome. Hum Reprod. 2005;20:1820–6.
90. de Vet A, Loven JS, de Jong FH, Themmen AP, Fauser BC. Anti-Mullerian hormone serum levels: a putative marker for ovarian aging. Fertil Steril. 2002;77:357–62.
91. La Marca A, Sighinolfi G, Giulini S, Traglia M, Argento C, Sala C, Masciullo C, Volpe A, Toniolo D. Normal serum levels of anti-Mullerian Hormone (AMH) in women with regular menstrual cycles. RBMonline. (in press).
92. Tehrani FR, Solaymani-Dodaran M, Azizi F. A single test of antimüllerian hormone in late reproductive-aged women is a good predictor of menopause. Menopause. 2009;16(4):797–802.
93. La Marca A, Sighinolfi G, Radi D, Argento C, Baraldi E, Artenisio AC, et al. Anti-Mullerian hormone (AMH) as a predictive marker in assisted reproductive technology (ART). Hum Reprod Update. 2010;16:113–30.
94. Seifer DB, MacLaughlin DT, Christian BP, Feng B, Shelden RM. Early follicular serum mullerian-inhibiting substance levels are associated with ovarian response during assisted reproductive technology cycles. Fertil Steril. 2002;77:468–71.

95. Van Rooij IA, Broekmans FJ, te Velde ER, Fauser BC, Bancsi LF, Jong FH, et al. Serum anti-Mullerian hormone levels: a novel measure of ovarian reserve. Hum Reprod. 2002;17:3065–71.
96. Fanchin R, Schonauer LM, Righini C, Guibourdenche J, Frydman R, Taieb J. Serum anti-Mullerian hormone is more strongly related to ovarian follicular status than serum inhibin B, estradiol, FSH and LH on day 3. Hum Reprod. 2003;18:323–7.
97. Muttukrishna S, Suharjono H, McGarrigle H, Sathanandan M. Inhibin B and anti-Mullerian hormone: markers of ovarian response in IVF/ICSI patients? BJOG. 2004;111:1248–53.
98. Hazout A, Bouchard P, Seifer DB, Aussage P, Junca AM, Cohen-Bacrie P. Serum antimullerian hormone/mullerian-inhibiting substance appears to be a more discriminatory marker of assisted reproductive technology outcome than follicle-stimulating hormone, inhibin B, or estradiol. Fertil Steril. 2004;82:1323–9.
99. Muttukrishna S, McGarrigle H, Wakim R, Khadum I, Ranieri DM, Serhal P. Antral follicle count, anti-mullerian hormone and inhibin B: predictors of ovarian response in assisted reproductive technology? BJOG. 2005;112:1384–90.
100. Eldar-Geva T, Ben-Chetrit A, Spitz IM, Rabinowitz R, Markowitz E, Mimoni T, et al. Dynamic assays of inhibin B, anti-Mullerian hormone and estradiol following FSH stimulation and ovarian ultrasonography as predictors of IVF outcome. Hum Reprod. 2005;20:3178–83.
101. Silberstein T, MacLaughlin DT, Shai I, Trimarchi JR, Lambert-Messerlian G, Seifer DB, et al. Mullerian inhibiting substance levels at the time of HCG administration in IVF cycles predict both ovarian reserve and embryo morphology. Hum Reprod. 2006;21:159–63.
102. Fiçicioglu C, Kutlu T, Baglam E, Bakacak Z. Early follicular antimüllerian hormone as an indicator of ovarian reserve. Fertil Steril. 2006;85:592–6.
103. Lekamge DN, Barry M, Kolo M, Lane M, Gilchrist RB, Tremellen KP. Anti-Müllerian hormone as a predictor of IVF outcome. Reprod Biomed Online. 2007;14:602–10.
104. La Marca A, Giulini S, Tirelli A, Bertucci E, Marsella T, Xella S, et al. Anti-Mullerian hormone measurement on any day of the menstrual cycle strongly predicts ovarian response in assisted reproductive technology. Hum Reprod. 2007;22:766–71.
105. Kwee J, Schats R, McDonnell J, Themmen A, de Jong F, Lambalk C. Evaluation of anti-Müllerian hormone as a test for the prediction of ovarian reserve. Fertil Steril. 2008;90(3):737–43.
106. Nakhuda GS, Sauer MV, Wang JG, Ferin M, Lobo RA. Müllerian inhibiting substance is an accurate marker of ovarian response in women of advanced reproductive age undergoing IVF. Reprod Biomed Online. 2007;14:450–4.
107. Macklon NS, Stouffer RL, Giudice LC, Fauser BC. The science behind 25 years of ovarian stimulation for in vitro fertilization. Endocr Rev. 2006;27:170–207.
108. Nelson SM, Yates RW, Fleming R. (2007) Serum anti-Müllerian hormone and FSH: prediction of live birth and extremes of response in stimulated cycles – implications for individualization of therapy. Hum Reprod. 2007;22:2414–21.
109. Elgindy EA, El-Haieg DO, El-Sebaey A. (2008) Anti-Müllerian hormone: correlation of early follicular, ovulatory and midluteal levels with ovarian response and cycle outcome in intracytoplasmic sperm injection patients. Fertil Steril. 2008;89:1670–6.
110. Lie Fong S, Baart EB, Martini E, Schipper I, Visser JA, Themmen AP, et al. Anti-Müllerian hormone: a marker for oocyte quantity, oocyte quality and embryo quality? Reprod Biomed Online. 2008;16:664–70.
111. Jee BC, Ku SY, Suh CS, Kim KC, Lee WD, Kim SH. Serum anti-Müllerian hormone and inhibin B levels at ovulation triggering day can predict the number of immature oocytes retrieved in in vitro fertilization cycles. J Korean Med Sci. 2008;23:657–61.
112. Jayaprakasan K, Campbell B, Hopkisson J, Johnson I, Raine-Fenning N. A prospective, comparative analysis of anti-Müllerian hormone, inhibin-B, and three-dimensional ultrasound determinants of ovarian reserve in the prediction of poor response to controlled ovarian stimulation. Fertil Steril. 2010;93(3):855–64.
113. Wunder DM, Guibourdenche J, Birkhäuser MH, Bersinger NA. Anti-Müllerian hormone and inhibin B as predictors of pregnancy after treatment by in vitro fertilization/intracytoplasmic sperm injection. Fertil Steril. 2008;90(6):2203–10.
114. Nelson SM, Yates RW, Lyall H, Jamieson M, Traynor I, Gaudoin M, et al. Anti-Mullerian hormone-based approach to controlled ovarian stimulation for assisted conception. Hum Reprod. 2009;24(4):867–75.
115. Broer SL, Mol BW, Hendriks D, Broekmans FJ. The role of antimullerian hormone in prediction of outcome after IVF: comparison with the antral follicle count. Fertil Steril. 2009;91(3):705–14.
116. Hendriks DJ, Mol BW, Bancsi LF, Te Velde ER, Broekmans FJ. Antral follicle count in the prediction of poor ovarian response and pregnancy after in vitro fertilization: a meta-analysis and comparison with basal follicle-stimulating hormone level. Fertil Steril. 2005;83:291–301.
117. Tarlatzis BC, Zepiridis L, Grimbizis G, Bontis J. Clinical management of low ovarian response to stimulation for IVF: a systematic review. Hum Reprod Update. 2003;9:61–76.
118. Tremellen KP, Kolo M, Gilmore A, Lekamge DN. Anti-mullerian hormone as a marker of ovarian reserve. Aust N Z J Obstet Gynaecol. 2005;45:20–4.
119. Peñarrubia J, Fábregues F, Manau D, Creus M, Casals G, Casamitjana R, et al. Basal and stimulation day 5 anti-Mullerian hormone serum concentrations as predictors of ovarian response and pregnancy in assisted reproductive technology cycles stimulated with gonadotropin-releasing hormone agonist – gonadotropin treatmen. Hum Reprod. 2005;20:915–22.

120. Ebner T, Sommergruber M, Moser M, Shebl O, Schreier-Lechner E, Tews G. Basal level of anti-Müllerian hormone is associated with oocyte quality in stimulated cycles. Hum Reprod. 2006;21:2022–6.
121. Fréour T, Mirallié S, Colombel A, Bach-Ngohou K, Masson D, Barrière P. Anti-mullerian hormone: clinical relevance in assisted reproductive therapy. Ann Endocrinol (Paris). 2006;67:567–74.
122. Smeenk JM, Sweep FC, Zielhuis GA, Kremer JA, Thomas CM, Braat DD. Antimüllerian hormone predicts ovarian responsiveness, but not embryo quality or pregnancy, after in vitro fertilization or intracyoplasmic sperm injection. Fertil Steril. 2007;87:223–6.
123. Gnoth C, Schuring AN, Friol K, Tigges J, Mallmann P, Godehardt E. Relevance of anti-Mullerian hormone measurement in a routine IVF program. Hum Reprod. 2008;23:1359–65.
124. Nardo LG, Gelbaya TA, Wilkinson H, Roberts SA, Yates A, Pemberton P, et al. Circulating basal anti-Müllerian hormone levels as predictor of ovarian response in women undergoing ovarian stimulation for in vitro fertilization. Fertil Steril. 2009;92(5):1586–93.
125. Practice Committee of American Society for Reproductive Medicine. Ovarian hyperstimulation syndrome. Fertil Steril. 2008;90:S188–93.
126. Tummon I, Gavrilova-Jordan L, Allemand MC, Session D. Polycystic ovaries and ovarian hyperstimulation syndrome: a systematic review. Acta Obstet Gynecol Scand. 2005;84:611–6.
127. Nakhuda GS, Chu MC, Wang JG, Sauer MV, Lobo RA. Elevated serum müllerian-inhibiting substance may be a marker for ovarian hyperstimulation syndrome in normal women undergoing in vitro fertilization. Fertil Steril. 2006;85:1541–3.
128. Lee TH, Liu CH, Huang CC, Wu YL, Shih YT, Ho HN, et al. Serum anti-Müllerian hormone and estradiol levels as predictors of ovarian hyperstimulation syndrome in assisted reproduction technology cycles. Hum Reprod. 2008;23:160–7.
129. Cupisti S, Dittrich R, Mueller A, Strick R, Stiegler E, Binder H, et al. Correlations between anti-müllerian hormone, inhibin B, and activin A in follicular fluid in IVF/ICSI patients for assessing the maturation and developmental potential of oocytes. Eur J Med Res. 2007;12:604–8.
130. Fanchin R, Mendez Lozano DH, Frydman N, Gougeon A, di Clemente N, Frydman R, et al. Anti-Müllerian hormone concentrations in the follicular fluid of the preovulatory follicle are predictive of the implantation potential of the ensuing embryo obtained by in vitro fertilization. J Clin Endocrinol Metab. 2007;92:1796–802.
131. Fanchin R, Taieb J, Lozano DH, Ducot B, Frydman R, Bouyer J. High reproducibility of serum anti-Mullerian hormone measurements suggests a multi-staged follicular secretion and strengthens its role in the assessment of ovarian follicular status. Hum Reprod. 2005;20:923–7.
132. La Marca A, Volpe A. Anti-Mullerian hormone (AMH) in female reproduction: is measurement of circulating AMH a useful tool? Clin Endocrinol (Oxf). 2006;64:603–10.

Evidence-Based Use of Progesterone During IVF

7

Elena H. Yanushpolsky

Abstract

It has been well demonstrated that luteal phase physiology is disrupted in IVF cycles conducted with either GnRH agonists or antagonists, and that supplementation of the luteal phase with exogenous progesterone is necessary to optimize IVF cycle outcomes. There is now sufficient evidence to state that intravaginal progesterone preparations in therapeutic doses are equally efficacious and better tolerated by patients compared to traditional intramuscular progesterone preparations. There is no need to monitor serum progesterone levels with vaginal supplementation as adequate endometrial maturation is achieved at relatively low serum progesterone levels because of superior local absorption.

In this chapter, we examine the evidence for efficacy, dosing, and timing of several progesterone preparations and also discuss as yet unclear issues of the ideal duration of progesterone support in early pregnancy and progesterone replacement in frozen embryo transfer cycles and donor/egg recipient cycles.

Keywords

Corpus luteum • Luteal phase support • GnRH agonists • GnRH antagonists • IVF • Intramuscular progesterone • Vaginal progesterone • Intravaginal progesterone • Oral progesterone • Pregnancy rates • Serum progesterone levels • Early pregnancy progesterone support

E.H. Yanushpolsky (✉)
Department of Obstetrics and Gynecology,
Brigham and Women's Hospital, Boston, MA , USA
e-mail: eyanushpolsky@partners.org

C. Racowsky et al. (eds.), *Biennial Review of Infertility: Volume 2*,
DOI 10.1007/978-1-4419-8456-2_7, © Springer Science+Business Media, LLC 2011

7.1 Introduction

Establishment of successful pregnancy in natural ovulatory cycles depends in large part on adequate endometrial development, which is induced by sequential and combined exposures to estrogen and progesterone, which are produced by the developing follicle prior to ovulation and by corpus luteum after ovulation. Both follicular estrogen production and corpus luteum function are governed by pulsatile GnRH output from the hypothalamus [1]. Stimulated in vitro fertilization (IVF) cycles are different from natural cycles in supraphysiological estrogen levels in the follicular phase and rapid changes in the estrogen and progesterone levels in the luteal phase after follicle aspiration. Removal of granulosa cells in the process of oocyte retrieval leads to depletion of the cell pool needed to produce progesterone in the luteal phase. In addition, since most IVF cycles currently involve administration of GnRH modulators, either agonists or antagonists, physiologic pulsatility necessary for adequate corpus luteum function and progesterone production is disrupted leading to well-described luteal phase foreshortening and dysfunction [2–4]. Exogenous supplementation of the luteal phase of IVF cycles with either progesterone or human chorionic gonadotropin (hCG) has been shown to result in better pregnancy rates and outcomes compared to no supplementation [5, 6]. However, data relative to the best method of luteal phase support in IVF have been insufficient until recently [7]. The best method for luteal phase support in IVF should be optimally efficacious, with minimal side effects, and with ease and convenience of administration. A 2004 Cochrane systematic review of 59 studies comparing intravaginal progesterone supplementation, intramuscular progesterone supplementation, and supplementation with hCG injections reported similar IVF pregnancy rates, but the odds for ovarian hyperstimulation (OHSS) complication were 20-fold higher with hCG than with progesterone supplementation [6]. They concluded that progesterone should be the preferred form of luteal phase support in IVF over hCG injections, yet oral progesterone preparation, which is the most convenient and easy for patients to self-administer has been shown to lack adequate efficacy [8, 9]. The question of the best parenteral progesterone preparation with respect to efficacy, convenience, and tolerability has been the focus of intense investigation in recent years.

7.2 What is the Evidence and How Should We Interpret it for Our Practice?

Practice of medicine in any field has not always been and is not always based on solid scientific data. This has not been for the lack of desire on the part of physicians to base their decisions on the best scientific methods and evidence, but rather because of the paucity of data that are derived from rigorously designed and properly powered studies. The strongest evidence is derived from prospective, randomized, double-blind, placebo-controlled trials involving homogeneous patient populations with adequate numbers to have the power to detect real differences in outcomes. Under ideal circumstances, confirming results from more than one such study should provide the best evidence for changing or adjusting clinical practice [10]. Prospective, randomized, adequately powered studies require substantial time and resources to complete, and the nature of some investigations often precludes the double-blinded design. Smaller prospective, randomized studies but with lower powers to detect effect of interest may be combined into meta-analyses in order to increase the overall validity of evidence. However, even results of the best designed studies and meta-analyses must be evaluated critically with respect to potential confounders, applicability to specific populations, and publication bias when clinical practice changes are in question [11]. Although retrospective studies are relatively inexpensive and easy to complete, we should exercise great caution in interpreting data derived from retrospective reviews and studies using nonconcurrent controls because bias and confounding that are inherent in such studies produce results with no internal or external validity [12]. A good example of such retrospective studies on the subject of progesterone support in IVF with either intramuscular or intravaginal progesterone preparations producing diametrically opposite conclusions are those of Papaleo et al. [13] and Ho et al. [14].

With the issues of proper methodology in mind, we examine the current evidence on the parenteral progesterone support in IVF-ET cycles with the main focus on prospective, randomized studies and meta-analyses.

7.3 Evolution and Accumulation of Evidence on Progesterone Support in IVF

The most common form of progesterone that has been used for luteal phase support in IVF has been progesterone in oil administered as intramuscular injections (IMP) at dose of 50–100 mg daily. While reasonably effective, IMP are painful for the patients, inconvenient to administer, usually requiring another person to help with administration, and associated with severe side effects, such as welts, infections, abscesses, allergic reactions, and even pulmonary complications requiring hospital admissions [15–17]. Not surprisingly, clinicians were interested in identifying other forms of progesterone support in IVF that will be at least equally efficacious and better tolerated by patients. Belgian researches led the way in investigations of luteal phase physiology, pathology, and corrective supplementation options related to optimal endometrial maturation and improved implantation in IVF cycles in the early 1990s [18, 19]. Using histopathological evaluations, they demonstrated that similar and appropriate luteal endometrial maturation can be achieved with either intramuscular progesterone 100 mg daily injections or with intravaginal micronized progesterone administration at doses between 300 and 600 mg daily. Oral micronized progesterone was ineffective in inducing secretory endometrial changes [20]. With this information on hand, Smitz et al. [21] set out a first prospective randomized study comparing pregnancy rates in IVF cycles supplemented with either intramuscular progesterone in oil or with micronized progesterone in vaginal capsules. They randomized 262 IVF, GIFT, and ZIFT patients into two groups to receive either intramuscular progesterone injections 50 mg daily, or micronized progesterone in capsules vaginally 600 mg in three divided doses starting on the day before oocyte retrieval. They also measured luteal phase and early pregnancy serum progesterone levels in pregnant and nonpregnant patients and found that, despite significantly higher serum progesterone levels observed in patients receiving intramuscular progesterone, those receiving intravaginal progesterone had a higher overall pregnancy rate as well as implantation rate.

Although original histopathologic studies [20, 22] demonstrating adequate secretory endometrial maturation utilized micronized progesterone capsules at doses between 300 and 600 mg daily, several randomized studies comparing intravaginal and intramuscular progesterone supplementation in IVF in the mid-to-late 1990s chose to use lower doses (100–200 mg daily) and in different and nonstandardized compounded preparations such as creams and suppositories [23–25]. Such doses and preparations are currently recognized as insufficient and inappropriate for luteal phase support in IVF.

An earlier meta-analysis of luteal phase support in infertility treatment that addressed comparison of intravaginal vs. intramuscular progesterone [5] preparations included five prospective studies, two of which [23, 24] contained the majority of patients included in the meta-analysis, all of whom used intravaginal progesterone preparations of 100–200 mg daily. The authors' conclusion was that intramuscular progesterone conferred the most benefit compared to intravaginal use. It is implicitly understood that the value of conclusions that can be drawn from any meta-analysis is dependent on the size and study design and quality of its individual components [10]. It is not surprising therefore that a meta-analysis that included the majority of patients receiving insufficient amounts of vaginal progesterone for luteal support would come to an unfavorable conclusion.

By the time Daya and Gunby [6] published their meta-analysis in 2004, five additional prospective studies comparing intravaginal and intramuscular progesterone preparations were eligible for inclusion. The authors admitted that methodological quality of the majority of the studies was only fair with an average validity score of only 51%. Three of the ten included studies utilized subtherapeutic vaginal progesterone doses of 100–200 mg daily [23–25] as described above. The authors concluded that there was significant statistical heterogeneity for the outcomes of clinical pregnancy, miscarriage, and ongoing pregnancy. Only two out of ten studies reported live births as an outcome, and statistical significance was reached in favor of intramuscular progesterone administration for the live birth parameter. However, authors of one of those two studies admitted to methodological flaws related to lack of stratification by age leading to a greater number of patients >40 years old in the intravaginal progesterone group, thus biasing results by the most important confounders of IVF outcome – age and ovarian reserve [26].

Given continued uncertainly of the comparative efficacy of intramuscular vs. intravaginal progesterone supplementation in IVF, there was a great need for rigorously designed and properly powered prospective randomized studies using proper therapeutic progesterone doses to resolve the issue. Two studies that fulfilled these requirements were published in 2008 [27, 28]. Both studies aimed at elimination of important confounders such as age and ovarian reserve by excluding patients over age 40, and those with day 3 FSH levels >15 mIU/mL. Dal Prato et al. [27] restricted enrollment to women <37 years old, and Yanushpolsky et al. [28] stratified women by age <35 years old and 35–39 years old prior to randomization to insure equal age distribution between treatment groups. In 1997, a new micronized vaginal progesterone bioadhesive gel preparation (Crinone 8% (90 mg) vaginal gel) became commercially available and FDA approved in the Unites States for progesterone supplementation at once-daily dose and for replacement at twice per day dosing in IVF treatments. Excellent transvaginal absorption and superior progesterone tissue levels achieved with Crinone 8% as compared with intramuscular progesterone were well demonstrated in several prior studies [29–31]. Dal Prato et al. [27] presented a noninferiority study design for three luteal phase treatment arms in IVF patients – intramuscular progesterone 50 mg/day, Crinone 8% (90 mg) vaginal gel once/day, and Crinone 8% vaginal gel twice/day starting the day after oocyte retrieval. They achieved their precalculated necessary sample size with 138 patients in the intramuscular progesterone group, 137 patients in Crinone 8% once-daily group, and 137 patients in the Crinone 8% twice-daily administration group. No statistical differences were found between the three groups with respect to pregnancy rates (hCG >5 mIU/mL), implantation rates, clinical pregnancy rates, miscarriages, and delivery rates. The authors concluded that vaginal gel can be successfully used as an alternative to intramuscular progesterone in luteal support in IVF, and that once-daily dose was sufficient for optimal results.

The "Correspondence" publication by Yanushpolsky et al. [28] was a report of an interim analysis of a larger study powered at 400 patients in two arms of either intramuscular progesterone supplementation starting the day after oocyte retrieval or Crinone 8% vaginal gel starting 2 days after oocyte retrieval. The rationale for a later start of Crinone was based on the known superior absorption data [29–31] as well as favorable results reported in preliminary studies by Schoolcraft et al. [32]. Similar results were observed between intramuscular progesterone and intravaginal progesterone arms with respect to positive beta-hCG rates, implantation rates, clinical and ongoing/delivered pregnancy rates, as well as failed pregnancies. In follow-up questionnaires, patients expressed significantly greater satisfaction with intravaginal route of progesterone administration [28].

The most recent and rigorous meta-analysis on the route of luteal progesterone administration in IVF [33] included both Dal Prato et al. [27] and Yanushpolsky et al. [28] studies with proper methodology and dosing and excluded three studies with subtherapeutic progesterone doses [23–25]. A total of nine studies met inclusion criteria with seven of nine using Crinone 8% vaginal gel and two using micronized progesterone capsules 600 mg (200 mg 3 times a day). All studies used intramuscular progesterone in oil 50 mg daily. The endpoints of analysis were clinical pregnancy and ongoing pregnancy rates. The Odds Ratio for these endpoints were 0.91 (95% CI 0.74–1.13) and 0.94 (95% CI 0.71–1.26), respectively. The authors concluded that daily administration of vaginal progesterone (90 mg bioadhesive gel or 600 mg [200 mg 3 times a day] progesterone capsules) is comparable to daily administration of 50 mg intramuscular progesterone in oil for luteal phase support in IVF. It should be noted that all publications included in the meta-analysis reported use of "long" GnRH downregulation regimens for patients enrolled in the studies.

As we have discussed earlier in the chapter, even the best intended, most rigorous meta-analyses have limitations because of nonhomogeneity of data in the studies on which meta-analyses are based. Therefore large, well-designed, adequately powered, prospective, randomized studies remain the gold standard evidence on which medical decisions should rely. Two such studies on the comparison of efficacy and patient tolerability of intramuscular progesterone and intravaginal gel for luteal phase support in IVF have become available in the literature in 2010. One of them by Yanushpolsky et al. [34] is a report of a completed, fully powered, prospective randomized study, the interim results of which at half point enrollment were included in the meta-analysis by Zarutski and Phillips [33]. All 407 patients in that study were on "long" GnRH downregulation protocol and were randomized to receive either intramuscular progesterone 50 mg daily starting the day after oocyte retrieval or Crinone 8% (90 mg) intravaginal gel starting 2 days after oocyte retrieval. All pregnant patients were supplemented with Crinone 8% gel daily until 10 weeks gestation.

There were no differences between the treatment arms with respect to patients' demographic and clinical characteristics. Likewise, there were no statistical differences with respect to pregnancy rates (beta hCG >5 IU/mL), implantation rates, clinical pregnancy and ongoing/delivered rates, or failed pregnancy rates between the groups. Ninety percent of enrolled patients were available to answer a questionnaire regarding product satisfaction with significantly higher satisfaction scores reported by those in the vaginal progesterone arm.

The other study by Kahraman et al. [35] included only those patients treated with the GnRH antagonist protocol, and it is the first prospective, randomized study of progesterone formulations for luteal support in IVF patients on antagonist protocols. With respect to methodology, this study was adequately powered at 209 and 217 patients in each of the treatment arms and important confounders were properly excluded. Older patients (>37 years old), those with diminished ovarian reserve according to their basal antral follicle counts and FSH levels, as well as patients who failed in at least three prior IVF cycle were excluded from enrollment to minimize confounders. Eligible patients were randomized into two groups to receive either intramuscular progesterone 100 mg daily, or Crinone 8% (90 mg) gel twice daily on the day after oocyte retrieval. Progesterone supplementation was extended up to the evidence of fetal heart activity on ultrasound examination. Investigators found no statistical differences between two arms relative to demographic and clinical parameters, and similar implantation, pregnancy, clinical and ongoing pregnancy rates as well as biochemical and miscarriage rates were observed in both arms.

The authors admitted that the rationale for using vaginal gel twice daily was not based on solid data, as they were aware of the data demonstrating equal efficacy of once-daily vs. twice-daily regimens [27], but more out of desire to reduce possible patient anxiety.

At this time in 2010, we can state with confidence that the body of scientific evidence confirms equal efficacy of intramuscular and intravaginal progesterone preparations in therapeutic doses for luteal phase support. Intravaginal progesterone preparations are more convenient and better tolerated by patients than intramuscular preparations and therefore should be the first line of progesterone supplementation in IVF.

Several other aspects of vaginal progesterone support deserve discussion:

1. What is the optimal dose?
2. How do various vaginal progesterone preparations compare with respect to efficacy and acceptance by patients?
3. What is the optimal timing of progesterone initiation within the IVF cycle?
4. How long should progesterone be continued in early pregnancy and should we monitor serum progesterone levels?
5. What about progesterone replacement in Frozen embryo transfer cycles and donor oocyte recipient cycles?

We will address each of these questions separately with respect to the evidence available at this time.

7.4 What is the Optimal Dose of Vaginal Progesterone Supplementation?

An optimal dose of any medication for any indication should be the dose that will be optimally effective, most convenient to administer, as well as cost effective. The body of literature that we have reviewed so far focused on comparison of intramuscular progesterone preparations from 50 to 100 mg daily with intravaginal preparations of micronized progesterone in oil capsules ranging from 100 to 600 mg daily in three divided doses, or micronized progesterone bioadhesive gel (Crinone 8% [90 mg]) inserts once or twice daily. It has been well demonstrated in histopathological studies [22], as well as clinical studies [21], that progesterone capsules in doses less than 300 mg/day are inferior in efficacy to intramuscular progesterone. Most studies demonstrating equal efficacy involved micronized progesterone capsules 600 mg (200 mg 3 times a day).

Crinone vaginal gel has been shown to have an excellent coefficient of absorption [29–31] into endometrial tissues and capable of inducing appropriate secretory endometrial changes necessary for luteal phase support [32]. A single daily dose (90 mg) was approved by FDA for progesterone supplementation in ART, while twice-daily dose was recommended for replacement in postmenopausal or agonadal women [36, 37]. Among prospective randomized studies comparing intramuscular progesterone to Crinone gel and demonstrating similar results, some involved once-daily gel administration, while others involved twice-daily doses [28, 35]. A study by Dal Prato el al contained three arms comparing intramuscular progesterone 50 mg daily, Crinone gel once a day, and Crinone gel twice a day. All three arms had similar results with respect to IVF outcomes [27].

We conclude that a safely effective dose of micronized progesterone in oil capsules is 600 mg daily (200 mg 3 times a day), while both single-dose as well as twice-daily dose of Crinone 8% gels are efficacious for luteal phase support.

With respect to convenience, single-dose medications are preferred by patients. Total costs have to be compared between preparations and weighed against convenience of administration. In most cases, these will be individual decisions that each patient will have to make for herself.

7.5 How Do Various Vaginal Progesterone Preparations Compare with Respect to Efficacy and Acceptance by Patients?

There are currently three standardized vaginal progesterone formulations commercially available for use in IVF. Micronized progesterone capsules (Utrogestan/Prometrium) are available and widely used in Europe and South America, but not FDA approved for use in IVF/ART in the United States. The two progesterone formulations approved by FDA for use in IVF are Crinone 8% vaginal gel, and more recently – Endometrin 100 mg (natural progesterone in capsules). The unique feature of Crinone bioadhesive gel is its property of sustained release delivery over time allowing for once-daily administration. Other formulations require multiple daily doses for optimal efficacy.

While both Utrogestan and Crinone have been compared in prospective, randomized trials to intramuscular progesterone and have been shown to be of equal efficacy in appropriate doses (as discussed above), no such comparison exists for Endometrin. Instead, Endometrin at twice-daily and 3 times daily doses has been compared to Crinone once-daily dose for luteal support in IVF in a prospective, randomized multicenter trial with noninferiority design [38]. The study had enough power to demonstrate noninferiority of Endometrin at twice a day and 3 times a day doses in women <35 years old with FSH <10 mIU/mL compared to Crinone 8% gel once daily. The authors stated that the study did not reach enough power for meaningful conclusions for women over age 35.

Three other prospective studies addressed comparison of Micronized progesterone capsules (Utrogestan 600 mg) in two or three doses a day with Crinone gel once daily [39–41] and Simunic et al. [39] also assessed patient preference for either of the preparations. All three studies concluded that pregnancy rates were similar between Utrogestan and Crinone groups, but patients expressed superior tolerability and acceptability of Crinone in Simunic's study.

A recent meta-analysis [42] pooled together results of seven randomized trials comparing once-daily or twice-daily Crinone vaginal gel with either twice or three times daily Endometrin, or 3 times daily Utrogestan. The authors concluded that all vaginal progesterone preparations in adequate doses were equally efficacious for luteal support in IVF cycles with respect to clinical pregnancy rates.

We conclude that all three available vaginal progesterone preparations – Crinone gel once a day, Utrogestan 200 mg 3 times a day, and Endometrin 100 mg twice or three times a day – are equally effective for luteal phase support in IVF cycles. However, data are insufficient for definite conclusion on the efficacy of Endometrin in women over age 35.

7.6 What is the Optimal Timing of Progesterone Initiation Within the IVF Cycle?

In stimulated IVF cycles, there is substantial endogenous progesterone production starting immediately after, and possibly even slightly before the hCG trigger. While progesterone supplementation in the luteal phase is important, it is similarly important not to advance endometrial maturation out of sink with embryo development. It has been demonstrated that administration of intramuscular progesterone early in the cycle, i.e., prior to oocyte retrieval compared to within 24 h after oocyte retrieval, will result in lower pregnancy rates [43]. Mochtar et al. [44] examined effects of timing of vaginal progesterone initiation (Micronized progesterone 400 mg twice daily) in a prospective randomized design ($n=385$). Progesterone was initiated either on the day of HCG trigger, or on the day of oocyte retrieval, or on the day of embryos transfer (day 3). While ongoing pregnancy rate was lower in the hCG group compared to two others, the difference was not statistically significant. If starting progesterone supplementation too early in the cycle has a negative effect on the outcome, starting progesterone too late could be equally detrimental. A prospective, randomized study by Williams et al. [45] comparing progesterone start 3 vs. 6 days after retrieval found higher pregnancy rates with earlier start. There was heterogeneity with the exact timing of progesterone start in prospective studies that we examined earlier in this chapter. Dal Prato et al. [27], Kahraman et al. [35], and Doody et al. [38] started supplementation on the day after retrieval, while Yanushpolsky et al. [28] and a smaller trial by Schoolcraft et al. [32] started supplementation with vaginal progesterone 2 days after retrieval, but all had similar results.

We conclude that there is an acceptable window of time – 24–48 h after oocyte retrieval for initiation of vaginal progesterone supplementation with optimal cycle results.

7.7 How Long Should Progesterone Be Continued in Early Pregnancy and Do We Need to Monitor Serum Progesterone Levels?

While it has long been established that luteal phase support with progesterone in IVF cycles leads to improved outcomes, and there is currently sufficient evidence to state that vaginal progesterone is equally efficacious and better tolerated form of luteal supplementation, there is still limited data and little consensus on the necessary duration for progesterone supplementation in early pregnancy, i.e., beyond first positive pregnancy test. Andersen et al. [46] conducted a prospective study in which patients enrolled in stimulated IVF cycles and receiving micronized progesterone 600 mg in the luteal phase were randomized to stopping progesterone support after first diagnosis of pregnancy vs. continuing for 3 more weeks ($n=303$). They found no differences in miscarriage rates and argued that progesterone supplementation can be safely withdrawn after the first positive beta-hCG result.

Aboulghar et al. [47] conducted a survey of 21 IVF programs with respect to progesterone support in early pregnancy after IVF. They found no uniform pattern or consensus, and then set out a prospective study where they randomized patients to either continuation or discontinuation of progesterone support on the day of first ultrasound demonstrating positive fetal heart activity ($n=257$). They found no significant differences in miscarriage rates or bleeding in early pregnancy rates between the groups. They concluded that there was no advantage to continuing progesterone support beyond the time of first ultrasound viability study. They also called for large, prospective, randomized trials to settle the issue of timing of progesterone support in early IVF pregnancies.

Since the first group of studies by Smitz et al. [21] showing lower serum progesterone levels but adequate endometrial maturation and similar pregnancy rates with vaginal progesterone preparations compared to intramuscular preparations, there has been little reason to be concerned with serum progesterone level monitoring. In addition, absorption and pharmacokinetic studies by Bulletti [29] and Ciccinelli [30] confirmed that there was no correlation between the desired endometrial maturation effect and serum progesterone levels, and that there is no reason to subject patients to unnecessary blood drawings and potentially unsubstantiated reasons for anxiety involved with serum level monitoring. None of the major randomized studies that demonstrated equal efficacy of intravaginal and intramuscular preparations reported serum progesterone levels because they were felt to be irrelevant to the outcomes [27, 28, 35].

There is no scientific evidence for monitoring serum progesterone levels during supplemented luteal phase of stimulated IVF cycles.

7.8 What About Progesterone Replacement in Frozen Embryo Transfer Cycles and Donor Oocyte Recipient Cycles?

Frozen embryo transfer cycles and Donor Oocyte recipient cycles are different from stimulated IVF cycle in that there is no endogenous progesterone production, and therefore, instead of luteal phase supplementation, there is a need for luteal phase "creation" or replacement.

Just as with stimulated cycles, intramuscular progesterone in doses of 50–100 mg daily has been the most common progesterone preparation used in these replacement cycles, and just as with stimulated cycles, there have been adverse reactions, complications, and inconveniences for the patients related to intramuscular progesterone administration; there is a need to find more tolerable but equally efficacious progesterone formulations for the replacement cycles. Unfortunately, there is a paucity of data addressing comparison of intramuscular and intravaginal progesterone preparations in frozen embryo transfer and donor egg/recipient cycles, and no definite conclusions can be drawn at this time. Crinone vaginal gel has been approved by FDA for supplementation at once-daily dose and for replacement at twice a day dose. There are only two small prospective studies comparing intramuscular progesterone to Crinone vaginal gel twice a day and once a day in donor egg/recipient cycles with similar results [37, 48]. Three other reports by Berger and Phillips [49, 50] and Williams et al. [51] are retrospective studies also showing equivalent pregnancy outcomes for frozen and donor egg/recipient cycles in intramuscular progesterone and Crinone gel groups at twice a day doses as well as once a day doses. As all retrospective studies, these cannot be relied upon as definite evidence of efficacy. Large and properly designed prospective, randomized trials are much needed to establish efficacy of vaginal progesterone replacement in Frozen embryo transfer cycles and donor egg/recipient cycles.

7.9 Is There Benefit of Adding Estradiol To Progesterone for Support of the Luteal Phase in the IVF Cycles?

The pattern of estrogen and progesterone decline in the luteal phase of IVF cycles has been well described in the literature and lower pregnancy rates have been observed with lower luteal phase estradiol to progesterone ratios [52, 53]. The question of causality vs. association, i.e., do the lower estradiol levels in the luteal phase cause lower pregnancy rates, or are lower estradiol levels the result of lack of implantation, could not be resolved without properly designed studies. Several small prospective randomized studies addressing addition of estradiol supplementation in doses between 2 mg and 6 mg/day suggested a benefit, while almost a similar number of small prospective randomized studies demonstrated no improvement in pregnancy rates with estradiol supplementation [7]. A meta-analysis assessment of the best available data was necessary for understanding of this issue. In 2008, Kolibianakis et al. [54] published a systematic review and meta-analysis of four prospective randomized studies ($n=587$ patients) addressing IVF cycle outcomes of patients who received estradiol supplementation in the luteal phase and those who did not. They concluded that the evidence available at the time suggested that the addition of estrogen to progesterone for luteal phase support does not increase the probability of pregnancy in IVF. A more recent meta-analysis of nine randomized studies was presented by Jee et al. [55] in January 2010. No statistically significant differences in IVF pregnancy rates were observed between the groups of patients who received additional estradiol in the luteal phase and those who received progesterone supplementation alone. Authors of both meta-analyses called for large, prospective randomized studies in order to confirm their findings. The largest prospective randomized study so far was published by Elgindy et al. [56] in May 2010. It included 270 patients undergoing ICSI cycles in long agonist protocols in three arms. All patients received intramuscular progesterone (100 mg daily). Patients in Group A received no additional estrogen, while patients in Group B received additional oral Estradiol valerate 6 mg daily, and patients in Group C received daily Estradiol valerate 6 mg per vagina. There were no differences in progesterone levels in the luteal phase among all three groups, and luteal estradiol levels were similar between Groups B and C. Likewise, there were no differences in pregnancy rates between progesterone only group (Group A), and oral Estradiol supplemented group (Group B), but higher pregnancy rates were observed in patients supplemented with vaginal Estradiol valerate 6 mg daily. The authors concluded that pregnancy rates in patients undergoing ICSI in long agonist protocols may be improved by addition of vaginal estradiol in the luteal phase.

While this prospective randomized study does not answer the question regarding benefits of luteal estradiol support definitively, it raises the possibility of greater benefit of vaginal estradiol supplementation over oral supplementation. Large prospective randomized studies will be needed to answer the question regarding potential benefits of vaginal estradiol supplementation for all IVF cycles.

7.10 Conclusions

Progesterone supplementation of luteal phase of stimulated IVF cycles leads to higher pregnancy rates and is necessary for optimal results. Vaginal progesterone supplementation is equally effective and better tolerated by patients than intramuscular preparations. There exists sufficient evidence of efficacy and tolerability to make vaginal supplementation the main route of progesterone support in stimulated IVF cycles.

Once-daily Crinone gel, or twice or three times daily Endometrin, or Micronized progesterone 200 mg 3 times a day are optimal doses of vaginal progesterone for luteal phase support in IVF. Patients should have a choice as to which preparation to use based on convenience and cost considerations.

There exists a window of time when vaginal progesterone should be initiated for optimal pregnancy results. Vaginal supplementation is best started within 24–48 h after oocyte retrieval.

There is no need for serum progesterone level monitoring with vaginal supplementation as there is little correlation between serum levels and local endometrial effects or pregnancy outcomes.

It is likely that continued progesterone support in early pregnancy beyond the first positive pregnancy test is of little value with respect to successful outcome, but there is insufficient data to date to establish the right time for discontinuing support. Large randomized, prospective studies are needed to establish parameters for discontinuation, but they may be complicated by difficulty in subject recruitment secondary to patients' anxiety.

Current evidence on progesterone replacement in frozen embryo transfer cycles and donor egg/recipient cycles with intravaginal progesterone is insufficient to establish equivalency with traditional intramuscular progesterone protocols. Large, prospective, randomized studies are needed to resolve this issue.

Benefits of adding estradiol to progesterone supplementation in the luteal phase of IVF cycles have not been demonstrated in the published meta-analyses of the data. However, the most recent prospective randomized study suggested potential benefit of vaginal, but not oral estrogen supplementation in long protocol ICSI cycles. More studies are needed to evaluate potential benefits of vaginal estradiol supplementation.

References

1. Filicori M, Butler JP, Crowley Jr WF. Neuroendocrine regulation of the corpus luteum in the human. Evidence for pulsatile progesterone secretion. J Clin Invest. 1984;73:1638–47.
2. Jones GS, Garcia J, Acosta A. Luteal phase evaluation in in-vitro fertilization. In: Edwards RG, Purdy JM, editors. Human conception in vitro. London: Academic Press; 1982. p. 297–310.
3. Tavaniotou A, Devroey P. Luteal hormone profile of oocyte donors stimulated with a GnRH antagonist compared with natural cycles. Reprod Biomed Online. 2006;13:326–30.
4. Beckers NG, Macklon NS, Eijkemans MJ, et al. Nonsupplemented luteal phase characteristics after the administration of recombinant human chorionic gonadotropin, recombinant luteinizing hormone, or gonadotropin-releasing hormone (GnRH) agonist to induce final oocyte maturation in in vitro fertilization patients after ovarian stimulation with recombinant follicle-stimulating hormone and GnRH antagonist cotreatment. J Clin Endocrinol Metab. 2003;88:4186–92.
5. Pritts EA, Atwood AK. Luteal phase support in infertility treatment: a meta-analysis of the randomized trials. Hum Reprod. 2002;17:2287–99.
6. Daya S, Gunby J. Luteal phase support in assisted reproduction cycles. Cochrane Database Syst Rev. 2004;3:CD004830.
7. Hubayter Z, Muasher S. Luteal supplementation in in-vitro fertilization: more questions than answers. Fertil Steril. 2008;894:749–58.
8. Licciardi FL, Kwiatkowski A, Noyes NL, et al. Oral versus intramuscular progesterone for in vitro fertilization: a prospective randomized study. Fertil Steril. 1999;71:614–8.
9. Friedler S, Raziel A, Schachter M, Strassburger D, Bukovsky I, Ron-El R. Luteal support with micronized progesterone following in-vitro fertilization using a down-regulation protocol with gonadotrophin-releasing hormone agonist: a comparative study between vaginal and oral administration. Hum Reprod. 1999;14:1944–8.
10. Scifres CM, Iams JD, Klebanoff M, Macones GA. Metaanalysis vs. large clinical trials: which should

guide our management? Am J Obstet Gynecol. 2009; 200:484.e1–e5.
11. Timmermans S, Mauk A. The promises and pitfalls of evidence-based medicine. Health Aff (Millwood). 2005;24(1):18–28.
12. Atkins D, Best D, Briss PA, et al. Grading quality of evidence and strength of recommendations. BMJ. 2004;328(7454):1490.
13. Papaleo E, Quaranta L, Molgora M. Intramuscular vs. intravaginal natural progesterone in patients undergoing in vitro fertilization-embryo transfer cycles. A retrospective observational, case-control study. Eur Rev Med Pharmacol Sci. 2010;14(2):103–6.
14. Ho CH, Chen SU, Peng FS, Chang CY, Yang YS. Luteal Support for IVF/ICSI cycles with Crinone 8% (90 mg) twice daily results in higher pregnancy rates than with intramuscular progesterone. J Clin Med Assoc. 2008;71(8):386–91.
15. Bouckaert Y, Robert F, Englert Y, De Backer D, De Vuyst P, Delbaere A. Acute eosinophilic pneumonia associated with intramuscular administration of progesterone as luteal phase support after IVF: case report. Hum Reprod. 2004;19:1806–10.
16. Veysman B, Vlahos I, Oshva L. Pneumonitis and eosinophilia after in vitro fertilization treatment. Ann Emerg Med. 2006;47:472–5.
17. Phy JL, Weiss WT, Weiler CR, Damario MA. Hypersensitivity to progesterone-in-oil after in vitro fertilization and embryo transfer. Fertil Steril. 2003; 80:1272–5.
18. Van Steirteghem AC, Smitz J, Camus M, Devroey P, Khan I, Staessen C, et al. The luteal phase after in-vitro fertilization and related procedures. Hum Reprod. 1988;3:161–4.
19. Smitz J, Devroey P, Camus M, Deschacht J, Khan I, Staessen C, et al. The luteal phase and early pregnancy after combined GnRH-agonist/HMG treatment for superovulation in IVF or GIFT. Hum Reprod. 1988;3:585–90.
20. Devroy P, Palermo G, Bourgan C, Van Waesberghe L, Smitz J, Van Steirteghem AC. Progesterone administration in patients with absent ovaries. Int J Fertil. 1989;34(3):188–93.
21. Smitz J, Devroey P, Faguer B, Bourgain C, Camus M, Van Steirteghem AC. A prospective randomized comparison of intramuscular or intravaginal natural progesterone as a luteal phase and early pregnancy supplement. Hum Reprod. 1992;7:168–75.
22. Bourgain C, Devroy P, Van Waesberghe L, Smitz J, Van Steirteghem AC. Effects of natural progesterone on the morphology of the endometrium in patients with primary ovarian failure. Hum Reprod. 1990;5(5):537–43.
23. Perino M, Brigandi A, Abate FG, Costabile L, Balzano E, Abate A. Intramuscular versus vaginal progesterone in assisted reproduction: a comparative study. Clin Exp Obstet Gynecol. 1997;24:228–31.
24. Artini PG, Volpe A, Angioni S, Galassi MC, Battaglia C, Genazzani AR. A comparative, randomized study of three different progesterone support of the luteal phase following IVF/ET program. J Endocrinol Invest. 1995;8:51–6.
25. Porcu E. Intramuscular versus vaginal progesterone in assisted reproduction. Fertil Steril. 2003;80 Suppl 3:S131.
26. Propst AM, Hill JA, Ginsburg ES, Hurwitz S, Politch J, Yanushpolsky EH. A randomized study comparing Crinone 8% and intramuscular progesterone supplementation in in vitro fertilization embryo transfer cycles. Fertil Steril. 2001;76:1144–9.
27. Dal Prato L, Bianchi L, Cattoli M, Tarozzi N, Flamigni C, Borini A. Vaginal gel versus intramuscular progesterone for luteal phase supplementation: a prospective randomized trial. Reprod Biomed Online. 2008; 16:361–7.
28. Yanushpolsky E, Hurwitz S, Greenberg L, Racowsky C, Hornstein MD. Comparison of Crinone 8% intravaginal gel and intramuscular progesterone supplementation for in vitro fertilization/embryo transfer in women under age 40: interim analysis of a prospective randomized trial. Fertil Steril. 2008;89: 485–7.
29. Bulletti C, de Ziegler D, Flamigni C, et al. Targeted drug delivery in gynecology: the first uterine pass effect. Hum Reprod. 1997;12:1073–9.
30. Cicinelli E, de Ziegler D, Bulletti C, Matteo MG, Schonauer LM, Galantino P. Direct transport of progesterone from vagina to uterus. Obstet Gynecol. 2000;95:403–6.
31. Miles RA, Paulson RJ, Lobo RA, Press MF, Dahmoush L, Sauer MV. Pharmacokinetics and endometrial tissue levels of progesterone after administration by intramuscular and vaginal routes: a comparative study. Fertil Steril. 1994;62(3):485–90.
32. Schoolcraft WB, Hesla JS, Gee MJ. Experience with progesterone gel for luteal support in highly successful IVF programme. Hum Reprod. 2000;15:1284–8.
33. Zarutskie P, Phillips J. A meta-analysis of the route of administration of luteal phase support in assisted reproductive technology: vaginal versus intramuscular progesterone. Fertil Steril. 2009;92:163–9.
34. Yanushpolsky E, Hurwitz S, Greenberg L, Racowsky C, Hornstein M. Crinone vaginal gel is equally effective and better tolerated than intramuscular progesterone for luteal phase support in in-vitro fertilization-embryo transfer cycles: a prospective randomized study. Fertil Steril. 2010;94:2596–9.
35. Kahraman S, Karagozoglu SH, Karlikaya G. The efficiency of progesterone vaginal gel versus intramuscular progesterone for luteal phase supplementation in gonadotropin-releasing hormone antagonist cycles: a prospective clinical trial. Fertil Steril. 2010;94:761–3.
36. Gibbons WE, Toner JP, Hamacher P, Kolm P. Experience with a novel vaginal progesterone preparation in a donor oocyte program. Fertil Steril. 1998; 69:96–101.
37. Jobanputra K, Toner JP, Denoncourt R, Gibbons WE. Crinone 8% (90 mg) given once daily for progesterone replacement therapy in donor egg cycles. Fertil Steril. 1999;72:980–4.

38. Doody KJ, Schnell VL, Foulk RA, et al. Endometrin for luteal phase support in a randomized, controlled, open-label, prospective in-vitro fertilization trial using a combination of Menopur and Bravelle for controlled ovarian hyperstimulation. Fertil Steril. 2009;91:1012–7.
39. Simunic V, Tomic V, Tomic J, Nizac D. Comparative study of the efficacy and tolerability of two vaginal progesterone formulations, Crinone 8% gel and Utrogestan capsules, used for luteal support. Fertil Steril. 2007;87:83–7.
40. Ludwig M, Schwartz P, Babahan B, Katalinic A, Weiss JM, Felberbaum R. Luteal phase support using either Crinone 8% or Utrogestan: results of a prospective, randomized study. Eur J Obstet Gynecol Reprod Biol. 2002;1003:48–52.
41. Gerber S, Moreira AC, de Calil Paula S, Sampaio M. Comparison between two forms of vaginally administered progesterone for luteal phase support in assisted reproduction cycles. Reprod Biomed Online. 2007;14(2):155–8.
42. Polyzos N, Messini C, Papanikolaou E, et al. Vaginal progesterone gel for luteal phase support on IVF/ICSI cycles: a meta-analysis. Fertil Steril. 2010;94:2083–7.
43. Sohn SH, Penzias AS, Emmi AM, Dubey AK, Layman LC, Reindollar RH, et al. Administration of progesterone before oocyte retrieval negatively affects the implantation rate. Fertil Steril. 1999;71:11–4.
44. Mochtar M, Van Wely M, Van der Veen F. Timing luteal phase support in GnRH agonist down-regulated IVF/embryo transfer cycles. Hum Reprod. 2006;21(4):905–8.
45. Williams SC, Oehninger S, Gibbons WE, Van Cleave WC, Muasher SJ. Delaying the initiation of progesterone supplementation results is decreased pregnancy rates after in vitro fertilization: a randomized, prospective study. Fertil Steril. 2001;76(6):1140–3.
46. Andersen NA, Popovic-Todorovic B, Schmidt KT, et al. Progesterone supplementation during early gestations after IVF or ICSI has no effect on the delivery rates: a randomized controlled trial. Hum Reprod. 2002;17:357–61.
47. Aboulghar MA, Amin Y, Al-Inany H, et al. Prospective randomized study comparing luteal phase support for ICSI patients up to the first ultrasound compared with an additional three weeks. Hum Reprod. 2008;3(4):857–62.
48. Toner J. Vaginal delivery of progesterone in donor oocyte therapy. Hum Reprod. 2000;15 Suppl 1:166–71.
49. Berger B, Phillips J. A retrospective analysis of pregnancy outcomes in recipients of anonymously donated oocytes at a large ART center. Fertil Steril. 2007;89:S11–2.
50. Berger B, Phillips J. Aretrospective analysis of pregnancy outcomes in recipients of frozen/thawed embryos (FET) from donated oocytes at a large assisted reproductive technology (ART) center. Fertil Steril. 2008;90:S459.
51. Williams SC, Donahue J, Muasher SJ. Vaginal progesterone therapy during programmed cycles for frozen embryo transfer: an analysis of serum progesterone levels and pregnancy rates. Fertil Steril. 2000;74 Suppl 1:S209.
52. Muasher S, Acosta AA, Garcia JE, Jones GS, Jones HW. Luteal phase serum estradiol level and progesterone in *in vitro fertilization*. Fertil Steril. 1984;41:838–43.
53. Sharara FI, McClamrock HD. Ratio of oestradiol concentration on the day of human chorionic gonadotrophin administration to mid-luteal-oestradiol concentration is predictive of in-vitro fertilization outcome. Hum Reprod. 1999;14:2777–82.
54. Kolibianakis EM, Venetis CA, Papanikolaou EG, et al. Estrogen addition to progesterone for luteal phase support in cycles stimulated with GnRH analogues and gonadotrophins for IVF: a systematic review and meta-analysis. Hum Reprod. 2008;23:1346–54.
55. Jee BC, Suh CS, Kim SH, Kim YB, Moon SY. Effects of estradiol supplementation during the luteal phase of in vitro fertilization cycles: a meta-analysis. Fertil Steril. 2010;93:428–36.
56. Elgindy EA, El-Haieg DO, Mostafa MI, Shafiek M. Does luteal estradiol supplementation have a role in long agonist cycles? Fertil Steril. 2010;93:2182–8.

8 Monozygotic Twinning and Perinatal Outcomes

Kenneth J. Moise Jr. and Ramesh Papanna

Abstract

The choice made by women to delay childbearing until later in their reproductive life coupled with the more widespread use of artificial reproductive techniques has contributed to an increasing incidence of multifetal gestations. When compared to dichorionic twins, monochorionic twins are at an increased risk for congenital anomalies as well as unique conditions including twin–twin transfusion syndrome (TTTS), selective intrauterine growth restriction (sIUGR), and twin reversed arterial perfusion (TRAP) sequence. Chorionicity can be accurately determined in the late first trimester through ultrasound examination of the interface between the intervening twin membrane and its attachment to the placenta. In the case of the monochorionic gestation, frequent ultrasound surveillance beginning at 16 weeks' gestation is important for the timely management of perinatal complications. The current standard treatment for severe TTTS is laser photocoagulation of placental anastomoses. Selective reduction is an option in an anomalous cotwin, previable sIUGR, or TRAP sequence in monochorionic twin gestations.

Keywords

Twin–twin transfusion syndrome • TTTS • Monochorionic twins • Twin reversed arterial perfusion sequence • TRAP • Acardiac twinning • Selective IUGR • Monoamniotic twins • Multifetal pregnancies

K.J. Moise Jr. (✉)
Department of Obstetrics and Gynecology,
Division of Maternal-Fetal Medicine, Baylor College of Medicine and the Texas Children's Fetal Center,
Texas Children's Hospital, Houston, TX, USA
e-mail: Kjmoise@bcm.edu

C. Racowsky et al. (eds.), *Biennial Review of Infertility: Volume 2*,
DOI 10.1007/978-1-4419-8456-2_8, © Springer Science+Business Media, LLC 2011

8.1 Background

Although the incidence of spontaneous twinning has been previously reported to be 1 in 80 pregnancies, the growing trend for women to postpone childbearing until later in their reproductive life along with the increased use of assisted reproductive technologies (ART) has led to a rise in the incidence of twinning. Data from the Centers for Disease Control from 2006 indicate that 3.25% of livebirths were twins (Fig. 8.1) [1]. The incidence of triplet and higher order gestations peaked in 2003 at 187/100,000 livebirths with a notable decreasing in the incidence since that time (Fig. 8.2). Voluntary guidelines for the number of embryos transferred at the time of in vitro fertilization have probably contributed to this change. However, although approximately 1% of all infants born in the United States are a product of ART, these infants account for 18% of all multiple births. In addition, these pregnancies continue to be a contributing factor to perinatal morbidity with 14% of ART singletons, 65% of ART twins and 97% of ART triplets, and higher order multiples born prematurely [2]. Finally, a threefold increase in monozygotic twinning, usually monochorionic, diamniotic (MC/DA), has been associated with assisted hatching, intracytoplasmic sperm injection, and the late transfer of cultured blastocysts [3].

8.2 Embryology

A dizygotic twin pregnancy results from the release of two zygotes within the same menstrual cycle which are each fertilized by separate spermatozoa. This process results in a dichorionic, diamniotic (DC/DA) twin pregnancy. Monozygotic twinning occurs when a single fertilized zygote divides into two embryos within the first 12 days after conception. If the embryo divides before the third day of life, DC/DA twins result, comprising 25% of monozygotic twins. Division of the embryo between the fourth and eighth day of life results in MC/DA twins which comprise 75% of monozygotic twins. Division of the blastocyst into two consepctuses between the ninth and the twelfth day will result in monochorionic, monoamniotic (MC/MA) twins. These represent <1% of monozygotic twins. Division after the twelfth day and up to sixteenth day of life will result in conjoined twins.

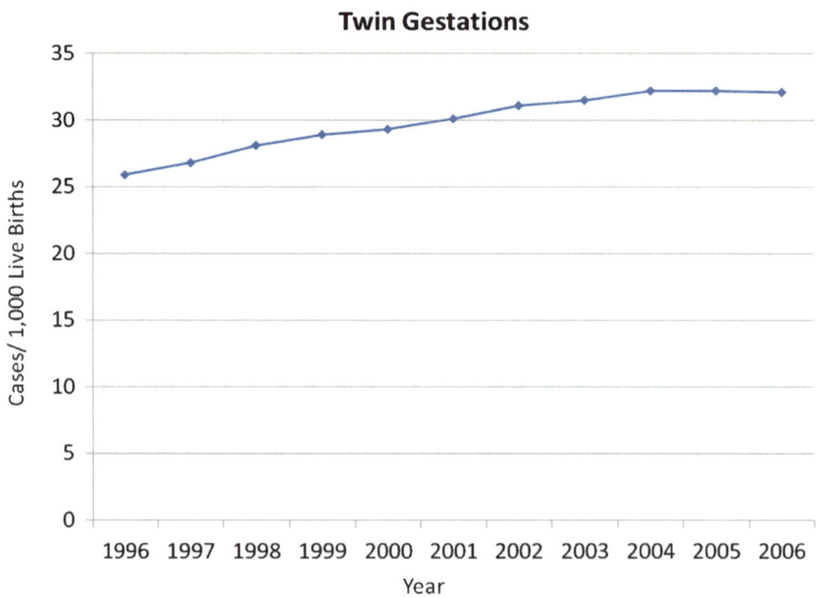

Fig. 8.1 Incidence of twin gestations in the United States between 1996 and 2006 [1]

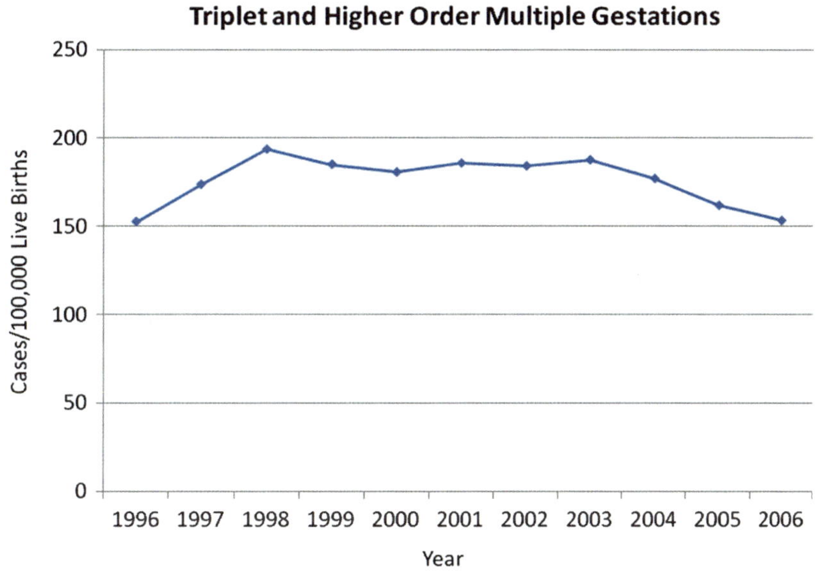

Fig. 8.2 Incidence of triplet and higher order multiple gestations in the United States between 1996 and 2006 [1]

Higher order multiples can result from fertilization of multiple ova, whether from spontaneous ovulation or ovulation induction, the transfer of multiple embryos in IVF, or the rare natural cleavage of a single fertilized conceptus.

8.3 Perinatal Risks

Identical twins are associated with a higher incidence of complications as compared to singleton pregnancies and even dizygotic twins.

Structural fetal anomalies are reported to occur in 0.6% of singletons, 1% of dizygotic twins, and 2.7% of monozygotic twins [4]. Even though the two embryos share a common genome, 82% of identical twins are discordant for structural abnormalities.

The shared placenta of monochorionic twins contains anastomotic vessels between the two fetal circulations in virtually all cases. These anastomoses lead to a unique situation where the death of one twin can result in compromise of its sibling. This can occur in cases of life-threatening congenital anomalies, twin–twin transfusion, or severe selective intrauterine growth restriction (sIUGR) (see below). Although originally thought to be the consequence of "bad humors" that passed from the dead fetus to its sibling, the rare ultrasound observation of the acute death of one monochorionic twin has helped to elucidate the true pathophysiology of the consequences of the death of one of the fetuses in a monochorionic twin gestation. As the compromised twin begins to die, it experiences hypotension. This leads to exsanguination of the normal cotwin into the "sink" of the abnormal twin's circulation through placental vascular anastomoses [5]. Acute anemia and hypotension then follow in the normal twin. This leads to the death of the normal twin in 12% of cases, while major neurologic deficit occurs in an additional 18% of cases when this twin survives [6].

8.4 Determining Amnionicity/Chorionicity

Historically, chorionicity was determined at the time of delivery by obtaining a histological cross-section of the intertwin membrane at its insertion into the placenta. This late diagnosis of chorionicity provided information to the parents as to whether their twins were "identical;" however, this practice did not allow for stratification of perinatal risks early in gestation.

The modern management of a twin gestation involves the diagnosis of chorionicity early in gestation. Current guidelines from the American College of Radiology and the American Institute of Ultrasound in Medicine recommend that chorionicity be determined and documented in all multiple gestations [7]. In late 2008, the Royal College of Obstetricians and Gynaecologists issued a *green top guideline* indicating that chorionicity should be determined in multiple gestations in the first trimester [8]. Similarly, the National French College in Obstetrics and Gynecology has made a similar recommendation [9].

Amnionicity of a twin gestation can usually be determined as early as 8 weeks of gestation by the presence of an intervening twin membrane identified by ultrasound. Although the presence of two separate yolks sacs is a good predictor of diamnionicity, a single yolk sac with two fetal poles may still result in a diamniotic pregnancy in 5–15% of cases [10].

Chorionicity can be determined at the time of a first trimester ultrasound at 10–13 weeks' gestation with a sensitivity and specificity of 90 and 100%, respectively, with both negative and positive predictive values of about 98% [11]. The presence of placental tissue between the combined chorion/amnion layers of the intervening twin membrane at its insertion into the placenta is indicative of a DC/DA gestation. This ultrasound finding is known as the "lambda" or "twin peak" sign. The absence of intervening placental tissue between the membranes is known as a "T sign" and indicates the presence of a single chorion – a MC/DA twin gestation (Fig. 8.3).

During the second trimester, determining chorionicity by ultrasound is less reliable than in the first trimester with a sensitivity, specificity, positive predictive value, and negative predictive value of 88, 95, 88, and 95%, respectively [12]. The presence of an intertwin membrane is first confirmed. The next step involves the determination of fetal gender – dichorionicity is confirmed if a male and a female fetus are both present. The presence of two separate placental masses also confirms dichorionicity. Finally, the thickness of the intervening membrane can be used if the twins are like sex and there is a single placenta mass. A membrane thickness of <2 mm thickness suggests a monochorionic gestation, while >2 mm suggests dichorionicity.

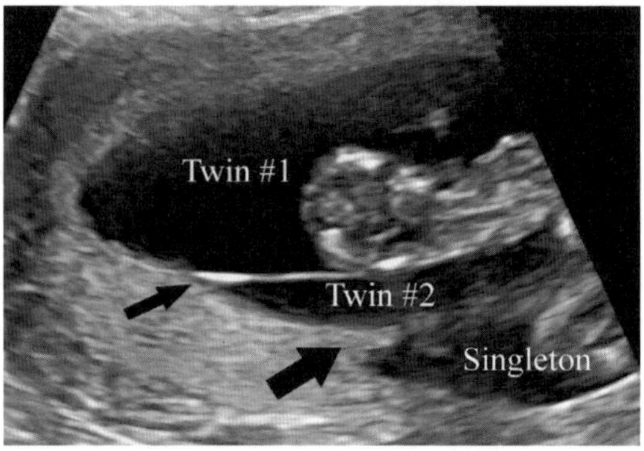

Fig. 8.3 Ultrasound detection of chorionicity in a triplet gestation at 12 weeks' gestation. *Smaller arrow* indicates a "T sign" indicative of a monochorionic, dichorionic intervening membrane between *Twin #1* and *Twin #2*. *Larger arrow* indicates a "lambda sign" between the *Twin #2* and the *Singleton* gestation. This gestation would therefore be classified as a dichorionic, triamniotic triplet gestation

8.5 Dichorionic, Diamniotic (DC/DA) Twins

More than two thirds of all spontaneous twins are DC/DA. Although one third of these are the result of early cleavage of a single zygote. The placentas of these identical twins lack vascular anastomoses; therefore all DC/DA twins are considered *low risk* for perinatal complications when compared to MC/DA twins. DC/DA twins, however, are associated with slightly higher risks of congenital anomalies and selective growth restriction when compared to singleton gestations.

8.5.1 Overall Clinical Management

Routine comprehensive ultrasound for anatomical assessment should be undertaken at 18–20 weeks of gestation and serial scans for fetal growth continued every 3–4 weeks until delivery. Delivery is generally recommended between 38 and 39 weeks of gestation with 40 weeks generally considered by most obstetrical experts as "postdatism." Growth restriction can occur in one or both fetuses and is usually related to a differential uterine blood flow to the separate placental masses. This is defined as a difference in estimated fetal weight by ultrasound of greater than 20% between the twin fetuses (larger twin's estimated weight minus the smaller twin's estimated weight divided by the larger twin's weight). However, this rule may not apply to all twin pairs as one twin may have an accelerated growth curve while the other grows normally. This has led some authorities to recommend that each fetus be assessed on its own growth curve with serial ultrasounds. A fetus found to have an estimated fetal weight of less than the 10% (usually using singleton ultrasound growth curves) is considered growth restricted. Antenatal testing using nonstress testing or biophysical profiles should be initiated by 30–32 weeks of gestation with delivery of the pregnancy planned if there is evidence of fetal compromise in the affected twin.

8.6 Monochorionic, Diamniotic (MC/DA) Twins

Approximately one third of spontaneous twin pregnancies are monozygotic, of which 75% are MC/DA. As mentioned earlier, these twin gestations should be stratified as *high risk* when compared to DC/DA twins.

8.6.1 Risk Assessment

Several authors have attempted to stratify the MC/DA twin gestation into *high risk* and *low risk* groups based on ultrasound parameters. Lewi et al. [13] prospectively followed 202 sets of MC/MA twins and attempted to predict a composite perinatal outcome of twin–twin transfusion syndrome (TTTS), sIUGR, and fetal death. In the first trimester, a discordance in the crown-rump length and/or amniotic fluid volume was associated with a worsening prognosis. Using a multiple logistic regression model and a threshold for complications of 50%, the sensitivity of their model was 29% with a positive predictive value of 70%. Similarly, a difference in the nuchal translucency in the first trimester of more than 20% has been associated with a >50% chance for the development of TTTS [14]. In another large series of 172 MC/DA twins, an absent or reversed wave in the ductus venosus in the first trimester proved to be a better predictor of TTTS than either a discrepancy in the nuchal translucency or the crown-rump length [15]. Finally, in the second trimester, composite poor perinatal outcome in MC/DA twins was calculated using a multiple logistic regression. A threshold of 50% chance for complications had a sensitivity of 48% and a positive predictive value of 73% [13]. These investigations would suggest that perinatal risks in the MC/DA twin gestation can be further refined with specific ultrasound parameters obtained in the late first and early second trimester. The clinical use of such data will await further trials to determine if these parameters can be incorporated into specific algorithms for subsequent ultrasound surveillance of these pregnancies.

8.6.2 Overall Clinical Management

Once monochorionicity is established, a limited ultrasound should be undertaken at 16 weeks' gestation to assess for discordance in fetal size and amniotic fluid volumes. A routine comprehensive ultrasound for anatomical assessment should then be performed at 18 weeks of gestation. Thereafter, limited ultrasound scans should be alternated with complete growth assessments every 2 weeks for the remainder of the pregnancy. A recent large Dutch trial of twin gestations with known chorionicity found that MC twins were at an 8.8-fold (95% CI: 2.7–28.9) increased risk for unexplained intrauterine fetal demise late in gestation [16]. Based on these data, the authors recommended consideration for delivery by 37 completed weeks of gestation.

8.6.3 Twin–Twin Transfusion Syndrome (TTTS)

TTTS complicates approximately 1 in 40–65 twin pregnancies so that approximately 2,500 cases occur in the U.S. each year. About 9–15% of MC/DA twin pregnancies ultimately develop TTTS [13].

The initial diagnostic criteria for "twin-twin transfusion" were based on pediatric parameters including discordance in birthweights and neonatal hemoglobin [17]. Many of these cases involved the acute transfusion of red cells through intraplacental anastomoses at the time of delivery. With the advent of routine prenatal ultrasound, these criteria have been abandoned in lieu of ultrasound parameters. True TTTS is now considered a second trimester entity with severe perinatal complications. In general, the smaller twin (usually with less amniotic fluid) is called the *donor* twin and the larger twin (usually with the greater amount of amniotic fluid) is referred to as the *recipient*.

The following ultrasound criteria are generally accepted for the diagnosis of TTTS:

- Polyhydramnios in the amniotic fluid compartment of the *recipient* twin: >8 cm maximum vertical pocket at <20 weeks' gestation or >10 cm vertical pocket at ≥20 weeks.
- Oligohydramnios in the amniotic fluid compartment of the *donor* twin: <2 cm maximum vertical pocket.

Five stages of TTTS have been proposed by Quintero et al. [18]. Stage I disease involves a discordance in amniotic fluid volumes as noted above. Stage II disease is defined as the absence of a visible fetal bladder by ultrasound in the *donor* twin. Stage III disease is present when Doppler ultrasound assessment of flow in the umbilical artery, umbilical vein, or ductus venosus of either twin is abnormal. Stage III disease encompasses a wide spectrum of presentations with more than 64 variations. In general, the *donor* twin in stage III exhibits Doppler abnormalities of absent or reversed diastolic flow in the umbilical artery. In the *recipient* twin, abnormalities of flow in the ductus venosus (absent or reversed "A" wave) or umbilical venous pulsations are seen. In stage IV disease, hydrops fetalis – the collection of fluid in extracellular compartments such as ascites and pleural effusions – is typically seen in the *recipient* twin. Finally, in stage V disease, fetal death has occurred in one or both twins.

Atypical presentations can occur such as an abnormal umbilical Doppler flow in the *donor* twin with a normal bladder seen on ultrasound (atypical stage III). In addition, although higher Quintero stages are generally associated with a worsening perinatal prognosis, the clinical presentation of a particular case does not always follow an orderly progression of stages. As an example, a stage I case may progress rapidly over several days to stage III. In addition, regression of disease can occur in as many as 41% of stage I cases [19].

The Quintero staging system has been criticized for its lack of ability to prognosticate perinatal survival after therapy. Other centers have proposed staging systems based on echocardiographic abnormalities of the fetal heart (more often seen in the *recipient* fetus) [20, 21]. However, a recent working group has recommended that the Quintero staging system continue to be used in the community due to its simplicity [17, 22].

8.6.3.1 Pathophysiology

There are four types of vascular connections in the monochorionic placenta. Arterio-venous (AV) and veno-arterial (VA) anastomoses consist of feeder vessels on the surface of the chorionic plate that descend into a common cotyledon capillary network. By convention, the anastomoses are named based on their directional flow from the *donor* to the *recipient* twin. In contrast, arterio-arterial (AA) and veno-venous (VV) anastomoses are seen exclusively on the surface of the placenta (Fig. 8.4). Flow in these latter two types of connections is bidirectional and net flow is related to opposing hydrostatic pressures of each fetus. Computer modeling has demonstrated that if the net number and diameter of connections are unbalanced, i.e., there are more AV connections between *donor* and *recipient* than there are VA connections between *recipient* and *donor*, then increasing hydrostatic and osmotic forces will result in the TTTS phenotype [23]. In contrast, if the connections are balanced, i.e., equal numbers of bidirectional anastomoses, then TTTS does not result. Postdelivery injection studies of the placenta have indicated that AA anastomoses tend to be protective against the development of TTTS [24].

This imbalance in vascular volume results in multiple endocrine and cardiovascular changes in

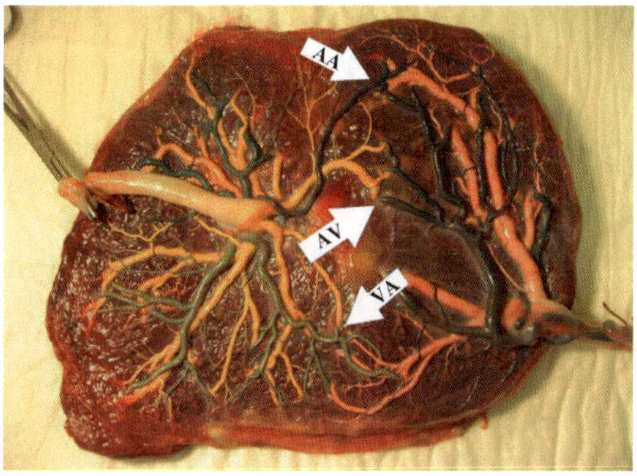

Fig. 8.4 Monochorionic twin placenta with the arterial system of both fetuses injected with *green dye* and the venous system of both fetuses injected with *orange dye*. *Arrows* indicate (*top* to *bottom*) – *AA* arterio-arterial; *AV* arterio-venous; *VA* veno-arterial anastomoses

both fetuses. Relative hypovolemia occurs in the *donor* twin leading to anuria and eventual anhydramnios (Quintero stage II). Relative hypervolemia in the *recipient* fetus leads to cardiomegaly with increased production of natriuretic hormones; subsequent polyuria leads to polyhydramnios in the *recipient*'s amniotic cavity [25]. As the disease progresses, the *donor* twin compensates by an up-regulation of its renin-angiotensin system leading to a shunting of these vasoactive substances through placental anastomoses to the *recipient* [26]. *Recipient* hypertension then dominates the clinical scenario leading to congestive heart failure (Quintero stage III) and eventually fetal hydrops (Quintero stage IV). Ultimately, fetal death occurs in one or both fetuses (Quintero stage V).

8.6.3.2 Clinical Management

Historically, the overall perinatal survival rate of untreated TTTS was 30% [27]. Attempts at amnioreduction to reduce the symptoms of polyhydramnios resulted in some increase in survival (78% at birth and 60% at 4 weeks of age); however, neurologic injury was evident in 25% of survivors [28]. Fetoscopic-guided laser photocoagulation of the problematic placental anastomoses was first proposed by De Lia [29]. Many perinatologists initially considered the therapy to be experimental. In 2004, the Eurofetus consortium randomized 142 patients between laser therapy and the gold standard for treatment, amnioreduction. The trial was stopped at 50% of the proposed sample size when the interim analysis indicated significant improvements in overall perinatal survival, gestational age at delivery, and 6-month survival without neurologic sequelae [30]. Since that time, both the Cochran library and a subsequent meta-analysis have reported laser to be more beneficial than amnioreduction in the treatment of TTTS [31, 32].

Fetoscopic laser ablation of placenta anastomoses is now accepted around the world as the standard of care for the treatment of TTTS. In the U.S., patients with extreme symptoms related to extensive polyhydramnios in stage I disease, or patients with stage II–IV disease, are considered candidates for therapy between 16 and 26 weeks of gestation. Today, a selective sequential ablation technique is used in which AV then VA then AA anastomoses are coagulated. In some centers, a "Solemnization" technique is then employed to coagulate placental tissue between these targeted vessels to prevent the patency of small anastomoses that can be difficult to visualize. Typically, an amnioreduction is performed at the end of the procedure to normalize the amount of amniotic fluid in the *recipient*'s sac.

Preterm premature rupture of the membranes complicates as many as 30% of laser cases. Preterm delivery is common with an average gestational age at delivery of 30–32 weeks in most U.S. studies. In experienced laser centers, survival of both fetuses occurs in approximately 70% of cases; survival of at least one fetus occurs in 90% of cases. In a 2-year study from Holland, greater than 80% of survivors were without neurologic deficits [33].

8.6.4 Selective Intrauterine Growth Restriction (sIUGR)

Growth discordance in twins is usually defined as greater than 20% discordance in the estimated fetal weight by ultrasound parameters. When one twin is noted to be at <10% estimated fetal weight, selective IUGR is diagnosed. This entity is as common as TTTS, complicating 10–15% of MC/DA twin gestations. The etiology is unclear but proposed to result from an unequal division of the inner cell mass early in embryonic life. This may then result in a decreased potential for fetal growth in the affected fetus. Alternatively, an unequal split in the cytotrophoblast that will ultimately form the placenta can result in disproportionate placental sharing. Recently, Gratacos et al. [34] classified the sIUGR in MC/DA twins based on the characteristics of the umbilical arterial Doppler in the smaller fetus. Type I (29%) had end-diastolic flow present on Doppler waveforms, type II (22%) had absent or reversed diastolic flow, and type III (49%) had intermittent absent or reversed end-diastolic flow. Type III sIUGR was found to be associated with a greater number of large AA placental anastomoses when compared to the other two types of sIUGR and controls. There was also a higher incidence of fetal demise of the smaller twin fetus in conjunction with cerebral lesions on neonatal head ultrasound in the surviving cotwin.

8.6.4.1 Clinical Management

The management of discordant growth depends on the gestational age at diagnosis. If detected at a previable gestational age, selective reduction should be considered for the premoribund sIUGR fetus in an attempt to prevent sequelae in the normally grown cotwin. This can be performed by occlusion of the umbilical cord through ultrasound-directed bipolar cautery or radiofrequency ablation [35]. Laser ablation of placental anastomoses for the treatment of sIUGR is offered by some centers in an effort to protect the normal twin from the complications of death of the growth-restricted twin. However, in one study, survival of both twins was 28% in the laser group compared to 81% in the observation group [36]. If discordant growth in a MC/DA pregnancy is detected after a viable gestational age has been attained, consideration for steroid administration to enhance fetal lung maturity, antenatal surveillance, and delivery should be undertaken.

8.6.5 Twin Reversed Arterial Perfusion (TRAP) Sequence

The incidence of twin reversed arterial perfusion (TRAP) sequence (*acardiac twinning*) is approximately 1 in 30,000 pregnancies or 1% of monochorionic twins [37]. Often the acardiac fetus is thought to represent a "vanishing twin" during a first trimester ultrasound only to find an amorphic mass that has increased in size at the time of a second trimester ultrasound. There are two important ultrasound findings that are consistently noted in TRAP sequence: one of the two fetal masses has a rudimentary or absent heart and there is reversed flow by Doppler in the umbilical artery into this fetal mass. Two thirds of cases are MC/DA, while the remainder are MC/MA. Umbilical cord insertions into the placenta are immediately proximate to one another. The most common phenotype is preservation of the lower fetal extremity structures with abnormal or absent structures in the upper half of the acardiac fetus (Fig. 8.5). This is thought to be related to perfusion with deoxygenated blood from the normal, or *pump* twin, to the acardiac twin via the umbilical arteries which course first through the lower portion of the fetus before flowing cephalad. Proposed theories for the development of TRAP sequence include abnormal cardiogenesis in the acardiac fetus and early reversal of flow through a large placental AA anastomosis leading to underdevelopment of the heart in the acardiac twin [38].

Progressive myocardial demand on the *pump* twin to perfuse its own circulation as well as that of the acardiac twin results in cardiac failure and polyhydramnios. Left untreated, fetal demise of the pump twin occurs in more than 55% of cases [39].

8.6.5.1 Clinical Management

Antenatal management of TRAP sequence involves a thorough ultrasound examination of the *pump* twin to exclude anatomical abnormalities. Earlier postnatal studies indicated that if the weight of the acardiac fetus was less than 50% of that of the normal fetus, the incidence of preterm delivery was only 35% and none of the *pump*

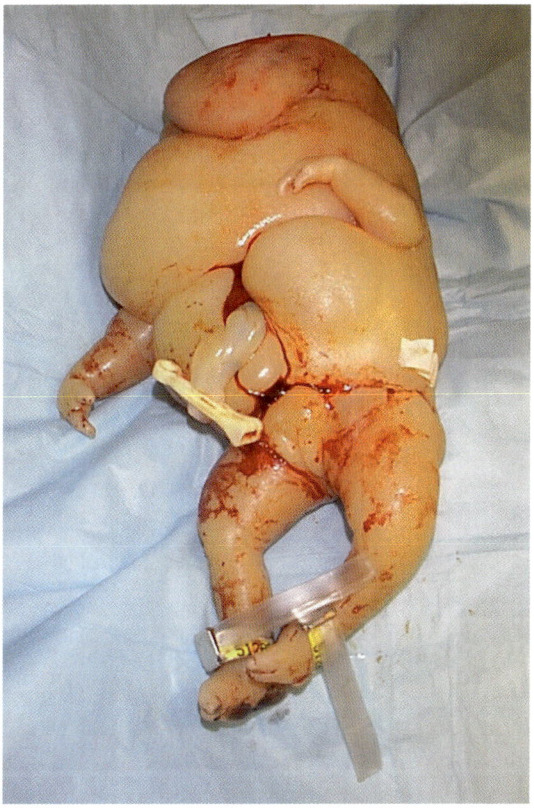

Fig. 8.5 Acardiac twin fetus

twins developed congestive heart failure [39]. Moore et al. went on to propose a formula for calculating the weight of the acardiac fetus based on its length. Many authorities, however, have abandoned this concept for deciding if the *pump* fetus is at risk. Wong and Sepulveda [38] have proposed that an abdominal circumference ratio of <50% should be considered indicative of a small to medium-sized acardiac fetus with little risk for compromise in the *pump* twin. A ratio of >50% warrants consideration of intervention particularly if there are signs of cardiac failure in the *pump* twin such as cardiomegaly or tricuspid regurgitation. Doppler ultrasound can also be used to assess the vascularity of the acardiac mass. A large amount of flow seen using power Doppler in conjunction with a low resistance to the arterial flow in the umbilical cord to the acardiac are also suggestive that it will increase in size. Should a decision be made to occlude the flow to the acardiac fetus, this is best accomplished by the use of a specialized radiofrequency ablation needle directed by ultrasound guidance to target the umbilical cord insertion into the abnormal fetal mass. A survival rate of greater than 85% can be expected in the *pump* twin, although PPROM and preterm delivery are still a risk factor [40].

8.6.6 Anomalous Cofetus

Discordance for a chromosomal or structural fetal abnormality can occur in both monochorionic and dichorionic twins. This discordance is not unexpected in the dichorionic gestation, given that the majority of these pregnancies are dizygotic. In the monozygotic gestation, however, this dissimilarity is thought to be the result of aberrancies after early cleavage of the embryo to form two separate cell lines. In the typical case of a heterokaryotypic defect, one embryo loses an X chromosome resulting in the usual phenotype of Turner's syndrome – cystic hygroma or hydrops. The cotwin appears normal on ultrasound. Assessment of the karyotype in the normal appearing twin is essential in these cases.

8.6.6.1 Clinical Management

Selective feticide for discordant abnormalities is usually undertaken in the dichorionic multiple gestation by injection of potassium chloride into the pericardial space of the anomalous twin. However, in the monochorionic twin gestation, this technique cannot be used as placental anastomoses will allow for passage of the noxious agent to the normal fetus resulting in a dual demise [41]. In these cases, selective feticide is performed using ultrasound-guided methods for umbilical cord ligation of the affected fetus. Originally undertaken using bipolar energy delivered by disposable forceps, this method has been replaced in most centers by radiofrequency energy delivered through special engineered needles. The latter technique offers the advantage of a smaller puncture of the amniotic cavity (17-gauge device vs. 3.3 mm cannula) and has been associated with a lower incidence of preterm premature rupture of the membranes [42]. Survival rates in the normal cofetus have been reported to be 85%.

8.7 Monochorionic, Monoamniotic (MC/MA) Twins

MC/MA twins account for about 1 in 8,000 pregnancies and 5% of monochorionic twins [43]. Although the majority of monoamniotic twins occur naturally, iatrogenic or spontaneous rupture of the intervening membrane in a MC/DA pregnancy can also lead to a monoamniotic condition. MC/MA twins are at risk for developing complications similar to MC/DA twins, although the incidence of TTTS is thought to be reduced by threefold due to the usual presence of large AA anastomoses [44]. The major risk for perinatal loss, however, is related to entanglement of the umbilical cords, which is seen in virtually all cases (Fig. 8.6). The perinatal mortality associated with cord compromise in these pregnancies was approximately 50% in early studies; however, a more recent series suggest that the perinatal mortality is ~15% after 20 weeks' gestation [45].

8.7.1 Clinical Management

In general, most centers in the U.S. now offer inpatient admission for intensive fetal monitoring several times daily when the patient and her obstetrician agree that a gestational age of fetal viability has been reached. In a series of 96 cases of MC/MA twins, outpatient fetal monitoring was associated with a perinatal mortality of 15% as compared to no perinatal losses when patients were hospitalized for fetal surveillance [44]. Antenatal steroids to enhance fetal lung maturity are indicated. Delivery by cesarean section at 32–34 weeks is generally accepted since approximately 1 in 25 MC/MA twins can be lost after this gestation [45].

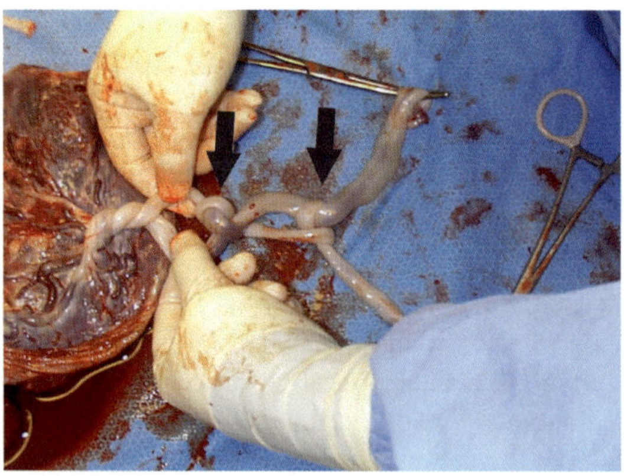

Fig. 8.6 Entangled umbilical cords seen at the time of Cesarean section in a monoamniotic twin gestation. Note the two true knots in the cords (*arrows*)

8.8 Conclusion

A recent lead editorial in the obstetrical literature was entitled "There is NO diagnosis of twins" [46]. The authors went on to advise that there are only monochorionic or dichorionic twins. Clearly, monochorionic multiple gestations are at significant risk for unique complications not seen in singleton pregnancies or dichorionic multiple gestations. Because there are now effective treatments for these conditions, ultrasound determination of chorionicity by reproductive endocrinologists and obstetrical providers should be part of routine prenatal care in multiple gestations.

References

1. Statistics NCfH. Final natality data for 2006. 2006. http://www.marchofdimes.com/peristats. Accessed 30 July 2010.
2. Sunderam S, Chang J, Flowers L, et al. Assisted reproductive technology surveillance – United States, 2006. MMWR Surveill Summ. 2009;58(5):1–25.
3. Saito H, Tsutsumi O, Noda Y, Ibuki Y, Hiroi M. Do assisted reproductive technologies have effects on the demography of monozygotic twinning? Fertil Steril. 2000;74(1):178–9.
4. Chen CJ, Wang CJ, Yu MW, Lee TK. Perinatal mortality and prevalence of major congenital malformations of twins in Taipei city. Acta Genet Med Gemellol (Roma). 1992;41(2–3):197–203.
5. Fusi L, McParland P, Fisk N, Nicolini U, Wigglesworth J. Acute twin-twin transfusion: a possible mechanism for brain-damaged survivors after intrauterine death of a monochorionic twin. Obstet Gynecol. 1991; 78(3 Pt 2):517–20.

6. Ong SS, Zamora J, Khan KS, Kilby MD. Prognosis for the co-twin following single-twin death: a systematic review. BJOG. 2006;113(9):992–8.
7. Medicine AIoUi. AIUM practice guideline for the performance of obstetrical ultrasound examinations. 2008. http://www.aium.org/publications/guidelines/obstetric.pdf. Accessed 25 July 2010.
8. Gynaecologists RCoOa. Monochorionic twin pregnancy, Management (Green-top 51). 2008. http://www.rcog.org.uk/womens-health/clinical-guidance/management-monochorionic-twin-pregnancy. Accessed 30 July 2010.
9. Gynecology NFCoOa. TWIN PREGNANCIES French 2009 Guidelines. 2009. http://www.doxtop.com/browse/e2bb04b6/twin-pregnancies-guidelines.aspx. Accessed 30 July 2010.
10. Shen O, Samueloff A, Beller U, Rabinowitz R. Number of yolk sacs does not predict amnionicity in early first-trimester monochorionic multiple gestations. Ultrasound Obstet Gynecol. 2006;27(1):53–5.
11. Shetty A, Smith AP. The sonographic diagnosis of chorionicity. Prenat Diagn. 2005;25(9):735–9.
12. Carroll SG, Soothill PW, Abdel-Fattah SA, Porter H, Montague I, Kyle PM. Prediction of chorionicity in twin pregnancies at 10–14 weeks of gestation. BJOG. 2002;109(2):182–6.
13. Lewi L, Lewi P, Diemert A, et al. The role of ultrasound examination in the first trimester and at 16 weeks' gestation to predict fetal complications in monochorionic diamniotic twin pregnancies. Am J Obstet Gynecol. 2008;199(5):493.
14. Kagan KO, Gazzoni A, Sepulveda-Gonzalez G, Sotiriadis A, Nicolaides KH. Discordance in nuchal translucency thickness in the prediction of severe twin-to-twin transfusion syndrome. Ultrasound Obstet Gynecol. 2007;29(5):527–32.
15. Maiz N, Staboulidou I, Leal AM, Minekawa R, Nicolaides KH. Ductus venosus Doppler at 11 to 13 weeks of gestation in the prediction of outcome in twin pregnancies. Obstet Gynecol. 2009;113(4):860–5.
16. Hack KE, Derks JB, Elias SG, et al. Increased perinatal mortality and morbidity in monochorionic versus dichorionic twin pregnancies: clinical implications of a large Dutch cohort study. BJOG. 2008;115(1):58–67.
17. Wenstrom KD, Tessen JA, Zlatnik FJ, Sipes SL. Frequency, distribution, and theoretical mechanisms of hematologic and weight discordance in monochorionic twins. Obstet Gynecol. 1992;80(2):257–61.
18. Quintero RA, Morales WJ, Allen MH, Bornick PW, Johnson PK, Kruger M. Staging of twin-twin transfusion syndrome. J Perinatol. 1999;19(8 Pt 1):550–5.
19. O'Donoghue K, Cartwright E, Galea P, Fisk NM. Stage I twin-twin transfusion syndrome: rates of progression and regression in relation to outcome. Ultrasound Obstet Gynecol. 2007;30(7):958–64.
20. Rychik J, Tian Z, Bebbington M, et al. The twin-twin transfusion syndrome: spectrum of cardiovascular abnormality and development of a cardiovascular score to assess severity of disease. Am J Obstet Gynecol. 2007;197(4):392.
21. Shah AD, Border WL, Crombleholme TM, Michelfelder EC. Initial fetal cardiovascular profile score predicts recipient twin outcome in twin-twin transfusion syndrome. J Am Soc Echocardiogr. 2008;21(10):1105–8.
22. Stamilio DM, Fraser WD, Moore TR. Twin-twin transfusion syndrome: an ethics-based and evidence-based argument for clinical research. Am J Obstet Gynecol. 2010;203(1):3–16.
23. van Gemert MJ, Sterenborg HJ. Haemodynamic model of twin-twin transfusion syndrome in monochorionic twin pregnancies. Placenta. 1998;19(2–3):195–208.
24. Denbow ML, Cox P, Taylor M, Hammal DM, Fisk NM. Placental angioarchitecture in monochorionic twin pregnancies: relationship to fetal growth, fetofetal transfusion syndrome, and pregnancy outcome. Am J Obstet Gynecol. 2000;182(2):417–26.
25. Bajoria R, Ward S, Chatterjee R. Natriuretic peptides in the pathogenesis of cardiac dysfunction in the recipient fetus of twin-twin transfusion syndrome. Am J Obstet Gynecol. 2002;186(1):121–7.
26. Mahieu-Caputo D, Salomon LJ, Le Bidois J, et al. Fetal hypertension: an insight into the pathogenesis of the twin-twin transfusion syndrome. Prenat Diagn. 2003;23(8):640–5.
27. Berghella V, Kaufmann M. Natural history of twin-twin transfusion syndrome. J Reprod Med. 2001;46(5):480–4.
28. Mari G, Roberts A, Detti L, et al. Perinatal morbidity and mortality rates in severe twin-twin transfusion syndrome: results of the International Amnioreduction Registry. Am J Obstet Gynecol. 2001;185(3):708–15.
29. De Lia JE, Cruikshank DP, Keye Jr WR. Fetoscopic neodymium:YAG laser occlusion of placental vessels in severe twin-twin transfusion syndrome. Obstet Gynecol. 1990;75(6):1046–53.
30. Senat MV, Deprest J, Boulvain M, Paupe A, Winer N, Ville Y. Endoscopic laser surgery versus serial amnioreduction for severe twin-to-twin transfusion syndrome. N Engl J Med. 2004;351(2):136–44.
31. Roberts D, Neilson JP, Kilby M, Gates S. Interventions for the treatment of twin-twin transfusion syndrome. Cochrane Database Syst Rev. 2008;1:CD002073.
32. Rossi AC, D'Addario V. Laser therapy and serial amnioreduction as treatment for twin-twin transfusion syndrome: a metaanalysis and review of literature. Am J Obstet Gynecol. 2008;198(2):147–52.
33. Lopriore E, Ortibus E, Acosta-Rojas R, et al. Risk factors for neurodevelopment impairment in twin-twin transfusion syndrome treated with fetoscopic laser surgery. Obstet Gynecol. 2009;113(2 Pt 1):361–6.
34. Gratacos E, Lewi L, Munoz B, et al. A classification system for selective intrauterine growth restriction in monochorionic pregnancies according to umbilical artery Doppler flow in the smaller twin. Ultrasound Obstet Gynecol. 2007;30(1):28–34.
35. Moise Jr KJ, Johnson A, Moise KY, Nickeleit V. Radiofrequency ablation for selective reduction in the complicated monochorionic gestation. Am J Obstet Gynecol. 2008;198(2):198.

36. Gratacos E, Antolin E, Lewi L, et al. Monochorionic twins with selective intrauterine growth restriction and intermittent absent or reversed end-diastolic flow (Type III): feasibility and perinatal outcome of fetoscopic placental laser coagulation. Ultrasound Obstet Gynecol. 2008;31(6):669–75.
37. James WH. A note on the epidemiology of acardiac monsters. Teratology. 1977;16(2):211–6.
38. Wong AE, Sepulveda W. Acardiac anomaly: current issues in prenatal assessment and treatment. Prenat Diagn. 2005;25(9):796–806.
39. Moore TR, Gale S, Benirschke K. Perinatal outcome of forty-nine pregnancies complicated by acardiac twinning. Am J Obstet Gynecol. 1990;163(3):907–12.
40. Lee H, T. C, Wilson D. Radiofrequency ablation for twin-reversed arterial perfusion: The North American Fetal Treatment Network (NAFTNET) experience. Am J Obstet Gynecol. 2008;199.
41. Benson CB, Doubilet PM, Acker D, Heffner LJ. Multifetal pregnancy reduction of both fetuses of a monochorionic pair by intrathoracic potassium chloride injection of one fetus. J Ultrasound Med. 1998;17(7): 447–9.
42. Roman A, Papanna R, Johnson A, et al. Selective reduction in complicated monochorionic pregnancies: radiofrequency ablation vs. bipolar cord coagulation. Ultrasound Obstet Gynecol. 2010;36(1):37–41.
43. Sebire NJ, Souka A, Skentou H, Geerts L, Nicolaides KH. First trimester diagnosis of monoamniotic twin pregnancies. Ultrasound Obstet Gynecol. 2000;16(3): 223–5.
44. Heyborne KD, Porreco RP, Garite TJ, Phair K, Abril D. Improved perinatal survival of monoamniotic twins with intensive inpatient monitoring. Am J Obstet Gynecol. 2005;192(1):96–101.
45. Hack KE, Derks JB, Schaap AH, et al. Perinatal outcome of monoamniotic twin pregnancies. Obstet Gynecol. 2009;113(2 Pt 1):353–60.
46. Moise Jr KJ, Johnson A. There is NO diagnosis of twins. Am J Obstet Gynecol. 2010;203(1):1–2.

9 Multiple Pregnancy Vanishing Twin Syndrome

Gabriel de la Fuente, Jose Manuel Puente, Juan A. García-Velasco, and Antonio Pellicer

Abstract

The vanishing twin syndrome is a relatively frequent finding, especially since the widespread use of assisted reproductive technology (ART). Both an earlier follow-up of pregnancy and the use of transvaginal ultrasound, providing a better ultrasound resolution, have brought us closer to the real incidence of this phenomenon, which was underestimated prior to the introduction of these techniques. Thanks to this, we can establish the real incidence of early embryonic loss, from its early ultrasound identification, as well as study the incidence of complications, clinical management, and perinatal prognosis associated with these pregnancies.

Keywords

Vanishing twin syndrome • Chorion • Amnion • Ultrasound • Zygosity

9.1 Incidence of Multiple Pregnancy

9.1.1 Incidence in Assisted Reproductive Technology (ART) and the Importance of Chorionicity and Amnionicity

Spontaneous twin pregnancies represent about 1–2% of all pregnancies. For practical purposes, the probabilities of twin, triplet and quadruplet pregnancies can be estimated at 1/80, 1/80 [1] (1/6,400), and 1/80 [2] (1/512,000), respectively. These data, however, refer to spontaneous pregnancies and not to the influence of assisted reproductive technology (ART). Said treatments have brought about a considerable increase in the number of both dichorionic and monochorionic twin pregnancies, as well as that of triplet and higher-order pregnancies. The reason lies both in ovulation induction treatments, leading to almost 30% of multiple pregnancies, and in the transfer of more than one embryo during in vitro fertilization (IVF) treatments. Scientific associations are currently committed to reducing these figures in view of the high number of perinatal complications entailed in comparison to singleton pregnancy, especially in relation to increased preterm birth; recommendation guides based on age and on the technique used have been prepared [3].

In cases of monozygotic pregnancy only, the influence of assisted reproduction treatments

G. de la Fuente (✉)
IVI Madrid & Rey Juan Carlos University,
Madrid, Spain
e-mail: gdelafuente@ivi.es

C. Racowsky et al. (eds.), *Biennial Review of Infertility: Volume 2*,
DOI 10.1007/978-1-4419-8456-2_9, © Springer Science+Business Media, LLC 2011

with IVF seems clear, with an estimated twofold increase in the relative risk compared to spontaneous pregnancy, and where the blastocyst transfer (RR = 4.25) and intracytoplasmic sperm injection (RR = 2.25) are the main associated factors [1].

All twin pregnancies in general entail increased complications. The most frequent are related to preterm birth (50% in twin pregnancies and 90% in triplet pregnancies). Preterm delivery, whether spontaneous or induced by pregnancy complications, accounts for the approximately fivefold increase in perinatal mortality associated with multiple pregnancies in comparison to singleton pregnancies. Moreover, other complications such as miscarriage or intrauterine loss of one of the twins, growth disorders, and a higher incidence of congenital abnormalities should be considered. Nevertheless, it is essential to differentiate chorionicity of twin pregnancies, as monochorionic twin pregnancies show an even higher risk of complications due to the potential blood shunting via intertwin vascular anastomoses that are present in all monochorionic placentas. This makes the follow-up protocol *completely different* in one and the other type of pregnancy and therefore extreme care should be taken in differentiating between both entities. The early and precise diagnosis of chorionicity and amnionicity is therefore an essential priority objective of the first trimester ultrasound examination, in order to establish an exhaustive action and follow-up protocol of these pregnant women leading to an early diagnosis of potential complications and eventually to appropriate therapies aimed at reducing morbidity and mortality.

Zygosity is determined by the genetic origin of the twins. Twins coming from fertilization of two separate oocytes are called *dizygotic*, and gestation will have two placentas (dichorionic) and two amniotic sacs (diamniotic); they can be of the same or different sex, since they are genetically different. On the other hand, twins coming from one single fertilized oocyte that divides into two embryos are called *monozygotic* and will be genetically identical. Monozygotic twins represent approximately 30% of twin pregnancies; they are of the same sex, and depending on the time of division, they can be completely independent, or share the placenta, amniotic sac, and even fetal structures in cases of late division.

From a practical standpoint, however, it is most important to establish chorionicity and amnionicity, given that the probability of fetal complications in *monochorionic* pregnancies is considerably higher in view of the presence in all cases of vascular anastomosis between the circulations of both twins. In cases of monoamniotic pregnancy, the risk of mortality is very high due to the possibility of intertwining of both umbilical cords, leading to a mechanical interruption of flow through the cords. A relevant fact in these types of pregnancies is that death after the first trimester of one of the fetuses in a monochorionic pregnancy is associated with a high probability of sudden death or severe neurological damage of the surviving twin; this should always be taken into account as it entails an important implication for the treatment of complications.

It should be noted that ultrasound diagnosis enables to establish the chorionicity of a twin pregnancy as of the fifth week of amenorrhea. In these early phases of gestation, transvaginal ultrasound is easier and more reliable, enabling to readily distinguish dichorionic twins through the presence of a thick septum between the sacs, with sensitivities and specificities close to 100% [2]. This septum, formed by two sheets of corium and two of amnion, becomes thinner as pregnancy progresses, but remains thicker and easier to identify at the base of the membrane, as an inverted "V" or lambda-shaped (*twin peak sign*) [4, 5] triangular projection of tissue. In monochorionic-diamniotic pregnancies, the separation membrane is made up of the fusion of two amnion membranes only. It is therefore thinner and forms an image similar to a "T" at its insertion to the placenta.

Similarly, we may resort to the determination of the intertwin membrane thickness. However, the latter is less reliable due to its variability and the inter-/intraobserver differences during assessment [5].

In ART pregnancies, ultrasound is conducted either 24 days after oocyte pick up or after insemination, or 21–23 days after embryo transfer, meaning in all cases a gestational age of about

5 weeks and 3 days. At that gestational age, it is simple to visualize both independent gestational sacs and the thick septum that separates them, in cases of dichorionic pregnancy.

Amnionicity: Every dichorionic pregnancy is diamniotic. The number of sacs in monochorionic pregnancies can be determined as of the eighth week of gestation, since before that, visualization is more difficult because the amnion and the embryo are very close to each other. Proximity of both cords at their placental insertion and the visualization of intertwined cords are typical signs of monochorionic monoamniotic pregnancies.

9.2 Early Embryonic Loss Associated with Multiple Pregnancy

9.2.1 Incidence and Associated Mechanisms

The incidence of embryonic loss is high and is estimated by some authors at ca. 40% [6, 7].

There are numerous causes for this early embryonic loss, with associated factors such as age [8–10], a high body mass index [11–15], and the occurrence of a multiple pregnancy.

With regard to recurrent embryonic loss, chromosomal and genetic causes [16] are the main etiological factors involved. The presence of antiphospholipid antibodies (lupus anticoagulant and anticardiolipin antibodies) has also been demonstrated as causes of recurrent pregnancy loss as well as some uterine abnormalities such as a septate uterus [17]. The importance of proper development of the endometrium and its correct decidualization, which would enable selection of the competent embryo, has recently become clear [18]. Some authors believe that endometrial stromal cells would therefore become "sensors" capable of detecting compromised embryos with severe chromosomal defects and would somehow prevent their implantation [19].

Maternal age is a widely studied factor, and the extensive experience gained shows that the miscarriage rate is higher in aged patients, mainly due to a higher frequency of chromosomal abnormalities. Similarly, the miscarriage rate is higher in obese patients, with several associated mechanisms. On the whole, total fertility of obese patients (BMI above 25 and particularly above 30) is reduced, due to affected oocyte quality, endometrial receptivity, and early and late embryonic loss.

Regarding multiple pregnancies, several authors claim a lower pregnancy loss rate for multiple pregnancy than for singleton pregnancy. In this sense, Tummers et al. [20] report a 23% miscarriage rate for singleton pregnancies, 12% miscarriage of one of the two embryos, and 5% cases of total embryonic loss. Glujovsky et al. [21] studying the rate of early spontaneous embryonic loss (before the ninth postmenstrual week) both in singleton and multiple pregnancies conceived by ART observed a lower rate of spontaneous loss for twin pregnancies (OR = 0.6 with 95% confidence intervals in 0.50–0.79). Singleton pregnancies showed a 23.7% miscarriage rate, whereas in 86.5% of the cases where two sacs were observed in the first ultrasound, pregnancy proceeded beyond the eighth week (period after which the patient was discharged); in 9.2% of the cases, a single viable embryo was observed, whereas in 4.2%, there was total embryonic loss. These figures remained the same for pregnancies with more than two embryos. These results cannot be explained using only a mathematical model of embryo implantation prediction; therefore, these and other authors claim the existence of an embryonic synergism in multiple pregnancies that would improve the local environment for implantation [22–24]. Matorras et al. [23] estimated that the probability of successful implantation of an embryo increases by 22% for every additional embryo transferred. Furthermore, the coexistence of other embryos improves not only the chances of implantation, but may also promote a more favorable environment for embryonic maintenance and development. Other variables associated with multiple implantation were a young maternal age, a greater endometrial thickness, a male sterility, and a high embryo score.

Lambers et al. [25] described an ongoing pregnancy rate for singleton and multiple pregnancies of 81.5 and 97.5% and the risk of loss per implanted gestational sac was 18.5 and 11.46% ($P<0.001$), respectively. This lower rate of loss per gestational sac found in multiple pregnancies represents a combination of both genetic and embryonic development factors and of an appropriate uterine environment. The occurrence of multiple implantation is predominantly dependent on (morphological) embryo quality, but the continuation of pregnancy seems to be more dependent on the combination of genetic (younger maternal age) and developmental potential of the embryo.

9.3 "Vanishing Twin" Syndrome

9.3.1 Definition

The vanishing twin (VT) syndrome refers to the loss of one of the twins during the first trimester. Definition of the syndrome varies among different authors. Either an empty gestational sac where no embryo grows, or an embryo without cardiac activity can be observed, while the other twin develops correctly. Since hematomas are frequent at early ages of pregnancy, we shall take care in differentiating them, considering that in early pregnancy there will be already the yolk sac and chorionic ring (Figs. 9.1 and 9.2).

9.3.2 Incidence in ART

The incidence of VT is variable, since neither the definition of the syndrome nor the population included in the different studies is homogeneous. Some authors report rates of 71% loss of at least one of the two twins in spontaneous pregnancies before the tenth week of gestation [26]. Others estimate the loss rate during the first trimester at 53% [27].

Data obtained from patients who became pregnant after assisted reproductive techniques offer the advantage that pregnancy is monitored from very early stages, allowing embryonic loss

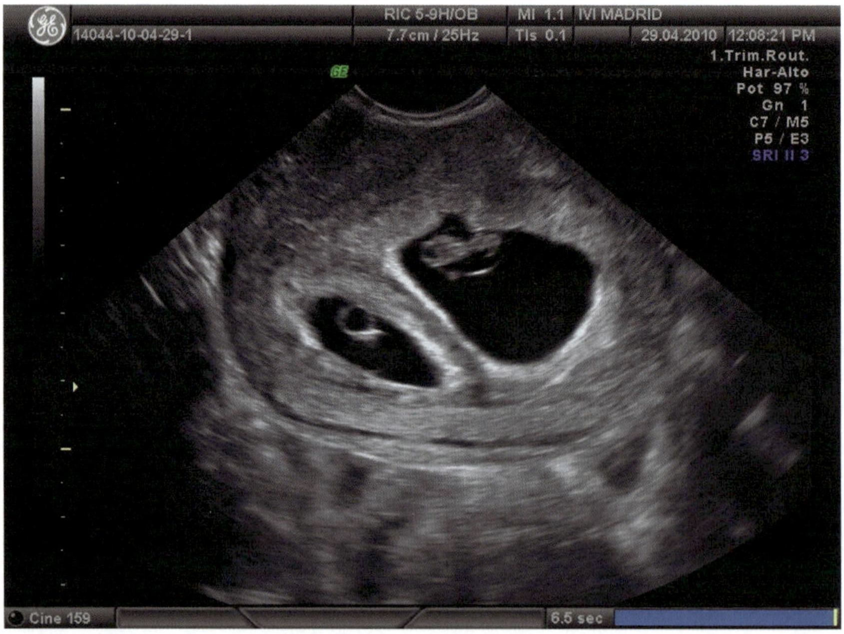

Fig. 9.1 Vanishing twin. Smaller sac without embryo development

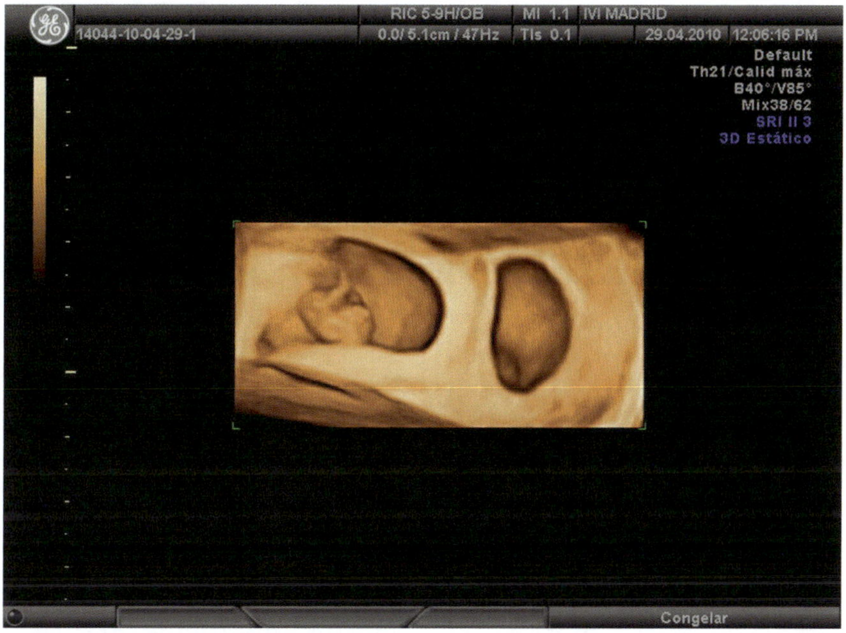

Fig. 9.2 Vanishing twin. Smaller sac without embryo development (3D Image)

to be diagnosed with considerable reliability. However, these patients are usually older, and in some cases, show disorders that could favor early pregnancy loss, resulting in values that could theoretically exceed those of the general population. Incidences reported by different authors are quite inconsistent; in general, approximate values can be estimated between 9% [28] and 20% [29], but could reach 50% in some cases of monochorionic twins [30]. High loss rates of 25–30% have been reported when the pregnancy is achieved through egg donation [31]. Hence, and in spite of the disparity found, we can conclude that for pregnancies conceived after ART, one every 8–10 singleton pregnancies originated initially from a twin pregnancy.

9.3.3 Ultrasound Diagnosis

As mentioned before, methodology is essential for appropriate diagnosis of a vanishing embryo (VE) and to avoid confusion with fluid collections located in the decidua or with hematomas, which are not uncommon in these stages of pregnancy. The real hematoma is located between the corium and the myometrium. In that sense, follow-up of patients conceiving pregnancy after ART is an advantage, as it is conducted from earlier stages.

At IVI, we perform a first ultrasound examination either 24 days after oocyte retrieval or insemination, or 21–23 days after embryo transfer, meaning in all cases a gestational age of about 5 weeks and 3 days; this study shows the gestational sac as an anechoic structure surrounded by a double hyperechogenic ring (double decidual sign). Its location is always eccentric, immersed in the decidua. The anechoic ultrasound image actually corresponds to the gestational sac's liquid content, which contains from the beginning the amnion, the yolk sac, and the embryonic pole. However, initially they are so small that visualization is impossible. The presence of the yolk sac is key to make sure it is a gestational sac and not a pseudosac. The yolk sac is visible for mean sac diameters (MSD) above 6 mm, but is *always* observed with a MSD of 10 mm. It corresponds to the secondary or definitive vitelline sac. It grows approximately 1 mm/week and its values range from 2 mm (week 5) to 6 mm (week 10). Nomograms of diameter and volume growth have been determined with considerable precision. As of week 12, it is usually no longer visible. Visualization of the yolk sac is key to early pregnancy diagnosis and its clear distinction from other entities such as fluid collections (pseudosacs), small adenomyotic foci, etc. Size and echogenicity of the yolk sac are also early prognostic factors of embryo health.

10 days later, we perform a second ultrasound examination aimed at assesing: (a) Pregnancy viability; and (b) Embryonic cardiac activity.

Identification of bad prognostic factors:

- Small gestational sac
- Early oligohydramnios
- Embryo crown-rump length (CRL) 1 week, lower than expected
- Yolk sac size <3 or >7 mm
- Embryonic bradycardia (<85 bpm)

The identification of bad prognostic factors may raise suspicion of upcoming embryonic loss. A weekly ultrasound follow-up may be important in these cases in order to diagnose the time of embryonic death, as death after the ninth week leads to a worse prognosis and may influence the results of the biochemical screening for aneuploidy [32]. In applying these bad prognostic markers, it should be noted that for pregnancies conceived through ART and being the conception date known, the limits of deviation from normality become significantly narrower. However, some variations – even in cases of good prognosis – attributed to variations in embryonic growth rate and/or possible intra- and interobserver measurement bias are observed. Finally, we perform a last ultrasound examination between menstrual weeks 8 and 9 where we assess early embryonic and placental development, and if this is adequate, we discharge the patient to the obstetrician's care. This protocol for early care of pregnancy based on three ultrasound controls allows us to diagnose all pregnancies with early VE (before 9 weeks) as well as to exclude the common complications of ART pregnancies (threatened miscarriage, miscarriage, and ectopic pregnancy).

9.3.4 Symptoms

The main symptom of the VT syndrome is bleeding, with a bleeding rate during the first trimester of up to 52.8% compared to 15.9% [33] in the pregnant control population after ART. Other authors [34] do not report any higher bleeding rates, whereas the literature refers to a great disparity in values that range from 7.8 to 76.5% [35–39].

9.3.5 Perinatal Results

Given that the presence of a VE is a frequent event in pregnancies after ART, it is important to advise the couple on the prognosis of these pregnancies, and if possible, to establish measures aimed at minimizing possible harmful effects. A general increase in the number of perinatal complications in ART pregnancies has been reported, even when distinguishing between singleton and multiple pregnancies. The cause may be, on occasions, age or the maternal pathology sometimes associated with these types of patients, but it is also true that on many occasions, the presence of a VE, whether spontaneous or product of embryo reduction (ER), may entail adverse consequences for both the duration and growth of the surviving fetus(es) [40–45].

Regarding *early complications* of pregnancies with VE, there seems to be no higher miscarriage rate for these pregnancies (twin converted to singleton) compared to initially singleton pregnancies [46]. For some authors as already shown, the miscarriage rate after the diagnosis of a VE might even be lower (5% as opposed to 20%) [27].

Regarding the course of pregnancy, we have found in our group a lower risk of preeclampsia and a higher rate of premature rupture of membranes (PROM), both preterm and term. The lower frequency of preeclampsia may be attributed to the immune tolerance induced by the twin that later stops developing, whereas the rupture of membranes may be attributed to the release into the bloodstream of proinflammatory substances that would facilitate medium- and long-term PROM. Although not statistical significant, Pinborg et al. [34] observed a slightly higher risk of preeclampsia in the VT survivors (OR 0.77 for singleton pregnancies compared to OR 1 for pregnancies with VE). This same study found a 1.4% rate of abruptio placentae in the survivor cohort, twice that of singleton pregnancies, which also affected the cases of early VE, although again statistical significance was not attained. However, this information should be considered insofar as recommendations and guidelines to reduce its incidence can be established.

A lower birthweight for the survivors of the VT syndrome has also been observed; the higher the gestational age at the time of vanishing, the higher the risk of the surviving newborn being small for gestational age.

In an extensive retrospective study of 642 cases of VT, 5,237 singleton pregnancies, and 3,678 twin pregnancies after ART, the difference between the early survivor and the singleton cohort in mean birthweight was 77 g.

Early survivors had a better outcome than intermediate and late survivors; however, they still had poorer birthweight outcome than singletons [34].

The rate of intrauterine growth restriction (IUGR) in singletons originating from a twin gestation was 3.8% compared to 3.6% in singleton pregnancies. These data are very important for reassuring the patient suffering from VE within the first 8 weeks. However, the rate of IUGR rose to 7.7% in cases of death between weeks 8 and 22, and to 12.5% as of week 22. The causes of this small difference in weight and growth in cases of early VE are difficult to explain, but possible hypotheses include inadequate placentation, the effect of embryo degradation products, or increased bleeding that could act as an independent factor [47].

Luke et al. [48] compared pregnancies conceived after ART where early ultrasound showed initially a higher number of gestational sacs with positive cardiac activity, but ending in singleton and twin pregnancies, with initially singleton and twin pregnancies. The presence of three fetal heartbeats was associated with a 47% increased odds of early preterm birth, a 28% increased risk of moderate preterm birth, and a 26% lower odds of a term birth. Likewise, three fetal heartbeats were associated with a 47% increased odds of low birthweight, as well as a 33% increased odds of preterm low birthweight and a 57% increased odds of term low birthweight. Therefore, early fetal loss in ART pregnancies that result in a twin live birth was associated with significantly increased risks for lowered birthweight and shortened gestation.

These authors do not specify the time of embryonic or fetal death, which, as mentioned before, is important for the prognosis [34].

Almong [49] also finds a higher rate both for very low weight (<1,500 g) 3.5 vs. 0.6% and for delivery before 28 weeks of pregnancy that reached 7% in pregnancies with VE and 1.2% in the remaining pregnancies. The study population was composed of a total of 228 patients, 57 with VE and 171 controls. However, these data were not confirmed by La Sala et al. [50] in a study conducted on 322 singleton pregnancies after IVF vs. 44 cases of VE during the first trimester and 320 singleton pregnancies after ICSI vs. 44 cases of VE during the first trimester. No significant statistical differences were found in the percentage of births before 28 weeks (no cases found in the VE group), nor in birthweight <1,500 g, nor in the IVF group or the ICSI group. Hence, the VT syndrome per se, according to La Sala, would not change the outcome of the survivors.

Based on 46 cases of VE and 96 controls, Shebl et al. [51] also found that the frequency of low birthweight (26.1 vs. 12.0%) and being small for gestational age (32.6 vs. 16.3%) was significantly higher in the VE group.

However, no significantly higher rate of preterm birth was found. The author insisted on informing the patients about the associated risks when transferring more than one embryo.

Hence, there seems to be a clear influence of VE on the perinatal result of pregnancy in terms of weight and gestational age. It should be noted, however, that almost 2/3 [34] and in other studies 80% [33] of VE occurred during the first trimester; therefore, the influence on weight and gestational age at birth, if any, is significantly lower. Moreover, as pointed out by La Sala et al. [50], VE is *sensu stricto* a phenomenon confined to the first trimester and we should therefore avoid increasing maternal anxiety of a patient experiencing a VE with pessimistic information about increased risk of preterm delivery or low birthweight.

Furthermore, some publications have shown concern for the neurological future of children born after a VE-complicated pregnancy. Although in many studies, small samples do not allow for definitive conclusions, the development of children born after an initially twin pregnancy with VE does not differ in general from that of children born after initially singleton pregnancies [52]. However, these same authors [53] later found developmental disorders in some cases of VE. Of great interest is the work published by Pinborg in 2005 where the incidence of cerebral palsy, neurological sequelae, and developmental disorders observed between the early VE pregnancies and the singleton pregnancies was not statistically significant. They observed that the number of neurological deficits grew as the gestational age at which the VE occurred increased. A possible explanation of this finding is the failure to establish the number of deaths in mono- or dichorionic pregnancies, each with very different neurological prognosis, being the case of monochorionicity the most unfavorable.

9.3.6 Trisomy 21 Screening and Vanishing Twin

Nowadays, there are numerous trisomy 21 screening strategies, both in the first and the second trimesters, with detection rates of up to 85–90% and 5% false positive rate [54]. The most widely accepted method in Europe is the one that combines maternal age with assessment of the free beta HCG and PAAP-A obtained between week 8 and 12+6 menstrual weeks, and nuchal translucency measurement obtained between weeks 11–13+6. CRL values should range between 45 and 84 mm.

The results of combined biochemical-ultrasound screening in pregnant women after ART (IUI, IVF, frozen embryo transfer, and oocyte donation) show no differences with results for the general population [55]; therefore, there is no need to make any adjustments, only to remember that maternal age in pregnancies after frozen embryo transfer is that of the freezing date, and maternal age after oocyte donation is the age of the donor.

In the biochemical screening of the second trimester, serum levels of free β-hCG, alpha-fetoprotein, and oestriol appear to be modified in pregnancies conceived after ART; this could increase the trisomy 21 false positive rate for these patients [56, 57], although this information has not been corroborated by other authors [58].

The presence of a VT could alter the results of the first trimester biochemical screening, given that production of free beta HCG and PAAP-A by the placenta of the embryo that stops developing could alter the results for the surviving twin, particularly in occasions where the biochemical determination is conducted in early stages (8–9 weeks). Moreover, if ultrasound control is not conducted at this early stage, the time of embryonic death will remain unknown (early or late); hence, the importance of conducting serial controls in this type of pregnancies.

However, results found in literature [33] do not seem to identify significant differences between free beta HCG and PAAP-A levels in VT pregnancies before 9 weeks compared to the control group in singleton pregnancies; authors expressed their doubt in cases of death at a later stage. In these cases, the screening recommended would use only maternal age and the value of the nuchal translucency.

9.3.7 Induced Vanishing Twin Embryo Reduction

ER consists in causing the death of one or several embryos or fetuses with the purpose of preventing the more severe consequences associated with multiple pregnancies: severe preterm birth and its associated neurological sequelae.

Fortunately, the use of this technique has fallen steadily since the gradual implementation of a policy to reduce the number of transferred embryos. In our center, the mean number of embryos transferred is lower than two, and we believe it is the right thing to do in order to reduce the rate of twin pregnancies and, what is worse, of triplet and higher-order pregnancies.

Among several possible ER situations, the most common is that after a triplet pregnancy, ER of one of the embryos is performed, resulting in the end in a twin pregnancy. Excluding early complications derived from the procedure, these cases have shown that the medium- and long-term prognosis is worse than that of a twin pregnancy, as the abortion rate [59] increases to 8% and the growth of the both surviving fetuses is also lower than in twin pregnancies, since after an ER, the fetal placentas of initially triplet twins are smaller than in the case of initially twins. The explanation of a higher abortion rate is given by the release of proinflammatory agents by the twin subject to ER, primarily cytokines that stimulate the production of prostaglandins; whereas the lower weight could be attributed to an inadequate placentation derived from the higher number of gestational sacs, which does not seem to improve after an ER.

The model that best describes the most common VE phenomenon is probably the few cases of ER from 2 to 1 fetus or from 3 to 1 fetus. Few literature cases allow for definitive conclusions, given that in this type of patients the ER is very often indicated due to a uterine problem (mullerian anomalies, myomas, previous cesareans) and therefore observations cannot be extrapolated to the general population. Some authors find the "take-home baby" rate would be higher than in initially twin pregnancies, although they express doubt about the ethical considerations that may arise when performing an ER in these cases [60].

9.4 Conclusions

9.4.1 Key Points

1. The VT syndrome is defined as the loss of one of the twins during the first trimester. Two thirds of the cases occur during the first 8–9 weeks.
2. The incidence is variable, with a mean value of about 12% (9–20%).
3. It is important to perform an accurate ultrasound diagnosis to avoid confusing the VE with hematomas or other type of fluid collections. Also, bad prognostic factors of pregnancy such as embryonic bradycardia, small gestational sac, and early oligohydramnios should be identified. Given that in general the prognosis worsens as gestational age increases, it is very important to determine adequately the probable date of VE in order to provide the patient with appropriate information regarding the perinatal prognosis and possible medium- and long-term impact.
4. Patients with VE show an increased bleeding frequency during the first trimester. However, the abortion rate does not increase and may be even lower according to some authors.
5. Some studies show a higher rate of PROM attributed to the release into the bloodstream of proinflammatory substances that would facilitate medium- and long-term PROM.
6. An increase in the rate of weight <1,500 g and of delivery before 28 and 32 weeks is reported, although these findings are primarily due to cases of VE beyond 8 weeks, which represent a minority of total VEs.
7. In cases of VE before 9 weeks, the possibilities of having weights <1,500 g and deliveries before 28 and 32 weeks are similar to those of singleton pregnancies.
8. In cases of VE before 9 weeks, no higher rate of neurological sequelae, cerebral palsy, or developmental disorders was found.
9. In cases of VE before 9 weeks, it is not necessary to adjust the biochemical parameters of trisomy 21 with nonconclusive results between weeks 9 and 12.
10. ER in multiple pregnancies is a model of iatrogenic VE that allows to determine the influence of early placentation on the growth of the other twins and on the abortion rate. However, the most frequent model of spontaneous VE, i.e., the reduction of two twins to a singleton pregnancy, is rare in the application of ER techniques and therefore the data obtained are less reliable.

Finally, the information given to a pregnant woman experiencing a VE during the first trimester, particularly before 9 weeks, should be positive and management should be expectant, with high possibilities of take-home baby and without major pregnancy complications in this group of pregnant women regarding preterm delivery, abortion, very low weight, and neurological deficits.

References

1. Vitthala S, Gelbaya TA, Brison DR, Fitzgerald CT, Nardo LG. The risk of monozygotic twins after assisted reproductive technology: a systematic review and meta-analysis. Hum Rep Update. 2009;15(1):45–55.
2. Gratacos E. Multiple pregnancy: general aspects and relevance in fetal medicine. In: Gratacos E, Gomez O, Nicolaides K, Romero R, Cabero L, editors. Fetal Medicine. 1st ed. Barcelona: Panamerican; 2007. p. 688–694.
3. Ricciarelli E. Marco de actitud ante las gestaciones múltiples: Legislaciones y recomendaciones. Rev Iberoamericana Fertilidad. 2007;24(6):405–10.
4. Monteagudo A, Timor-Tritsch I, Sharma S. Early and simple determination of chorionic and amniotic type in multifetal gestations in the first 14 weeks by high frequency transvaginal ultrasound. Am J Obstet Gynecol. 1994;170:824–9.
5. Carroll SG, Soothill PW, Abdel-Fattah SA, Porter H, Montague I, Kyle PM. Prediction of chorionicity in twin pregnancies at 10–14 weeks of gestation. BJOG. 2002;109(2):182–6.
6. Wilcox AJ, Weinberg CR, O'Connor JF, Baird DD, Schlatterer JP, Canfield RE, et al. Incidence of early loss of pregnancy. N Engl J Med. 1988;319:189–94.
7. Wilcox AJ, Baird DD, Weinberg CR. Time of implantation of the conceptus and loss of pregnancy. N Engl J Med. 1999;340:1796–9.
8. Dickey RP, Taylor SN, Lu PY, Sartor BM, Storment JM, Rye PH, et al. Spontaneous reduction of multiple pregnancy: incidence and effect on outcome. Am J Obstet Gynecol. 2002;186:77–83.
9. Abdalla HI, Burton G, Kirkland A, Johnson MR, Leonard T, Brooks AA, et al. Age, pregnancy and miscarriage: uterine versus ovarian factors. Hum Reprod. 1993;8:1512–7.
10. Andersen N, Wohlfahrt J, Christens P, Olsen J, Melbye M. Maternal age and fetal loss: population based register linkage study. Br Med J. 2000;320:1708–12.
11. Wang JX, Davies MJ, Norman RJ. Obesity increases the risk of spontaneous abortion during infertility treatment. Obes Res. 2002;10:551–4.
12. Fedorcsak P, Storeng R, Dale PO, Tanbo T, Abyholm T. Obesity is a risk factor for early pregnancy loss after IVF or ICSI. Acta Obstet Gynecol Scand. 2000;79:43–8.
13. Bellver J, Busso C, Pellicer A, Remohi J, Simon C. Obesity and assisted reproductive technology outcomes. Reprod Biomed Online. 2006;12:562–8.
14. Maheshwari A, Stofberg L, Bhattacharya S. Effect of overweight and obesity on assisted reproductive technology – a systematic review. Hum Reprod Update. 2007;13:433–44.
15. Bellver J, Ayllon Y, Ferrando M, Melo M, Goyri E, Pellicer A, et al. Female obesity impairs in vitro fertilization outcome without affecting embryo quality. Fertil Steril. 2010;93:447–54.
16. Vanneste E, Voet T, Le Caignec C, Ampe M, Konings P, Melotte C, et al. Chromosome instability is common in human cleavage-stage embryos. Nat Med. 2009;15:577–83.
17. Christiansen OB, Steffensen R, Nielsen HS, Varming K. Multifactorial etiology of recurrent miscarriage and its scientific and clinical implications. Gynecol Obstet Invest. 2008;66:257–67.
18. Regan L, Macklon NS, Brosens JJ. Natural selection of human embryos: impaired decidualization of endometrium disables embryo-maternal interactions and causes recurrent pregnancy loss. PLoS One. 2010;5:e10287.
19. Brossens J, Gellersen B. Something new about early pregnancy: decidual biosensoring and natural embryo selection. Ultrasound Obstet Gynecol. 2010;36:1–5.
20. Tummers P, De Sutter P, Dhont M. Risk of spontaneous abortion in singleton and twin pregnancies after IVF/ICSI. Hum Reprod. 2003;18:1720–3.
21. Glujovsky D, Shamonki MI, Bergh PA. Embryonic synergism may reduce pregnancy loss: a multivariate regression analysis. Fertil Steril. 2007;87:509–14.
22. Torsky SP, Amato P, Cisneros PL, Sangi-Haghpeykar H, Trukhacheva EV, Carson SA. Algorithm to predict assisted reproductive technology pregnancy outcome reveals minimal embryo synergy. Fertil Steril. 2005;83:782–4.
23. Matorras R, Matorras F, Mendoza R, Rodriguez M, Remohi J, Rodriguez-Escudero FJ, et al. The implantation of every embryo facilitates the chances of the remaining embryos to implant in an IVF programme: a mathematical model to predict pregnancy and multiple pregnancy rates. Hum Reprod. 2005;20:2923–31.
24. La Sala G, Nicoli A, Vilani LT, Gallinelli A, Nucera G, Blickstein I. Spontaneous embryonic loss rates in twin and singleton pregnancies after transfer of top-versus intermediate-quality embryos. Fertil Steril. 2005;84:1602–5.
25. Lambers MJ, Mager E, Goutbeek J, Homburg R, et al. Factors determining early pregnancy loss in singleton and multiple implantations. Hum Reprod. 2007;22(1): 275–9.
26. Levi S. Ultrasonic assessment of the high rate of human multiple pregnancy in the first trimester. J Clin Ultrasound. 1976;4:3.
27. Robinson HP, Caines JS. Sonar evidence of early pregnancy failure in patients with twin conceptions. Br J Obstet Gynaecol. 1977;84:22.
28. Mansour R, Serour G, Aboulghar M, Kamal O, Al-Inany H. The impact of vanishing fetuses on the outcome of ICSI pregnancies. Fertil Steril. 2010;94:2430–2.
29. Cano F, Simon C, Remohi J, et al. Effect of aging on the female reproductive system: evidence for the role of uterine senescente in the decline in female fecundity. Fertil Steril. 1995;64:584–9.
30. Benson CB, Doubilet PM, Laks MP. Outcome of twin gestations following sonographic demonstration of

two heart beats in the first trimester. Ultrasound Obstet Gynecol. 1993;3(5):343–5.
31. Remohi J, Gartner B, Gallardo E, et al. Pregnancy and birth rates alter oocyte donation. Fertil Steril. 1997;67:717–23.
32. Gjerris AC, Loft A, Pinborg A, Christiansen M, Tabor A. The effect of a "vanishing twin" on biochemical and ultrasound first trimester screening markers for Down's syndrome in pregnancies conceived by assisted reproductive technology. Hum Reprod. 2009;24:55–62.
33. Rodriguez-Gonzalez M, Serra V, Garcia-Velasco JA, Pellicer A, Remohi J. The vanishing embryo phenomenon in an oocyte donation programme. Hum Reprod. 2002;17:798–802.
34. Pinborg A, Lidegaard O, Freiesleben NC, Andersen AN. Vanishing twins: a predictor of small-for-gestational age in IVF singletons. Hum Reprod. 2007;22(10):2707–14.
35. Landy HJ, Keith LG. The vanishing twin: a review. Hum Reprod Update. 1998;4(2):177–83.
36. Goldman GA, Dicker D, Feldberg D, et al. The vanishing fetus: a report of 17 cases of triplets and quadruplets. J Perinat Med. 1989;17:157–62.
37. Jackson J, Benirschke K. The recognition and significance of the vanishing twin. J Am Board Fam Pract. 1989;2:58–63.
38. Jeanty P, Rodesch F, Verhoogen C, et al. The vanishing twin. Ultrasonics. 1981;2:25–31.
39. Sampson A. Ch. (1992) Vanishing twins: the frequency of spontaneous fetal reduction of a twin pregnancy. Ultrasound Obstet Gynecol. 1992;2:107–9.
40. Daniel Y, Ochshorn Y, Fait G, Geva E, Bar-Am A, Lessing JB. Analysis of 104 twin pregnancies conceived with assisted reproductive technologies and 193 spontaneously conceived twin pregnancies. Fertil Steril. 2000;74:683–9.
41. Lambalk CB, van Hooff M. Natural versus induced twinning and pregnancy outcome: a Dutch nationwide survey of primiparous dizygotic twin deliveries. Fertil Steril. 2001;75:731–6.
42. Helmerhorst FM, Perquin DAM, Donker D, Keirse MJNC. Perinatal outcome of singletons and twins after assisted conception: a systematic review of controlled studies. Br Med J. 2004;328:261.
43. Jackson RA, Gibson KA, Wu YW, Croughan MS. Perinatal outcomes in singletons following in vitro fertilization: a meta-analysis. Obstet Gynecol. 2004; 103:551–63.
44. Wang YA, Sullivan EA, Black D, Dean J, Bryant J, Chapman M. Preterm birth and low birth weight after assisted reproductive technology-related pregnancy in Australia between 1996 and 2000. Fertil Steril. 2005;83:1650–8.
45. Schieve LA, Cohen B, Nannini A, Ferre C, Reynolds MA, Zhang Z, et al. A population-based study of maternal and perinatal outcomes associated with assisted reproductive technology in Massachusetts. Matern Child Health J. 2007;11:517–25.
46. Pinborg A, Lidegaard O, la Cour Freiesleben N, Andersen AN. Consequences of vanishing twins in IVF/ICSI pregnancies. Hum Reprod. 2005;10: 2821–9.
47. Weiss JL, Malone FD, Vidaver J, Ball RH, Nyberg DA, Comstock CH. Threatened abortion: a risk factor for poor pregnancy outcome, a population-based screening study. Am J Obstet Gynecol. 2004;190:745–50.
48. Luke B, Brown MB, Grainger DA, Stern JE, Klein N, Cedars MI. The effect of early fetal losses on twin assisted-conception pregnancy outcomes. Fertil Steril. 2009;91(6):2586–92.
49. Almog B, Levin I, Wagman I, Kapustiansky R, Lessing JB, Amit A, et al. Adverse obstetric outcome for the vanishing twin syndrome. Reprod Biomed Online. 2010;20(2):256–60.
50. La Sala GB, Villani MT, Nicoli A, Gallinelli A, Nucera G, Blickstein I. Effect of the mode of assisted reproductive technology conception on obstetric outcomes for survivors of the vanishing twin syndrome. Fertil Steril. 2006;86(1):247–9.
51. Shebl O, Ebner T, Sommergruber M, Sir A, Tews G. Birth weight is lower for survivors of the vanishing twin syndrome: a case-control study. Fertil Steril. 2008;90(2):310–4.
52. Anand D, Platt MJ, Pharoah PO. Comparative development of surviving co-twins of vanishing twin conceptions, twins and singletons. Twin Res Hum Genet. 2007;10(1):210–5.
53. Anand D, Platt MJ, Pharoah PO. Vanishing twin: a possible cause of cerebral impairment. Twin Res Hum Genet. 2007;10(1):202–9.
54. Spencer K. Aneuploidy screening in the first trimester. Am J Med Genet C Semin Med Genet. 2007;145:18–32.
55. Bellver J, Lara C, Soares SR, Ramirez A, Pellicer A, Remohi J, et al. First trimester biochemical screening for Down's syndrome in singleton pregnancies conceived by assisted reproduction. Hum Reprod. 2005;20(9):2623–7.
56. Maymon R, Shulman A. Serial first- and second-trimester Down's syndrome screening tests among IVF-versus naturally-conceived singletons. Hum Reprod. 2002;17(4):1081–5.
57. Hui PW, Lee CP, Tang MH, Ho PC. Nuchal translucency in pregnancies conceived after assisted reproduction technology. Curr Opin Obstet Gynecol. 2006;18(3):319–24.
58. Rice JD, McIntosh SF, Halstead AC. Second-trimester maternal serum screening for Down syndrome in in vitro fertilization pregnancies. Prenat Diagn. 2005;25(3):234–8.
59. Papageorghiou AT, Avgidou K, Bakoulas V, Sebire NJ, Nicolaides KH. Risks of miscarriage and early preterm birth in trichorionic triplet pregnancies with embryo reduction versus expectant management: new data and systematic review. Hum Reprod. 2006;21(7):1912–7.
60. Evans MI, Kaufman MI, Urban AJ, Britt DW, Fletcher JC. Fetal reduction from twins to a singleton: a reasonable consideration? Obstet Gynecol. 2004;104(1): 102–9.

Part II

Male Infertility

The Effect of Cancer Therapies on Sperm: Current Guidelines

10

Akanksha Mehta and Mark Sigman

Abstract

Advances in treatments and improved survival for young men with cancer have led to attempts to preserve or restore fertility in these patients. Baseline fertility is often impaired at the time of cancer diagnosis and is often worsened by subsequent cancer therapies. Fertility is most commonly impaired in testicular cancer followed by Hodgkin's lymphoma, non-Hodgkin's lymphoma, and leukemia, and even in those with other solid tumors. Sperm banking prior to therapy remains the most important tool for fertility preservation. Recovery of spermatogenesis may take months to years following chemotherapy or radiation therapy. Attempts to protect spermatogenesis from the effects of these therapies remain experimental and largely unsuccessful. Both chemotherapy and radiation therapy cause damage to sperm DNA with temporary increased rates of aneuploidy. Despite this, most studies show no increase in the rates of congenital anomalies in children born to men following cancer therapies. Future efforts are being directed at protection of spermatogenic cells from damage and germ cell transplantation and in vitro maturation.

Keywords

Leukemia • Hodgkin's lymphoma • Chemotherapy • Radiation therapy • Cancer • Gonadotoxic • Type Ad spermatogonia • Type Ap spermatogonia • Type B spermatogonia • Spermatocytes • Spermatids • Testicular cancer • Alkylating agents • Bone marrow transplantation • Retroperitoneal lymph node dissection • Retrograde ejaculation • Sperm banking • Sperm cryopreservation • Testicular sperm retrieval • Germ cell transplantation • Sperm aneuploidy • Congenital anomalies • Testicular allograft

---

M. Sigman (✉)
Division of Urology, Rhode Island Hospital,
Warren Alpert Medical School at Brown University,
Providence, RI, USA
e-mail: msigman@lifespan.org

C. Racowsky et al. (eds.), *Biennial Review of Infertility: Volume 2*,
DOI 10.1007/978-1-4419-8456-2_10,

10.1 Introduction

During the last two decades, the survival rates of young men suffering from various types of cancers have improved dramatically, due to advanced diagnostic techniques and better treatment modalities. Greater attention is therefore being paid to patients' quality of life. Testicular cancer, lymphoma, and leukemia remain the most common malignancies diagnosed in men of reproductive age, and infertility problems stemming from cancer diagnosis as well cancer therapy are a growing concern for cancer survivors.

In many cancer patients, sperm quality is already impaired before receiving any form of treatment. Further deterioration in semen parameters and endocrine parameters typically ensues due to the damaging effects of chemotherapy or radiotherapy, and this deterioration may be temporary or permanent. Many of these patients are young men who have either not started, or not completed their families. While our understanding of the gonadotoxic effects of specific cancer therapy regimens is improving, it is impossible to predict with any degree of certainty which patients will have impaired spermatogenesis and which patients will have improvement in their gonadal function to reestablish normal spermatogenesis. As such, preservation of fertility potential and the use of assisted-reproductive techniques have become increasingly important in the long-term management of cancer patients of reproductive age.

This chapter discusses the effects of the cancer disease process as well as the associated therapies, including surgery, chemotherapy, and radiation therapy on gonadal function and sperm quality in male cancer patients. The availability of assisted-reproductive techniques has undoubtedly improved the chances of a successful pregnancy for these patients, but there is some controversy as to the safety of these techniques when using sperm from irradiated or postchemotherapeutic patients.

10.2 Overview of Spermatogenesis

Spermatogenesis is an elaborate cell-differentiation process that takes place in the seminiferous tubules of the testes, starting with the spermatogonial stem cell and terminating with a fully differentiated and highly specialized male gamete called the spermatozoa. In humans, spermatogenesis requires approximately 64 days.

On histologic examination of the seminiferous tubules, spermatogonia are located along the base of the seminiferous epithelium and consist of two classes: Type A and Type B cells. The Type A spermatogonia, in turn, consist of the pale type (Ap) and dark type (Ad) cells. The Ap spermatogonia are mitotically active cells, which divide into Ap spermatogonia and type B spermatogonia. The Type B spermatogonia undergo mitotic division to produce primary spermatocytes, which then undergo two meiotic divisions to form spermatids. Thus, Ap spermatogonia are primarily responsible for replenishing their own populations, as well as the entire spermatogenic process. This process is summarized in Fig. 10.1.

Ad spermatogonia rarely divide and are believed to represent dormant reserve germ cells. When the number of Ap spermatogonia is diminished, for example, after irradiation, Ad spermatogonia become active, transform into Ap spermatogonia, and then start to proliferate [1].

The hormonal regulation of spermatogenesis is via the hypothalamic-pituitary-gonadal axis, which is based on hormonal feedback mechanisms. Pulsatile release of gonadotropin-releasing hormone (GnRH) from the hypothalamus regulates the pulsatile release of follicle-stimulating hormone (FSH) and luteinizing hormone (LH) from the anterior pituitary. LH acts on Leydig cells to regulate testosterone (T) secretion, while FSH acts on Sertoli cells to initiate and sustain spermatogenesis, in the presence of testosterone.

Elevated serum levels of LH and FSH, as well as depressed levels of testosterone, have been associated with impaired spermatogenesis.

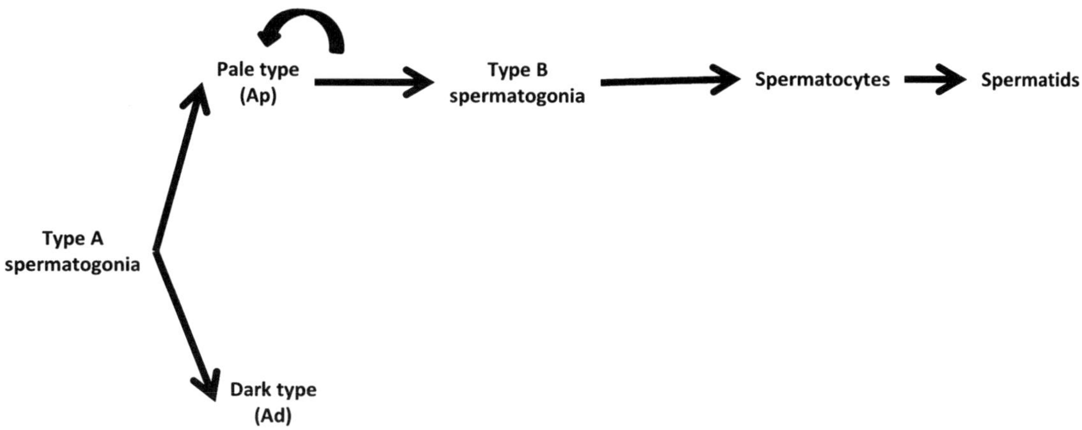

Fig. 10.1 Overview of spermatogenesis

In particular, elevated FSH has been used as a marker for impaired Sertoli-cell function. Recently, Inhibin B, secreted by Sertoli cells, has been proposed as a marker for Sertoli-cell function, especially in prepubertal boys and male adolescents [2, 3]. Bordallo et al. compared Inhibin B/FSH ratios in 21 males after chemotherapy for Hodgkin's lymphoma with 20 healthy, matched controls. There was no significant difference in LH, T, Inhibin B concentrations, or T/LH ratio between the two groups, but serum Inhibin B was correlated with serum FSH levels and Inhibin B/FSH ratio was positively correlated with sperm count [2]. The authors concluded that serum Inhibin B levels may be an important marker of seminiferous tubule function in men treated with chemotherapy and should be interpreted in the context of serum FSH.

Each Sertoli cell supports a defined number of germ cells, and therefore, spermatogonia. It is evident that reduction in the Sertoli cell population directly impairs spermatogenesis. Hormonal cues are equally important. FSH plays a major role in the regulation of spermatogenesis, although the mechanism of action of FSH on the Sertoli cell is unknown. Several animal studies have indicated that Type A spermatogonia are affected by the withdrawal of FSH [4], or by the administration of GnRH antagonists [5], indicating that the first mitotic division is a site of hormone action. The role of testosterone in spermatogonial development is less obvious. Normal spermatogenesis requires high intratesticular testosterone concentrations. However, the role of intratesticular testosterone in return of spermatogenesis in impaired testes is more complicated. Animal studies have shown that high intratesticular testosterone concentrations can be detrimental to spermatogonial differentiation, and suppression of testosterone is required to promote spermatogonial development in irradiated rodents and mouse models of juvenile spermatogonial depletion [6]. During normal early pubertal development, when spermatogonial divisions are very active, testosterone levels are very low [1]. Fine regulation of intratesticular hormone concentrations during the spermatogenesis cycle appears key to normal sperm production and differentiation.

10.3 Cancer

The most common cancers in men of reproductive age are leukemia, lymphoma, and testicular germ cell tumors. In past years, patients suffering from these cancers were most concerned about disease recurrence and treatment side effects. As survival rates after treatment have improved, there is growing concern about quality-of-life issues, such as preserving fertility potential. A recent study on semen quality in 205 adolescent males with various solid and hematologic cancers found that semen parameters such as sperm count, motility, and semen volume were significantly lower in cancer patients compared to healthy controls [7]. It is important to determine patients' pretreatment fertility potential, in order to better understand how their cancer disease and its treatment will affect their fertility potential in the future.

It is well accepted that malignant disease, in and of itself, can lead to impaired gonadal function, through hormonal alterations and metabolic conditions [8]. Reproductive hormones may be low in some patients as a result of physiologic stress associated with the cancer state, or downregulation by endocrine substances produced by some tumors, or even direct tumor invasion of endocrine organs. Malignancy may also result in malnutrition, with deficiencies in vitamins, minerals, and trace elements needed for optimal gonadal function. Hematologic malignancies such as Hodgkin's lymphoma are often accompanied by constitutional symptoms, especially fevers, which negatively influence spermatogenesis. Some authors have described the development of antisperm antibodies as a result of disruption of the blood–testis barrier by cancer, leading to poor semen analysis results [9]. Lastly, tumor-released cytokines such as interleukins and tumor necrosis factor can affect spermatozoal function, resulting in low sperm motility. This effect may be local, as demonstrated by the observation that the number of spermatogenesis defects in testicular tissue is highest in the tissue closest to the tumor, while spermatogenesis is uniform in orchiectomy samples that have benign tumors [10, 11].

There is no concrete evidence to support the hypothesis that pretreatment spermatogenic function predicts posttreatment spermatogenic function. Rather, the purpose of studying pretreatment fertility potential and sperm quality is to determine whether semen cryopreservation prior to initiation of therapy can provide sperm of adequate quality to allow for use with assisted-reproductive techniques in the event that fertility potential is not restored at the conclusion of cancer therapy. Improvement in and increased availability of in vitro fertilization (IVF) and intracystoplasmic sperm injection (ICSI) techniques have allowed for successful pregnancy outcomes even in instances of severe male factor infertility.

10.3.1 Testicular Cancer

The incidence of testicular cancer has increased worldwide over the past five decades [12]. There is controversial evidence of a concurrent decline in male reproductive health, as manifest by decreasing semen parameters and increasing frequency of other genital abnormalities such as hypospadias and cryptorchidism, and it has been suggested that the development of testicular cancer is etiologically linked to these genital abnormalities.

Several studies have documented lower sperm counts in patients with testicular germ cell carcinoma compared to controls. Based on sperm concentrations, a striking 50–75% of patients with unilateral testicular carcinoma are subfertile at the time of diagnosis, with sperm concentrations below 10 million/mL [12]. It is well known that approximately 10% of patients with testicular cancer will have a history of cryptorchidism, and this may explain in part, but not entirely, the effect on spermatogenesis. Previous histologic studies have shown severe abnormalities in 24% of the biopsies from contralateral testes in men who underwent orchiectomy for unilateral testicular germ cell tumor. Eight percent had no sperm production, 16% showed varying degrees of spermatogenesis, and 5% had carcinoma in situ (CIS) [13].

The question of whether Leydig cell dysfunction preexists in patients with testicular cancer remains unresolved, but evidence from current literature does support this notion. Men who undergo orchiectomy for testicular cancer have lower testosterone and higher serum LH levels than men who undergo orchiectomy for benign causes [14]. Petersen et al. [15] compared gonadal function between two groups of men who underwent orchiectomy for unilateral testicular carcinoma with or without CIS of the contralateral testicle. Significantly higher LH levels and lower testosterone levels were found in the group with CIS, indicative of markedly altered Leydig cell function in this group. Additionally, patients with CIS had significantly lower sperm concentration and total sperm count. Similar results were reported by Jacobsen et al. who studied gonadal function in 63 men with bilateral testicular cancer after their first orchiectomy and before additional treatment. Results were compared with those from 174 patients with unilateral cancer after orchiectomy [16]. Although testosterone levels did not differ between the two groups, LH levels were significantly higher in the subset of patients who developed a contralateral testicular tumor. Taken together, the above results indicate that abnormal serum testosterone and LH profiles after orchiectomy are not simply a result of removal of the testis, but rather may be attributed to some inherent impairment of Leydig cell function in the contralateral testis.

Patients who develop testicular carcinoma in one testis are 500–1,000 times more likely to develop carcinoma in the contralateral testis, compared to the general population. Metachronous tumors are far more common than bilateral synchronous tumors [17]. While bilateral radical orchiectomy remains the standard of care for these patients, there is growing enthusiasm for testis-sparing surgery, which has been supported by the publication of specific guidelines from the German Testicular Cancer Study Group [18]. In theory, testis-sparing surgery should be associated with improved fertility and endocrine function. However, a major concern when sparing a tumor-bearing testis is the high prevalence of adjacent foci of CIS. Given the exquisite radiosensitivity of CIS, supporters of organ-preserving surgery for testicular carcinoma generally recommend that every patient undergoing partial orchiectomy be treated with adjuvant local radiation therapy to the testicular parenchyma, regardless of whether the tumor was seminoma or nonseminoma. Such treatment, intended to minimize the risk of local recurrence, invariably arrests spermatogenesis and culminates in infertility [16].

CIS is found in the contralateral testis of 5% of patients with testicular germ cell cancer [19]. The management of CIS is important because the majority – if not all – cases of CIS will eventually progress to invasive disease. Seminiferous tubules containing CIS are devoid of spermatogenesis, and the neighboring tubules often demonstrate severely impaired spermatogenesis as well. This explains the frequent finding of oligospermia or azoospermia, in combination with elevated serum LH and FSH levels in patients with CIS [15].

10.3.2 Lymphoma

Hodgkin's lymphoma affects patients of all ages, but has a first incidence peak between 18 and 40 years. Presently, 5-year survival from the disease is around 90%. Infertility is one of the most significant side effects in long-term survivors of Hodgkin's lymphoma, as treatment usually involves chemotherapy, radiation, or a combination of both.

To this end, several authors have investigated the pretreatment fertility status of Hodgkin's lymphoma patients. In a large observational study, Lass et al. [20] demonstrated no difference in semen parameters such as sperm count and motility between patients with lymphoma vs. leukemia, but patients with Hodgkin's lymphoma had significantly lower sperm quality compared with non-Hodgkin's lymphoma. Rueffer et al. [21] investigated semen quality in 158 Hodgkin's lymphoma patients, classified as having either early-, intermediate-, or advanced-stage disease and found that 70% of patients had inadequate semen quality at baseline, with 21% of patients demonstrating severe damage such as azoospermia or oligoasthenoteratozoospermia. Advanced stage of disease was associated with a greater likelihood of having semen abnormalities, possibly because advanced Hodgkin's lymphoma is a biologically active disease, often presenting with systemic symptoms and elevated ESR, which may have a significant impact on spermatogenesis. These results are in agreement with those of the German Hodgkin Study group trial, wherein only 20% of patients had normozoopermia in pretreatment analysis, with 11% of patients having azoospermia and 69% other dyspermia [22].

FSH and Inhibin B have both been proposed as markers of gonadal function in patients with Hodgkin's lymphoma [22, 23]. A prospectively randomized trial of the German Hodgkin Study group examined pre- and posttreatment fertility parameters in groups of 202 and 112 patients, respectively, and found a significant difference in FSH levels between patients with azoospermia and those with preserved spermatogenesis [22]. However, some authors have argued that FSH is not a reliable marker for fertility in postchemotherapy patients, as the frequency of elevated FSH levels after chemotherapy varies from 35 to 100% and depends on the cumulative doses of alkylating agents used [24]. Van Beek et al. showed that male survivors of Hodgkin's lymphoma treated in childhood with alkylating chemotherapy agents have significantly lower levels of inhibin B, when compared to men not treated with these agents. Additionally, they found Inhibin B to be a stronger and more independent determinant of sperm concentration compared to FSH and recommended Inhibin B be used as a screening tool to detect gonadal damage in men treated for Hodgkin's lymphoma in childhood.

10.3.3 Leukemia

Like patients with testicular carcinoma and Hodgkin's lymphoma, patients with leukemia also appear to have significant pretreatment impairment of spermatogenesis. Hallak et al. [25] examined semen characteristics in 25 men with acute or chronic leukemia and compared them with 50 healthy controls and found that patients with leukemia had significantly lower prefreeze and postthaw sperm motility, motile sperm count, and curvilinear velocity. In this analysis, the type of leukemia did not have an effect on prefreeze or postthaw semen quality. Most importantly, the quality of the postthaw sperm was sufficient for use with ICSI, and therefore, cryopreservation of sperm was recommended for leukemia patients despite the abnormalities noted in the analysis.

10.3.4 Other Solid Tumors

Although much less frequent than testicular germ cell tumors and hematologic malignancies, fertility impairment is nevertheless present in solid tumors involving other organ systems, ranging from carcinomas and sarcomas to CNS tumors. Lass et al. [20] evaluated 231 men diagnosed with malignant disease, categorized as testicular tumors, hematologic malignancy, or other cancers. Men with testicular tumors had significantly lower sperm concentration and motility than the other two groups of patients. Men with other solid tumors had semen quality abnormalities similar to patients with hematologic malignancies, but significantly better than testicular cancer patients.

10.4 Cancer-Associated Therapies

Treatment options for cancer patients consist of surgical intervention, chemotherapy, radiotherapy, or multimodal therapy, depending on the type of malignancy. Both chemotherapy and radiation therapy act by interfering with rapidly dividing cells. Germ cells are also rapidly dividing, and thus become a target for these therapies. Recovery for surviving germ cells can happen, but is unpredictable and is often a lengthy process. Leydig cells, with their slower rate of turnover, are more resistant to gonadotoxic therapy, resulting in preservation of androgen production even when patients are infertile.

Because of their high mitotic activity, spermatogonia are more vulnerable to DNA damaging agents such as radiation and chemotherapy, compared to Sertoli and Leydig cells and spermatids. Spermatogonia have also been shown to be more vulnerable than spermatocytes, which carry out meiotic divisions only [1].

As previously mentioned, spermatogenesis is already impaired to some degree in men with cancer, even prior to cancer therapy. Interestingly, some patients who are azoospermic prior to cancer therapy do go on to have normal sperm parameters after treatment. This observation has led some authors to suggest that the mechanism of infertility before treatment is reversible and distinct from the mechanism following treatment for cancer [26]. Therefore, even in patients with preexisting impairment of spermatogenic function, it is still worthwhile to select the least gonadotoxic treatments possible.

For patients with testicular cancer, treatment typically consists of radical orchiectomy, followed by retroperitoneal lymph node dissection (RPLND), chemotherapy, or radiation therapy, based on the histopathology and stage of the germ cell tumor. Patients with lymphoma and leukemia are primarily candidates for chemotherapy, with or without radiation therapy, with a variety of regimens. Patients who undergo bone marrow transplantation (BMT) for hematological malignancies are subject to a combination of chemotherapy and total body irradiation (TBI), significantly increasing their risk of gonadotoxicity compared to patients who do not undergo multimodal therapy.

10.4.1 Surgery

Radical orchiectomy remains the gold standard for surgical treatment of testicular germ cell carcinoma, followed by RPLND or chemotherapy or radiotherapy, as indicated by tumor histopathology. Radical orchiectomy for testicular cancer is associated with a decrease in postoperative sperm concentrations. Petersen et al. [12] noted a decrease from 20 million/mL before orchiectomy to 10 million/mL after orchiectomy in a group of 29 patients. This observation is in agreement with other investigators who found azoospermia in 10–56% of men after orchiectomy [26]. Fertility is nevertheless possible in men after orchiectomy. Jacobsen et al. [16] compared fertility in 63 patients with bilateral and 174 patients with unilateral testicular cancer and found that 74% of men with unilateral disease and 40% patients with bilateral disease were able to achieve paternity after their first orchiectomy, with or without the use of assisted-reproductive techniques.

The most common complications of RPLND are loss of ejaculation and retrograde ejaculation, due to interruption of the retroperitoneal sympathetic nerves. During the past two decades, the frequency of these complications has been reduced from approximately 75% to approximately 33%, with the introduction of a modified right- and left-sided template for RPLND, with no effect on relapse rate [12]. The introduction of nerve-sparing techniques has allowed for even greater preservation of ejaculatory function. While surgical treatment for testicular germ cell tumors can certainly impact fertility, the impact is not as great as that of chemotherapy and radiation therapy.

10.4.2 Chemotherapy

Chemotherapy agents are divided into classes, each with specific mechanisms of action (Table 10.1) [8, 26, 27]. Because these cytotoxic agents interfere with cell division cycle, rapidly dividing cells are more susceptible to their effects. During spermatogenesis, chemotherapeutic agents most severely affect Type B spermatogonia [26]. Recovery of spermatogenic function therefore depends on survival of Type A spermatogonia. If cytotoxic therapy destroys both Type A spermatogonia in addition to Type B spermatogonia, permanent azoospermia results. The time to impairment of spermatogenesis after initiation of chemotherapy can be a few weeks, but recovery of spermatogenesis after cessation of therapy can take a few years [16].

Maymon et al. [28] have argued that Sertoli-cell damage may be a contributory factor to chemotherapy-induced azoospermia, in addition to germ cell damage. By staining testicular biopsy specimens for specific cell-differentiation factors, the authors found a mixed histologic pattern consistent with dedifferentiation of Sertoli cells in a patient who had undergone chemotherapy for testicular carcinoma [28]. Because Sertoli cells are involved in maintaining the blood–testis barrier, damage to even a fraction of Sertoli cells in a given tubule can have a disproportionately larger impact on spermatogenesis.

The testes are highly sensitive to alkylating agents. Chemotherapy regimens that include alkylating agents are more gonadotoxic than

Table 10.1 Classes of chemotherapeutic agents and risk for impairment of spermatogenesis

Group	Drug names	Risk
Alkylating agents		
Nitrogen mustards	mechlorethamine chlorambucil cyclyphosphamide melphalan ifosfamide	High High High High High
Nitrosureas	carmustine lomustine	Medium Medium
Others	busulphan	High
Antimetabolites		
Folate antagonists	methotrexate	Low
Pyrimidine analogs	cytarabine fluorouracil gemcitabine	Medium Low Low
Purine analogs	mercaptopurine thioguanine	Low Low
Cytotoxic antibiotics		
Anthracyclines	doxorubicin	Medium
Others	bleomycin dactinomycin	Low Low
Plant alkaloids		
Vinca alkaloids	vincristine vinblastine	Low Low
Topoisomerase inhibitors	etoposide	Low
Others		
Platinum compounds	cisplatin carboplatin	Medium Medium
Miscellaneous	procarbazine dacarbazine	High High
MOPP	nitrogen mustard, vincristine, procarbazine, and prednisone	High
BEP	bleomycin, etoposide, and cisplatin	Medium
ABVD	adriamycin, bleomycin, vinblastine, and dacarbazine	Medium

those that do not contain alkylating agents. After six cycles of MOPP (nitrogen-mustard, vincristine, procarbazine, and prednisone) or a comparable regimen, 90–100% of patients experience prolonged azoospermia. In sharp contrast, regimens like ABVD (adriamycin, bleomycin, vinblastine, and dacarbazine) cause transient azoospermia in a third of patients, who usually go on to make a full recovery [29]. For this very reason, chemotherapy cocktails used in the treatment of non-Hodgkin's lymphoma are much less gonadotoxic than those used for Hodgkin's lymphoma [30].

A large study by the European Organization for Research and Treatment of Cancer (EORTC) analyzed FSH levels as a measure of fertility in men treated with chemotherapy or nonpelvic radiotherapy [26]. FSH was elevated in 60% of patients treated with alkylating chemotherapy, compared to 8% of patients treated with nonalkylating chemotherapy and 3% of patients treated with radiotherapy. Recovery of spermatogenesis is, however, often associated with a normalization of FSH level. Patients treated with alkylating agents were less likely to return to normal FSH levels than those treated with nonalkylating agents. In addition, recovery, if it did occur, took considerably longer in patients treated with alkylating vs. nonalkylating chemotherapy and was dependent on the dose of alkylating agents received.

Standard treatment for testicular cancer consists of platinum-based combination chemotherapy including bleomycin, etoposide, and cisplatin (BEP). The cytotoxic effects of cisplatin are mediated by induction of DNA cross-linking, while etoposide causes toxicity due to its interaction with Topoisomerase II. Shortly after initiation of chemotherapy, semen analysis demonstrates oligospermia, decreased sperm motility, decreased chromatin integrity, and increased abnormal morphology [31]. Not surprisingly, the gonadotoxicity of the BEP regimen for testicular cancer is thought to be less than that of regimens that include alkylating agents. While individual responses may be quite variable following chemotherapy for testis cancer, spermatogenesis, if it recovers, will do so in the majority of patients within 4 years.

The risk of permanent azoospermia after chemotherapy is drug-specific and dose-dependent. Pont and Albrecht concluded in their review that cumulative doses of >400 mg/m^2 of Cisplatin given to testicular cancer patients led to irreversible impairment of gonadal function [30]. Similarly, gonadal dysfunction is well documented in over 80% of patients who receive >300 mg/m^2 of cyclophosphamide [30].

10.4.3 Radiation Therapy

The testis is one of the most radiosensitive tissues in the body. Radiotherapy produces lethal cell damage to most tissues, including the male gonad, by inducing double-strand DNA breaks not amenable to repair. Like chemotherapy-induced damage, radiotherapy-induced damage is dose-dependent; the speed of onset of this damage, chance of reversal, and time to recovery of spermatogenesis are all related to the testicular dose of irradiation [30]. Spermatogonia can be affected by doses as small as 0.15 Gy, although spermatogenesis has been shown to recover at doses of up to 1–3 Gy. Permanent azoospermia can be seen at doses exceeding 4 Gy [32]. It is possible that men with germ cell neoplasia might be more vulnerable to the effects of irradiation because spermatogenic function in these individuals is already abnormal before irradiation.

In contrast, Leydig cells are more resistant to radiation, and doses exceeding 20 Gy are usually needed to produce hypogonadism [8]. Graded doses of radiation therapy (14–20 Gy) in patients with testicular germ cell neoplasia have been linked to a gradual and continued decline in testosterone levels at a rate of approximately 3.6% per year [33]. In one study, this decline lasted over 5 years, irrespective of the treatment, and 40% of the patients required androgen supplementation [33].

Men with testicular germ cell cancer are treated with radiotherapy given in fractionated doses, which is known to be more gonadotoxic than the bioequivalent dose given in one single sitting. In men with CIS in the contralateral testis, treatment with fractionated radiotherapy (20 Gy given in ten fractions of 2 Gy) led to eradication not only of the CIS, but also of germ cells [34]. Sertoli and Leydig cells were preserved in this patient population.

Several studies have confirmed that subdiaphragmatic irradiation can cause profound, dose-dependent impairment of spermatogenesis due to radiation reaching the testis. The effect is due to scatter, more so than direct irradiation of the testes, and the use of a gonadal shield have been shown to be beneficial even in cases of radiotherapy focused on, and limited to, the para-aortic region [35]. In the absence of a testicular shield, the median testicular dose received has been calculated to be as high as 1.7 Gy [36].

Radiotherapy has a much more deleterious effect on fertility than chemotherapy. In a large, retrospective study of 451 patients with testicular germ cell tumors, patients were divided into two groups, based on whether they were treated with orchiectomy and chemotherapy, or orchiectomy and radiotherapy [37]. Only two thirds of the couples who attempted a pregnancy after treatment for testicular cancer were successful, echoing the data from other studies that have shown a 30% decrease in fertility in testicular cancer patients compared to the general population [37–39]. With respect to specific treatment modalities, the authors found that cumulative conception rates were much lower for patients treated with radiotherapy compared to those treated with chemotherapy [37]. The recovery of sperm production following radiotherapy can take up to 60–80 weeks after a dose of 0.32 Gy [38], but has been reported to take up to 9 years in some cases [36]. However, most patients can expect spermatogenic recovery within 2 years of radiation.

10.4.4 Multimodal Therapy

Over the last two decades, BMT has become an important treatment modality for hematological malignancies, and a combination of high-dose chemotherapy and TBI is frequently used in preparative regimens for BMT. The primary aims of the preparative regimens are myeloablation in order to enable grafting of donor bone marrow and the eradication of malignant cells that might have survived previous therapy [40]. Bakker et al. investigated pubertal development in 21 prepubertal boys treated with TBI and BMT. The majority of boys had elevated serum LH and FSH, with concomitant low testicular volumes, suggestive of severe impairment of reproductive gonadal function [40]. A second group of authors has examined semen parameters in BMT patients conditioned with a single alkylating agent, two alkylating agents, or an alkylating agent plus irradiation. Recovery of spermatogenesis was best in patients receiving single or dual-agent chemotherapy (90 and 50%, respectively), followed by patients receiving chemotherapy and irradiation (17%) [41]. Patients treated with a single alkylating agent also had better sperm quality and faster recovery of spermatogenesis compared to the other two groups of patients. In patients receiving a combination of chemotherapy and radiation, recovery of spermatogenesis was delayed as much as 9 years after cessation of therapy in some cases [41].

Recently, nonmyeloablative stem cell transplantation has been introduced, which employs conditioning regimens of reduced intensity, in an effort to reduce gonadotoxicity. Kyriacou et al. have compared the impact of myeloablative and nonmyeloablative regimens on the germ cell and Leydig cell compartments in 32 men. Study results showed that the nonmyeloablative regimen was gonadotoxic and affected both the germ cell and Leydig cell compartments, but damage to the germ cell compartment was more severe with myeloablative regimens that included TBI [42].

Even when multimodal therapy is used, the irradiation component of therapy appears to have impact of a greater magnitude and longer duration on the spermatogenesis cycle. Limiting the radiation dose in multimodal therapy may improve posttreatment gonadal function in these patients.

10.5 Fertility Following Cancer Treatment

Although cancer treatment can induce azoospermia in many men, fortunately, this effect is usually temporary and recovery of spermatogenesis to some extent can be seen months to years after end of treatment. However, sperm quality may be reduced compared with pretreatment levels, as reported in the case of testicular cancer and hematological malignancies [43, 44]. In a large French study of 451 testicular cancer survivors, the fertility rate was found to be 30% lower after cancer treatment, but was nevertheless significant at 67% [37]. Other authors have reported similar fertility rates of 71–82%, with a small proportion of these pregnancies achieved using assisted-reproductive techniques [32]. Brydoy et al. have reported a 15-year actuarial posttreatment paternity rate of 71% among survivors of unilateral testicular cancer, without the use of cryopreserved semen [44]. Not surprisingly, patients with the highest intensity of treatment had the longest time to conception.

Among survivors of lymphoma, posttreatment fertility rates of 49–71% have been reported, depending on the treatment modality and chemotherapy cocktail used [26]. For Hodgkin's lymphoma patients, use of the ABVD regimen has been associated with a lower incidence of gonadotoxicity compared to the MOPP regimen, with 90% of patients recovering normal sperm counts 12 months after cessation of therapy [8].

Posttreatment fertility is lowest among leukemia survivors, especially those who undergo chemotherapy in combination with TBI. This regimen has been shown to result in permanent azoospermia in 83% of patients, severe oligospermia in the remainder, with spontaneous conceptions rare [41].

Although conception is unlikely while patients are on cytotoxic therapy, contraception is recommended for at least 6 months following therapy, given the theoretical risk of teratogenic effects of treatment. Tempest et al. used fluorescence in situ hybridization analysis to evaluate aneuploidy in sperm DNA from testicular cancer and Hodgkin's lymphoma patients and found increased aneuploidy frequency prior to, and up to 2 months from the start of, chemotherapy [45]. They therefore recommended delayed attempts at conception 2 years after the end of treatment. Most authors recommend a waiting period between 6 and 24 months.

10.6 Fertility Preservation

Any discussion of fertility in cancer survivors must involve both biologic and psychosocial considerations. Survivors may be less likely to find a partner, or less inclined to want children because of the psychological effects of the disease or treatment, or because of fear of an increased risk of congenital malformation in the offspring of parents who have received cytotoxic therapy. Nevertheless, a recent report by Schover et al. revealed that 51% of men with cancer expressed their wish to preserve their capacity for procreation in the future, including 77% of men who were still childless when their cancer was diagnosed [46]. Strategies of fertility preservation can be broadly divided into two categories: pre- and postcytotoxic therapy. Semen cryopreservation prior to initiation of cancer therapy remains the cornerstone for fertility preservation in the majority of patients. Recent research has focused on methods of improving posttreatment fertility. However, the alternatives to semen cryopreservation, such as testicular stem cell transplantation or testicular tissue transplantation, are experimental at present.

10.6.1 Pretreatment Options

Patient counseling and access to sperm banking should be a standard component of patient education and decision-making before the initiation of cytotoxic cancer therapy. Yet, a significant percentage of patients do not bank sperm before undergoing treatment. Based in part on the type of malignancy, the treatment modality, the availability of resources, the urgency to treat, and the knowledge of the oncologist regarding reproductive technology, the options of sperm cryopreservation are not always discussed with patients. Furthermore, in patients who are prepubertal or young adolescents, obtaining mature sperm for cryopreservation is not always possible or appropriate [47]. Even patients who chose cryopreservation are not always able to pursue it, if spermatogenesis is sufficiently impaired due to the underlying malignancy. Nevertheless, pretreatment sperm cryopreservation remains the only means of ensuring semen availability for future use, and studies have documented the use of cryopreserved sperm with good result up to 15 years after initial preservation [27].

In order to compensate as best as possible for tumor-induced impairment of spermatogenesis, Schrader et al. have described the use of testicular sperm extraction (TESE) prior to the onset of cancer therapy [48]. The authors noted successful sperm retrieval in 8 of 17 azoospermic patients (47%), with no delay in initiating cancer treatment. Two patients chose to use the cryopreserved sperm; there was one successful pregnancy.

Down-regulation of spermatogenesis prior to the initiation of cytotoxic therapy has been proposed as a means of preventing the deleterious effects of cancer therapies on sperm production. However, given the length of the spermatogenesis cycle in humans, hormonal inhibition may require several weeks to completely inhibit sperm production, thereby delaying cancer therapy for weeks as well. Therefore, such a strategy, although logical, may not be technically feasible [27].

10.6.2 Posttreatment Options

Men who remain azoospermic long after undergoing chemotherapy have traditionally been considered sterile. However, sperm retrieval in these patients is possible using microdissection TESE. Even in men previously treated for testicular germ cell tumors, despite the presence of a solitary testis, the sperm retrieval rate with TESE is 67% [49]. Chan et al. reported on the success rate of TESE followed by ICSI in a cohort of 17 patients. Sperm retrieval was accomplished in 45% of the patients, with biochemical pregnancy in four couples, clinical pregnancy in three couples, and live deliveries in two couples [50]. In a separate study, Mesegue et al. showed that sperm recovery rates were higher in patients with testicular cancer than with hematological malignancies (67% vs. 20%), and that sperm were more often retrieved from patients treated with chemotherapy alone or with RPLND, compared to those receiving chemotherapy and radiation therapy [51]. From a histopathological point of view, sperm were retrieved from patients with Sertoli cell-only syndrome, severe hypospermatogenesis, and maturation arrest [51]. Data from other studies report similar success rates [52]. For patients suffering from persistent azoospermia after cytotoxic cancer therapy, the combination of TESE and ICSI has certainly introduced new opportunities for fertility.

Spermatogenesis restoration by hormone treatment after cytotoxic therapy has been studied in animal models using GnRH agonists. The resulting suppression of FSH and testosterone secretion has been shown to remove the block in spermatogenesis [53]. However, only one of seven trials using hormone suppression to prevent gonadotoxicity in humans showed a positive result. The value of application of this treatment is currently uncertain.

Germ cell transplantation is being considered as a new tool for fertility preservation in cancer patients [54] and has been applied to restore spermatogenesis in mice. However, when the technique was applied in primates, no recovery of sperm counts was noted [55]. Although promising in theory, at present, germ cell transplantation remains very much an experimental technique in humans.

In the same vein, testicular tissue allograft has been proposed as a treatment to restore fertility if no recovery of spermatogenesis can be established after cessation of cytotoxic therapy. The technique has been successfully performed in animal models [54], but human studies to date are lacking. One concern with this approach has been the possibility, albeit small, of reintroducing malignant cells via the transplanted testicular issue. For example, as few as five reintroduced cells are sufficient for leukemia to recur [8].

In vitro culture and maturation of spermatogonial cells in specific stages of development have also been described. Tesarik et al. previously cultured primary spermatocytes in premeiotic arrest to produce morphologically abnormal but developmentally competent gametes, which were then used for successful micromanipulation-assisted fertilization [56].

Although considerable research effort is being directed to evaluate new options for fertility restoration in cancer patients, the majority of these options are not currently tangible or reproducible. Use of ART still remains the leading option for interested patients.

10.6.3 Ethical Considerations

While the availability of assisted-reproductive techniques has enabled some cancer patients with azoospermia to father children, concerns have been raised about the safety of IVF and ICSI in patients who have received chemotherapy or radiation therapy. DNA damage induced by cytotoxic cancer therapies may result in genetic errors that cannot be repaired in late-stage spermatids and spermatocytes. These germ cell mutations might increase the risk of congenital malformations, growth disturbances, and even cancer in the offspring of cancer patients.

DNA and chromosomal aberrations that can be transmitted by sperm include aneuploidy, structural aberrations, epigenetic modifications, nucleotide repeats, and gene mutations. Controversy exists as to the degree and reversibility of DNA damage secondary to chemotherapy and radiation therapy. Unfortunately, most studies addressing this topic are very limited in size. In testicular cancer patients treated with BEP chemotherapy, an abnormally high percentage of DNA-damaged sperm has been found by Spermon et al. [57]. The same chemotherapy regimen has also been linked with altered chromatin quality in sperm from a mouse model [31]. Similarly, increased rates of human sperm aneuploidy have been reported for up to 18–24 months following initiation of chemotherapy [58]. On the contrary, Thomson et al. have shown that, despite a reduction in sperm concentration, the sperm produced by cancer patients carries as much healthy DNA as the sperm produced by healthy, age-matched controls [59]. Other authors have reported chromosomal aneuploidies after alternative chemotherapy regimens, but these anomalies have been transient and self-limited [60]. Most recently, Thomas et al. have reiterated the absence of long-term effects of chemotherapy or radiation therapy on sperm aneuploidy rates, based on a cohort of 38 patients [61]. Based on current evidence, recommending a delay from the cessation of treatment to attempt pregnancy of 18–24 months is prudent.

To date, epidemiologic studies have not shown an increased risk of congenital anomalies, genetic diseases, or chromosomal abnormalities in the offspring of male cancer survivors, compared to the offspring of age-matched, healthy controls [45, 62, 63]. These studies do have shortcomings. The majority of reports were individual case studies or had small sample sizes, and thus would only have been able to detect a three- to fivefold increase in abnormalities. It should also be emphasized that most of the children in these studies were conceived spontaneously. With the use of IVF and ICSI, the chance of passing on a defective genetic material to the next generation may be higher because the mechanism of natural selection no longer applies with these technologies. The available data from offspring of cancer survivors are limited, representing diverse cancers, therapies, time to pregnancies, and reproductive outcomes. Long-term follow-up of these children is needed to better answer the concern for genetic transmission of germline mutations.

10.7 Summary

Current cancer therapies have significantly improved survival rates for young patients suffering from a variety of malignancies, including testicular cancer, Hodgkin's lymphoma, and leukemia. However, cancer therapies are often aggressive, and side effects are common. Most patients demonstrate pretreatment impairment of spermatogenesis. Further harmful effects of cytotoxic therapy depend on the agents used and the dose delivered. It is not possible to predict with certainty if spermatogenesis will return to normal after therapy [64]. Therefore, greater attention needs to be paid to the treatment modalities used, in order to prevent gonadotoxity to the extent possible. Sperm cryopreservation should be discussed with all men of reproductive age prior to the onset of cytotoxic therapy. Fertility rates in these patients have already improved with the use of TESE and ICSI. Based on current evidence, there appears to be no increased biologic or genetic risk to offspring of cancer survivors. With ongoing research, a better understanding of fertility preservation in these men is expected.

References

1. De Rooij DG, Russell LD. Everything you wanted to know about spermatogonia but were afraid to ask. J Androl. 2000;21:776–98.
2. Bordallo MA, Guimaraes MM, et al. Decreased serum inhibin B/FSH ratio as a marker of Sertoli cell function in male survivors after chemotherapy in childhood and adolescence. J Pediatr Endocrinol Metab. 2004;17(6):879–87.
3. Crofton PM, Thomson AB, et al. Is inhibin B a potential marker of gonadotoxicity in prepuberal children treated for cancer? Clin Endocrinol. 2003;58(3):296–301.
4. Schlatt S, Arslan M, et al. Endocrine control of testicular somatic and premeiotic germ cell development in the immature testis of the primate *Macaca mulatta*. Eur J Endocrinol. 1995;113:235–47.
5. Schlatt S, Weinbauer GF. Immunohistochemical localization of proliferating cell nuclear antigen as a tool to study cell proliferation in rodent and primate testes. Int J Androl. 1994;17:214–22.
6. Matsumiya K, Meistrich ML, et al. Stimulation of spermatogonial differentiation in juvenile spermatogonial depletion (jsd) mutant mice by gonadotropin releasing hormone antagonist. Endocrinology. 1999;140:4912–5.
7. Bahadur G, Ling KL, et al. Semen quality and cryopreservation in adolescent cancer patients. Hum Reprod. 2002;17:3157–61.
8. Dohle GR. Male infertility in cancer patients: review of the literature. Int J Urol. 2010;17:327–31.
9. Foster RS, Rubin LR, et al. Detection of anti-sperm antibodies in patients with primary testicular cancer. Int J Androl. 1991;14:179–85.
10. Ho GT, Gardner H, et al. The effect of testicular nongerm cell tumors on local spermatogenesis. Fertil Steril. 1994;62:162–6.
11. Ho GT, Gardner H, et al. Influence of testicular carcinoma on ipsilateral spermatogenesis. J Urol. 1992;148:821–5.
12. Petersen PM, Skakkebaek NE, Giwercman A. Gonadal function in men with testicular cancer: biological and clinical aspects. APMIS. 1998;106:24–36.
13. Berthelsen JG, Skakkebaek NE. Gonadal function in men with testicular cancer. Fertil Steril. 1983;39:68–75.
14. Willemse PHB, Sleiffer DT, et al. Altered Leydif cell function in patients with testicular cancer: evidence for a bilateral testicular defect. Acta Endocrinol. 1983;102:616–24.

15. Petersen PM, Giwercman A, et al. Impaired testicular function in patients with carcinoma in situ of the testis. J Clin Oncol. 1999;17(1):173–9.
16. Jacobsen KD, Fossa SD, et al. Gonadal function and fertility in patients with bilateral testicular germ cell malignancy. Eur Urol. 2002;42:229–38.
17. Che M, Tamboli P, et al. Bilateral testicular germ cell tumors: twenty-year experience at M.D. Andersen Cancer Center. Cancer. 2002;95:1228–33.
18. Heidenreich A, Weissbach L, et al. Organ sparing-surgery for malignant germ cell tumor of the testis. J Urol. 2001;166:2161–5.
19. Dieckmann KP, Loy V. Prevalence of contralateral testicular intraepithelial neoplasia in patients with testicular germ cell neoplasms. J Clin Oncol. 1996;14:3121–5.
20. Lass A, Akagbosu F, et al. A programme of semen cryopreservation for patients with malignant disease in a tertiary infertility center: lessons from 8 years' experience. Hum Reprod. 1998;13(11):3256–61.
21. Rueffer U, Breuer K, et al. Male gonadal dysfunction in patient's with Hodgkin's disease prior to treatment. Ann Oncol. 2001;12:1307–11.
22. Sieniawski M, Reineke T, et al. Assessment of male fertility in patient's with Hodgkin's lymphoma treated in the German Hodgkin Study Group (GHSG) clinical trials. Ann Oncol. 2008;19:1795–801.
23. Van Beek RD, Smit M, et al. Inhibin B is superior to FSH as a serum marker for spermatogenesis in men treated for Hodgkin's lymphoma with chemotherapy during childhood. Hum Reprod. 2007;22(12):3215–22.
24. Kulkarni SS, Sastry PS, et al. Gonadal function following ABVD therapy for Hodgkin's disease. Am J Clin Oncol. 1997;20:354–7.
25. Hallak J, Kolletis PN, et al. Cryopreservation of sperm from patients with leukemia: is it worth the effort? Cancer. 1999;85(9):1973–8.
26. Van der Kaaij MAE, Heutte N, et al. Sperm quality before treatment in patients with early stage Hodgkin lymphoma enrolled in EORTC-GELA lymphoma group trials. Haematologica. 2009;94:1691–7.
27. Puscheck E, Philip PA, Jeyendran RS. Male fertility preservation and cancer treatment. Cancer Treat Rev. 2004;30:173–80.
28. Maymon BB, Yogev L, et al. Sertoli cell inactivation by cytotoxic damage to the human testis after cancer chemotherapy. Fertil Steril. 2004;81(5):1391–4.
29. Lampe H, Horwich A, et al. Fertility after chemotherapy for testicular germ cell cancer. J Clin Oncol. 1997;15:239–45.
30. Howell SJ, Shalat SM. Testicular function following chemotherapy. Hum Reprod Update. 2002;7:363–9.
31. Delbes G, Hales BF, Robaire B. Effects of chemotherapy cocktail used to treat testicular cancer on sperm chromatin integrity. J Androl. 2007;28(2):241–9.
32. Schmidt KLT, Carlsen E, Andersen AN. Fertility treatment in male cancer survivors. Int J Androl. 2007;30:413–9.
33. Peterson PM, Giwercman A, et al. Effect of graded testicular doses of radiotherapy in patients treated for carcinoma in situ of the testis. J Clin Oncol. 2002;20:1537–43.
34. Giwercman A, von der Maase H, et al. Localised irradiation of testis with carcinoma in situ: effects on Leydig cell function and eradication of malignant germ cells in 20 patients. J Clin Endocrinol Metab. 1991;73:596–603.
35. Bieri S, Rouzaud M, Miralbell R. Seminoma of the testis: is scrotal shielding necessary when radiotherapy is limited to the para-aortic nodes? Radiother Oncol. 1999;50(3):349–53.
36. Hansen PV, Trykker H, et al. Long-term recovery of spermatogenesis after radiotherapy in patients with testicular cancer. Radiother Oncol. 1990;18:117–25.
37. Huyghe E, Matsuda T, et al. Fertility after testicular cancer treatments: results of a large multicenter study. Cancer. 2004;100:732–7.
38. Hahn EW, Feingold SM, et al. Recovery from aspermia induced by low-dose radiation in seminoma patients. Cancer. 1982;50:337–40.
39. Fossa SD, Kravdal O. Fertility in Norwegian testicular cancer patients. Br J Cancer. 2000;82:737–41.
40. Bakker B, Massa GG, et al. Pubertal development and growth after total-body irradiation and bone marrow transplantation. Eur J Pediatr. 2000;159:31–7.
41. Anserini P, Chiodi S, et al. Semen analysis following allogeneic bone marrow transplantation. Bone Marrow Transplant. 2002;30:447–51.
42. Kyriacou C, Kottardis PD, et al. Germ cell damage and Leydig cell insufficiency in recipients of nonmyeloablative transplantation for hematological malignancies. Bone Marrow Transplant. 2003;31:45–50.
43. Bahadur G, Ozturk O, et al. Semen quality before and after gonadotoxic treatment. Hum Reprod. 2005;20:774–81.
44. Brydoy M, Fossa SD, et al. Paternity following treatment for testicular cancer. J Natl Cancer Inst. 2005;97:1580–8.
45. Tempest HG, Ko E, et al. Sperm aneuplody frequencies before and after chemotherapy in testicular cancer and Hodgkin's lymphoma patients. Hum Reprod. 2008;23(2):251–8.
46. Schover LR, Brey K, et al. Knowledge and experience regarding cancer, infertility, and sperm banking in younger male survivors. J Clin Oncol. 2002;20:1880–9.
47. Bahadur G, Ling KLE, et al. Semen production in adolescent cancer patients. Hum Reprod. 2002;17(10):2654–6.
48. Schrader M, Muller M, et al. "Onco-TESE": testicular sperm extraction in azoospermic cancer patients before chemotherapy – new guidelines? Urology. 2003;61:421–5.
49. Meacham RB. Testicular sperm retrieval in the management of chemotherapy-induced azoospermia. J Androl. 2003;24(6):807.
50. Chan PTK, Palermo GD, et al. Testicular sperm extraction combined with intracytoplasmic sperm injection in the treatment of men with persistent azoospermia postchemotherapy. Cancer. 2001;92:1632–7.
51. Meseguer M, Garrido N, et al. Testicular sperm extraction (TESE) and ICSI in patients with permanent

azoospermia after chemotherapy. Hum Reprod. 2003;18(6):1281–5.
52. Damani MN, Master V, et al. Post-chemotherapy ejaculatory azoospermia: fatherhood with sperm from testis tissue with intracytoplasmic sperm injection. J Clin Oncol. 2002;20:888–90.
53. Meistrich ML. Restoration of spermatogenesis by hormone treatment after cytotoxic therapy. Acta Paediatr Suppl. 1999;88(433):19–22.
54. Meacham S, von Schonfeld V, et al. Spermatogonia: stem cells with a great perspective. Hum Reprod. 2001;12:825–34.
55. Schlatt S, Foppiani L, et al. Germ cell transplantation into X-irradiated monkey testes. Hum Reprod. 2002;17(1):55–62.
56. Tesarik J, Bagceci M, et al. Restoration of fertility by in-vitro spermatogenesis. Lancet. 1999;353:555–6.
57. Spermon JR, Ramos L, et al. Sperm integrity pre and post chemotherapy in med with testicular cancer. Hum Reprod. 2006;21(7):1781–6.
58. Tempest HGT, Ko E, Chan P, Robaire B, Rademaker A, Martin RH. Sperm aneuploidy frequencies analysed before and after chemotherapy in testicular cancer and Hodgkin's lymphoma patients. Hum Reprod. 2008;23:251–8.
59. Thomson AB, Campbell AJ, et al. Semen quality and spermatozoal DNA integrity in survivors of childhood cancer: a case-control study. Lancet. 2002;360(9330): 361–7.
60. Robbins WA, Meistrich ML, et al. Chemotherapy induces transient sex chromosomal and autosomal aneuploidy in human sperm. Nat Genet. 1997;16(1):74–8.
61. Thomas C, Cans C, et al. No long-term increase in sperm aneuploidy rates after anticancer therapy: sperm fluorescence in situ hybridization analysis in 26 patients treated for testicular cancer or lymphoma. Clin Cancer Res. 2004;10:6535–43.
62. Dodds L, Marrett LD, et al. Case-control study of congenital anomalies in children of cancer patients. Br Med J. 1993;307(6897):164–8.
63. Senturia YD, Peckham CS. Children fathered by men treated with chemotherapy for testicular cancer. Eur J Cancer. 1990;26(4):429–32.
64. Naysmith TE, Blake DA, et al. Do men undergoing sterilizing cancer treatments have a fertile future? Hum Reprod. 1998;13:3250–5.

Environmental Insults on Spermatogenesis

11

Stefan S. du Plessis and Ashok Agarwal

Abstract

The frequency of defective spermatogenesis and accompanying decreases in sperm parameters such as sperm count and motility appears to be on the increase. Arguably one of the most compelling reasons for this phenomenon is the influence of environmental factors on male reproduction. Despite spermatogenesis being a function of only the mature testis, environmental insults during maternal, perinatal, and prepubertal phases can indirectly influence eventual sperm production in the adult male. It is believed that exposure during these phases of the developing testis leads to irreversible effects on spermatogenesis, while the accompanying effects of adulthood exposure are in all probability reversible.

This chapter explores the various environmental factors that can influence spermatogenesis, both directly and indirectly (i.e., exposure during all the stages from the developing fetus all the way up to and in the adult male). In this overview, not only are the effects of environmental chemicals and toxins discussed, but the focus is also on several lifestyle factors and occupational exposure that can impinge on the process of sperm production. Furthermore, the role of epigenetic defects that can result in defects in transgenerational inheritance due to environmental insults is also investigated briefly.

Despite the lack of conclusive studies, it is evident from this overview that there are enough compelling reasons to believe that the future of male gamete production may be actively affected by the environment.

Keywords

Spermatogenesis • Environmental • Chemical • Lifestyle factors • Epigenetics • Oxidative stress • Endocrine disrupting • Maternal exposure • Testis

A. Agarwal (✉)
Center for Reproductive Medicine, Cleveland Clinic,
Cleveland, Ohio, USA
e-mail: agarwaa@ccf.org

C. Racowsky et al. (eds.), *Biennial Review of Infertility: Volume 2*,
DOI 10.1007/978-1-4419-8456-2_11, © Springer Science+Business Media, LLC 2011

11.1 Introduction

Production of gametes in the male occurs as a process known as spermatogenesis and occurs in the testes. This stepwise progression from diploid spermatogonia to ultimately turn into haploid spermatozoa is a truly remarkable process that requires delicate control and takes approximately 64 days to complete in humans. Spermatogenesis is a highly synchronized event that involves stage- and testis-specific gene expression, mitotic and meiotic division, and histone-protamine substitution [1]. Sperm production starts at puberty and continues uninterrupted until death, unlike oogenesis in females. Due to the complexity of germ cell development, spermatogenesis is dependent on optimal conditions. It is a critical period during which many things can go wrong, making spermatogenesis inherently more susceptible to disruption by external factors [2].

In recent decades, couple infertility has been on the increase with male factor infertility identified as one of the most common causes thereof. It is estimated that paternal factors contribute 30–50% towards all infertility cases [1]. Male reproductive health and semen quality seem to be on the decline with Toppari et al. [3] reporting that mean sperm counts in the general population has decreased by 50% in the past 50 years [4–8]. The incidence of testicular cancer and cryptorchidism increased in parallel to defective spermatogenesis. This decline in male fertility is proposed to be the result of a variety of environmental factors that impact both directly and indirectly the process of spermatogenesis [9, 10]. The key motivation for this argument is that significant lifestyle and environmental changes have occurred during this same period of time. This is substantiated by the rapid expansion of the chemicals industry in both the developed and developing worlds during the latter part of the twentieth century which has resulted in the release of a plethora of toxins and xenobiotics into the environment [11]. These foreign molecules, including pesticides, herbicides, cosmetics, preservatives, cleaning materials, municipal and private waste, pharmaceuticals, and industrial by-products have worked their way into our lives in a variety of forms [11]. Changes in male reproductive neuroendocrine function in response to environmental challenges have also been implicated to affect reproductive function and spermatogenesis. This phenomenon is more evolutionary by nature and does not have acute effects on sperm production [12].

The disruption of spermatogenesis seems to involve two fundamentally different routes of exposure. As spermatogenesis only occurs in the mature testis, environmental insults can directly affect male germ cells throughout adulthood. The second route by which environmental insults exert an influence on spermatogenesis is less direct. It can act on events preceding gamete production through exposure of women during pregnancy and subsequent disruption of testicular development in the male fetus as well as during infancy [11, 13].

The evidence for and against environmental insults as key factors in decreased spermatogenesis and male infertility is not very clear-cut, but nonetheless evidence indicates that this is a serious health issue requiring closer scrutiny [11]. This chapter will therefore aim to highlight and address various environmental insults which can directly impede the process of spermatogenesis in the mature testis, while it will also briefly refer to and discuss any preceding events influencing spermatogenesis indirectly. For the purpose of this review, both lifestyle and occupational factors will be included under the umbrella term of environmental factors.

11.2 Maternal and Perinatal Exposure to Environmental Insults Affecting Future Spermatogenesis in the Offspring

Spermatogenesis occurs in the male gonads only during adulthood. All the cells and structures involved in this process differentiate during fetal development. Initially, the embryo has bipotential structures that can develop into male or female gonads. The medullary region of this sexually indifferent ridge starts to differentiate into the testes, with the Sertoli cells being the first recognizable testicular cell type. During this process, the Sertoli cells enfold the germ cells to form seminiferous tubules, while the mesenchymal cells differentiate into Leydig cells in the interstitial spaces.

Spermatogonia and Sertoli cells are crucial to allow normal spermatogenesis during adulthood. It is important that germ cells multiply and differentiate normally during fetal development to ensure a sufficient pool of spermatogonia [14]. This involves proliferation of the fetal germ cells, before loss of their pluripotency. They subsequently become quiescent for a period of time before migrating to the basal lamina of the seminiferous tubules [15]. In humans, the latter phase might only occur and be finalized just prior to the onset of puberty [16].

Sertoli cell number and function play a major role in regulation of spermatogenesis and altering rates of sperm production in the adult testis [17, 18]. It is well recognized that the number of Sertoli cells is related to the level of spermatogenesis as measured by daily sperm production per testis because each Sertoli cell can only support a finite number of developing spermatozoa [19, 20]. Functions of Sertoli cells include providing nutrition and structural support to developing germ cells, phagocytosis of degenerating germ cells, production of protein hormones (e.g., inhibin), and finally release of the spermatids [17, 21–28]. According to Sharpe et al. [29], increase in Sertoli cell numbers occurs during fetal development, immediately postnatal and again near puberty. Testosterone secreted by the newly developed Leydig cells appear to regulate the first two phases of proliferation [30], while follicle-stimulating hormone (FSH) is more likely involved in the prepubertal phase [29, 31, 32].

Therefore, any exposure of these developing structures to environmental insults, while the basis for sperm production is set in place, can impact indirectly spermatogenesis during adulthood (Fig. 11.1). Sharpe [2] advocates that exposure during any of the three Sertoli cell proliferation periods, as well as during the first and last phases of germ cell differentiation, could delimit the final number of these cells and impact sperm count. The testicular dysgenesis syndrome (TDS) hypothesis furthermore suggests that these and other disorders such as cryptochidism, hypospadias, and testicular germ cell cancer have a universal fetal precursor triggered by malformation of the testis [33].

There is very little concrete evidence to prove that a relationship exists between maternal exposure to environmental insults and impaired spermatogenesis in humans. One of the problems faced with such studies is the long periods of time that may have elapsed between maternal exposure and the appearance of a condition such as offspring infertility [11]. However, results from many animal studies are reason enough to support the theory that exposure to environmental insults during development can determine spermatogenesis and fertility in adulthood [2].

In utero exposure of the male fetus to maternal lifestyle factors and environmental insults can be an important determinant of its future fertility profile. The result of these insults on male testicular development and adult spermatogenesis is likely to be irreversible [2]. This is evidenced by a study of Mocarelli et al. [34] stating that dioxin exposure, from infancy through puberty, affects semen quality while adult exposure showed no effect.

From the aforementioned information, it is clear that hormones, specifically testosterone, are important role players in promoting testicular differentiation. Maternal lifestyle or exposure to any environmental chemicals with endocrine-disrupting properties, especially antiandrogenic activity, can therefore impinge on testicular development and spermatogenesis in the adult testis. Maternal smoking and obesity have both been implicated in causing reduced sperm counts in developing male offspring. A significant decrease in total sperm count was reported in male offspring whose mothers smoked substantially during pregnancy [35–38]. In all probability it was the effect of polycyclic aromatic hydrocarbons (PAHs) or other components in the cigarette smoke which activate the aryl hydrocarbon (Ah) receptor and antagonize the androgen receptor (AR)-mediated action. Ultimately, this manifests as reduced Sertoli cell numbers [2, 39, 40].

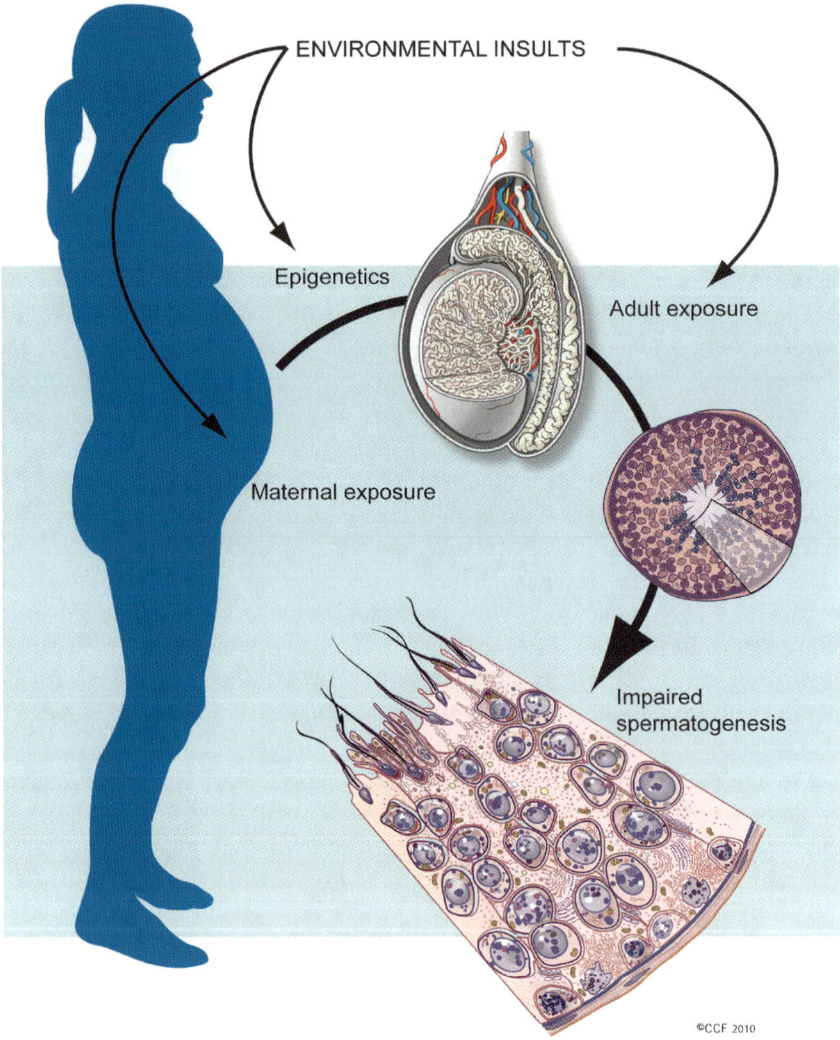

Fig. 11.1 Both maternal and adult exposure to environmental insults together with epigenetics can have an influence on spermatogenesis in the mature testis

On the other hand, maternal obesity can theoretically encroach on testicular development via increased aromatization, thereby disrupting the testosterone: estrogen ratio in the developing fetus. Various organochlorines, including many herbicides/pesticides and polychlorinated biphenyls (PCBs), are lipophilic and accumulate in fat of obese expectant mothers. During pregnancy and lactation, these accumulated compounds can be delivered to the fetus and neonate [41]. Anabolic steroids present in meat consumed by expectant mothers have also been linked to reduced spermatogenesis in the mature testis of their sons [42].

Xenobiotics (environmental estrogens) can have long-term impacts on male fertility as they are associated with reduced sperm counts. One explanation involves the capacity of these environmental estrogens to suppress production of FSH by the fetal pituitary gland, consequently leading to decreased Sertoli cells [43]. Alternatively, the xenobiotics impair Leydig cell development or function, thereby affecting testosterone production and germ cell differentiation

Table 11.1 A list of the most common environmental chemicals, including xenobiotics, which can possibly impact on future spermatogenesis in the offspring due to maternal exposure

Environmental chemicals	References
Polychlorinated biphenyl (PCB) (used as coolants and dielectric fluids in transformers)	[64]
Dioxin (by-product of combustion)	[34]
Polycyclic aromatic hydrocarbon (PAH) (constituent of exhaust fumes, smoke, and cooking processes)	[2]
Diesel exhaust fumes (mixture of particulate and gas phase pollutants)	[238]
Polybrominated compounds (used as flame retardants)	[239]
Phthalates (present in cosmetics, toiletries, and medications)	[240]
Organochlorine compounds (pesticides such as dichlorodiphenyltrichloroethane (DDT); 1,2-dibromo-3-Chloropropane)	[241]
Nonylphenol (industrial surfactant)	[61, 234]
Genistein (plant-derived phytoestrogens present in, e.g., soybeans)	[61, 242]
Bisphenol A (BPA) (used to improve polycarbonate plastics)	[52, 243]
Arsenic (used as pesticides, herbicides, insecticides, and in various alloys)	[226]
Vinclozolin (common fungicide used in vineyards)	[237]

accordingly. The action of androgen receptors may also be inhibited by these environmental estrogens within the fetal testes. Another possible mechanism is that some of these environmental estrogens are metabolized and converted to quinones. These molecules can cause cellular damage by either generating reactive oxygen species (ROS) or by binding to DNA [43]. A list of environmental chemicals, including xenobiotics, which can possibly impact spermatogenesis due to maternal exposure is given in Table 11.1.

A marked change in the testicular thermal environment postnatally is an additional factor that might influence the outcome of adult spermatogenesis [44]. Partsch et al. [45] reported the effect of reusable cotton vs. plastic-lined disposable diapers on scrotal temperature during infancy and early childhood. Significant lower recto-scrotal temperature differences, as well as higher mean 24-h scrotal skin temperatures, were observed in all boys wearing plastic-lined nappies. They subsequently hypothesized that increased scrotal temperatures in boys, as a result of disposable diaper use, could be an important contributor towards a decline in sperm production observed in recent years [3].

11.3 Environmental Insults Impinging on Spermatogenesis in the Mature Testis

Males have the capacity to reproduce continuously, unless inhibited by environmental factors. On average, men produce around 200 million sperm cells daily, which would have taken between 9 and 10 weeks to pass through the various stages of development. To allow for continual sperm production throughout adult life, a subpopulation of primordial germ cells remains as part of the stem cell pool at the outer edge of the seminiferous tubule during mitotic division. One of the daughter spermatogonia moves towards the lumen to continue the process of spermatogenesis. Spermatogonia undergo a finite number of mitotic divisions to form primary spermatocytes which enter the first meiotic division. The second meiotic division of secondary spermatocytes results in the production of haploid spermatids. Following meiosis II is the developmental phase known as spermiogenesis. This involves the differentiation and transformation of round spermatids into elongated spermatozoa. Spermatids undergo restructuring of the chromatin architecture, replacing the majority of histones first by transitional proteins and then protamines which are required for nuclear compaction. Thereafter, the spermatozoa are released into the lumen of the seminiferous tubules during spermiation and can then enter the epididymis [46]. Transit through the epididymis takes about 12 days as spermatozoa complete their final developmental stages. Spermatogenesis is under hypothalamic-pituitary-gonadal control and appears to require FSH, luteinizing hormone (LH), and testosterone, with FSH acting as the primary agent responsible for stimulating sperm maturation.

Evaluation of the results of environmental insults on spermatogenesis in human sperm studies is hampered by inconsistencies in biological analytical methods, in controlling for confounding factors, and in weakness of study design [47]. It is also recognized that documentation of cause and effect in human studies is exceedingly more difficult than in laboratory animals because of ease of intervention and measurement in animal studies, as well as the shorter gestation and development in animal studies [2]. Furthermore, animals vary less with regard to their spermatogenesis profile than humans [48]. Sharpe also emphasizes that, in reality, males are constantly exposed to a mixture of environmental chemicals that may lead to additive or interactive effects on spermatogenesis. This may confound interpretation of studies in which only one factor is evaluated [2]. Even so, there is reason to suggest that human spermatogenesis in the mature testis is affected by environmental factors during adulthood as it is becoming increasingly apparent from analysis of the biological fallout from environmental pollution that a major target of this chemical barrage is the reproductive system, particularly in the male [11, 47].

Furthermore, dramatic changes in Western lifestyle, diet, and exercise suggest that one or more of these factors appear to be involved in the etiology of declining male fertility and the impairment of sperm production. In addition, spermatogenesis in normal men is badly organized and extremely inefficient, making men highly susceptible to these environmental and lifestyle insults [2].

The remainder of this section will highlight and deal with a few environmental chemicals, lifestyle factors, and occupational exposures during adulthood that can contribute to impaired spermatogenesis (Fig. 11.1).

11.3.1 Environmental Chemicals, Toxins, and Endocrine Active Compounds

Many environmental chemicals contribute to increased toxic load and have the potential to disrupt fertility. Some have estrogenic properties and are toxic because they affect the endocrine system (endocrine disruptors). Some of these compounds affect LH-stimulated Leydig cell function, which in turn influence androgen secretion and interrupt the endocrine regulation of spermatogenesis. Not only can endocrine disruptors affect the testosterone:estradiol ratio and their respective roles in the feedback and regulation of the hypothalamus-pituitary-gonadal axis, but it can also disturb the prooxidant/antioxidant system of the cells. This can lead to the generation of free radicals and ROS. These free radicals are harmful to cells once they destabilize the electrolytic balance within the cells. As spermatozoa contain a large amount of polyunsaturated fatty acids (PUFA's) in their membranes, they are more susceptible to ROS attack and lipid peroxidation.

11.3.1.1 Chemicals Produced in the Plastics Industry

Plasticizers are polyphenolic chemical additives used to enhance the flexibility and toughness of plastic. They are found in all clear, heat-resistant, and unbreakable plastics. A few of these compounds are reportedly toxic to the male reproductive system and in specific spermatogenesis.

Bisphenol A (BPA) is used to improve polycarbonate plastics and can be found in most disposable plasticware, especially in the coverings of food containers (e.g., milk, water, and infant bottles), as well as in dental materials. Potential human exposure occurs due to migration of BPA from food containers into food or migration from dental sealants and composites (fillings), ultimately ending up in the systemic circulation [49, 50]. It is estimated that 90% of Americans have BPA present in their blood. Due to it being so common, BPA is one of the more harmful known chemicals that reduce sperm count, motility, and viability in a time- and dose-dependant manner. Chitra et al. [51] reported that BPA generates ROS in various rat tissues including the reproductive organs. BPA was shown to increase the levels of H_2O_2 and TBARS (thiobarbituric acid reactive substance) in rat testicular tissue. This subsequently leads to the depletion of the antioxidant defense system. Kabuto also reported that BPA administration induces overproduction of H_2O_2 in the kidneys, liver, and testes of rats [52, 53].

Phthalate esters are also used in the plastics industry to provide flexibility and resilience to various plastic products and commonly occur in many consumer products such as plastic bags, inflatable recreational toys, blood storage bags, plastic clothing, soaps, and shampoo. One of the most commonly used and best studied phthalate esters in the plastics industry is Di(2-ethyhexyl) phthalate (DEHP) [54–57]. Animal studies provided clear evidence of reproductive toxicity due to DEHP; however, human studies lack to provide similar effects. DEHP and its most toxic metabolite mono (2-ethylhexyl) phthalate (MEHP) were shown to induce testicular atrophy and impinge on spermatogenesis in laboratory animals. Administration of phthalate esters to rats increased ROS generation within the testis with a simultaneous decrease in antioxidant levels, culminating in impaired spermatogenesis [58]. DEHP leads to the depletion of zinc in the testis that can cause the induction of oxidative stress and germ cell apoptosis. This is possibly the mechanism via which it can exert its negative effect on reproductive function [59, 60]. It is also speculated that germ cell apoptosis can be the result of redox-mediated activation of nuclear factor-kB and up-regulation of Fas ligand on Sertoli cells by MEHP [59].

Nonylphenol, another synthetic plastic additive, has estrogenic properties and can accumulate in tissues due to its lipophylic nature. It is commonly used in detergents, paints, personal care products, food processing, and the packaging industry. Adult exposure to nonylphenol has been shown to decrease sperm count [61, 62].

Despite studies reporting a link between phthalate exposure and decreased sperm counts, it is suggested that more conclusive studies are needed [2, 63, 64].

11.3.1.2 Heavy Metal Toxicity

Several studies reported impaired spermatogenesis and decreased sperm counts due to heavy metal (e.g., lead, cadmium, mercury) toxicity in men even after moderate exposure [65–68]. Metals such as aluminum and vanadium are believed to also have effects on male fertility.

Occupational lead exposure negatively affected fecundity of male workers [69]. Inorganic lead can disturb the prooxidant and antioxidant balance and cause development of oxidative stress [65]. Before being banned, lead was commonly used as an additive in paint and petroleum, leading to widespread exposure via fumes. However, due to its nature it can accumulate in fish, providing for an alternative source and form of exposure [70]. Lead has an inhibitory effect on the delta amino levulanic acid (ALA) synthase enzyme. The subsequent accumulation of ALA causes ROS generation and peroxidation of PUFA's in plasma membranes. Spermatozoa are more susceptible to lead-induced oxidative stress due to the high content of PUFA's in their plasma membrane. Another target of lead is the enzymatic antioxidant systems of the cell [65]. Lead has also been shown to hinder the activity of superoxide dismutase (SOD), catalase, and glutathione peroxidase by inhibiting the functional sulfhydril group of these enzymes [65, 71].

The toxic effect of Cadmium on the reproductive system is well established. It has been shown to be present at significantly higher levels in both the seminal plasma and blood of infertile men when compared to that of the normal population [72], while a negative correlation exists between cadmium and sperm concentrations. First, it has been shown to have antisteroidogenic effects. It lowers testosterone production due to reducing the expression of steroidogenic acute regulatory protein in the adult rat testes [73]. Yang et al. [74] reported that cadmium has direct toxic effects on the Leydig cells and thereby on testosterone levels. Furthermore, cadmium is regarded as a prooxidant and exposure causes alterations in transcription of genes and expression of L type voltage-dependent calcium channels [75]. These channels regulate calcium as well as cadmium entry into the cell. The negative effects of cadmium may be mediated by indirect generation of hydroxyl radical, superoxide anion, H_2O_2 or NO, and reduction of the zinc content. Chronic zinc deficiency is associated with increased sensitivity to oxidative stress, mainly because it serves as an antioxidant and has a protective effect on spermatogenesis [75]. In support of this theory, it was shown that chronic low-dose cadmium exposure produced a time- and dose-dependent reduction in sperm motility. Finally, it was recently discovered that cadmium impinges on spermatogenesis by disruption of the inter-Sertoli cell tight junctions and thus disrupting the blood-testis barrier [76].

Oxidative damage to sperm DNA due to inhalation of metal fumes by battery and paint factory workers/welders has been blamed for the increase in infertility and miscarriage observed in their partners [77, 78]. An assessment of heavy metal status may be necessary during infertility treatment depending on the lifestyle and occupational exposures of the couples affected [79–81].

11.3.1.3 Agriculture Fertilizers, Pesticides, and Herbicides

Due to the extensive use of chemical fertilizers in agricultural areas, nitrogen and ammonia soil saturation is occurring. Plenty of research has been performed on the effect thereof on crops, grasslands, and surrounding areas or the impact of nitrogen loading on aquatic ecosystems [82–84]. These fertilizers can stimulate NO production, and when in excess, it negatively affects spermatogenesis as seen by the decrease in motility, viability, acrosome reaction as well as ability to penetrate the oocytes [85].

Results from a study by Jurewicz et al. [86] suggest that there are consistent indications that some pesticides like dichlorodiphenyltrichloroethane (DDT), ethylenedibromide, and organophosphates affect sperm count. Studies from Wong et al. [87] and Oliva et al. [88] support these findings by reporting that men exposed to pesticides, e.g., farmers, have a higher incidence of infertility.

Various pesticides and herbicides such as lindane, methoxychlor, and dioxin-TCDD have all been linked with testicular oxidative stress and decreased sperm counts [89–92]. Lindane exposure can damage the morphology of the seminiferous tubule by affecting both gap and tight junction proteins in Sertoli cells, resulting in decreased spermatogenesis [93]. Not only does lindane lead to testicular oxidative stress, but it also decreased activity of steroidogenic enzymes and steroidal regulatory and transport proteins (e.g., androgen-binding protein), resulting in decreased circulating testosterone levels [94].

Carbendazim (methyl-2-benzimidazole carbamate) is a systemic broad-spectrum fungicide, but is also used as a preservative for fruits, paint, textiles, and leather [95]. Its detrimental effects on male reproduction include decreased mean testes weight, low sperm count, reduced seminiferous tubule diameters [96], decreased sperm motility, and increased abnormal sperm morphology [97]. A study done in rats revealed that carbendazim's deleterious effects on male reproduction are mediated via its ability to increase oxidative stress, by impairing steroidogenic enzymes and antioxidant cellular defenses. It also enhanced H_2O_2, hydroxyl radicals, and lipid peroxidation in the Leydig cells [98]. Chlorpyrifos, an organophosphate pesticide, is another agricultural chemical that can lead to ROS-induced DNA strand breaks and lipid peroxidation of spermatozoa [99].

11.3.1.4 Solvents

Humans are primarily exposed to toluene, a widely used organic solvent, via vapor inhalation. Toluene is found in paint, rubber, gasoline, adhesives, and various cleaning fluids [100]. Recent investigations have shown that toluene may induce reproductive dysfunctions. In a study done in male rats, toluene administration led to a decrease in epididymal sperm count and serum testosterone levels [101]. It mediates reproductive toxicity via oxidative damage by either inducing excessive ROS generation [101] or decreasing the antioxidant status [100].

Abnormally high concentrations of another solvent, xylene, have been found to be present in the blood and semen of workers exposed to a working environment where the air concentration of xylene exceeded the maximum allowable concentration. These men experienced decreased sperm vitality, motility, and acrosin activity [102]. Studies have shown that xylene is capable of inducing complete inhibition of mitochondrial respiration and is known to usually enhance mitochondrial ROS generation [103, 104]. This propensity of xylene to generate ROS is more than likely the basis of its harmful effects on male reproduction.

11.3.2 Lifestyle and Occupational Exposure

Exposure to certain lifestyle and occupational factors can influence the adult testis directly and lead to impaired spermatogenesis. A few of the most common issues will be subsequently discussed.

11.3.2.1 Smoking

It is well established that smoking has detrimental effects on spermatogenesis as it has been correlated with significantly lower sperm counts (10–17%), decreased motility, and impaired morphology [105–108]. A meta-analysis performed by Vine et al. [109] substantiates this association.

Smoking not only interferes with oxygen supply, but also exposes smokers to thousands of potentially harmful substances (e.g., alkaloids, nitrosamines, nicotine, hydroxycotine). Several of these toxins can lead to the generation of ROS and reactive nitrogen species, ultimately leading to oxidative stress when reaching pathophysiological concentrations [110, 111].

Saleh et al. [107] demonstrated that cigarette smoking leads to an increase in ROS levels and decreases in ROS-TAC scores in semen of smokers showing a 100-fold increase in oxidative stress and up to 5× higher cadmium levels. Furthermore, it was reported that smokers have high levels of leukocytospermia and suggested that oxidative stress develops due to ROS generation by activated leukocytes [107]. Smoke metabolites and several compounds of cigarette smoke may act as chemotactic stimuli, thereby inducing an inflammatory response, recruitment of leukocytes, and subsequent ROS generation [107, 112]. It was furthermore reported that smokers have decreased levels of seminal plasma antioxidants such as Vitamin C [113] and Vitamin E [114].

Approximately half of the arterial blood supply to the testes is drained off via arterio-venous anastomoses in the spermatic cord. This, coupled with the evidence that the testes have high metabolic requirements due to the ongoing process of spermatogenesis, translates to the testis being regarded as physiologically on the verge of being hypoxic [2, 115, 116]. Sharpe [2] speculated that any factors which compromise oxygen supply to the testis, including smoking, would have detrimental effects on spermatogenesis.

An alternative route whereby components of cigarette smoke might affect spermatogenesis is through the interaction of PAH with the Ah receptor and the subsequent effects on the AR [2, 39, 40].

A recent study showed that motility is one of the first sperm parameters affected and asthenozoospermia may be an early indicator of reduced semen quality in light smokers. This study also found the incidence of teratozoospermia to be significantly higher in heavy smokers when compared to nonsmokers [117].

11.3.2.2 Alcohol Consumption and Drugs

There is a growing body of evidence suggesting that alcohol is a lifestyle factor that impacts spermatogenesis. Moderate alcohol consumption did not show a significant impact on sperm count [118, 119]; however, chronic alcoholism appears to harm spermatogenesis and male fertility [120, 121]. Not only are impotence, testicular atrophy, and loss of sexual interest associated with alcoholism, but it is often accompanied by reduced FSH, LH, and testosterone levels [122]. Goverde et al. furthermore reported that semen volume, sperm count, motility, and number of morphologically normal sperm were significantly decreased in alcoholics when compared to nonalcoholics [123]. Excessive alcohol consumption has also been linked to oxidative stress in the testis as a significant reduction in testosterone, increase in lipid peroxidation by-products, and a drop in antioxidants were observed [124].

Many processes and factors are involved in alcohol-induced oxidative stress. One possible mechanism is the generation of ROS molecules in response to the metabolism of ethanol by the microsomal ethanol-oxidizing system (MEOS) [125, 126]. Alcohol metabolism results in NADH formation which enhances activity of the respiratory chain, including heightened oxygen use and excessive ROS formation [127]. ROS are natural cellular renegades and wreak havoc in biological systems through tissue damage, alteration of biochemical compounds, corrosion of cell membranes, and killing outrightly [128]. Alcohol also induces hypoxia that results in tissue damage. In addition, many alcohol abusers follow diets deficient in protective antioxidants [129, 130].

The association between alcohol and infertility is of great concern because the use of alcohol is widespread. In many countries, alcohol usage is extensive, especially in the teenager. The evidence regarding moderate alcohol intake is less clear, but most experts agree it is best to avoid more than 1 or 2 drinks/day.

Certain drugs, whether therapeutic, recreational, or performance enhancing, can have adverse effects on spermatogenesis. Several prescription drugs used for therapeutic purposes, especially when used chronically, can impact on spermatogenesis. Antibiotics and cancer chemotherapy usually damage the germinal epithelium [131, 132]. Some drugs may cause spermatogenic arrest (mechlorethamine) (U49), while many antimicrobials (e.g., tetracycline derivatives, sulfa drugs) impair spermatogenesis and chronic use can lead to infertility [132–134]. In a very interesting study by Hayashi et al. [135], it was shown that men who switched or stopped treatment of the most common medications (allergy relief, antiepileptics, antibiotics) had a 93% improvement in semen quality. In general, the severity of testicular influence is related to the class of therapeutic agent used, as well as the dose and duration of therapy [136].

Concrete evidence for the effect and mechanism of recreational drug abuse, such as marijuana and cocaine, on sperm production is still lacking. Several articles report that it does have detrimental effects and that the mode of action is more than likely via receptor binding and endocrine disruption or direct effect on the spermatozoa.

The use of anabolic steroids, predominantly used to enhance body image or improve performance among athletes, is on the increase and reaching epidemic proportions [136]. This can result in oligozoospermia as spermatogenesis is reduced because steroids cause suppression of LH secretion and consequently suppress intratesticular testosterone levels. Hypogonadotropic hypogonadism is therefore the most common cause for impairment of sperm production in this group [137, 138]. These defects can be reversed in the mature testis within a couple of months after discontinuation of anabolic steroid use [138].

11.3.2.3 Diet and Obesity

Diet and obesity are important lifestyle factors that can influence spermatogenesis. Accompanying modern Westernized lifestyles are changes in diets and eating habits. Not only are people eating more highly refined carbohydrate-rich food, but they are simultaneously consuming less fresh fruit and vegetables [139].

The importance of fresh fruits and vegetables in the diet was suggested in a study where decreased intake of these nutritional substances was correlated with subfertility [87]. Apart from containing antioxidants, essential nutrients like micronutrients, vitamins, and folate are found in fruit and vegetables and these substances play an important role in spermatogenesis as they are involved in DNA and RNA synthesis. It is not clear if the mechanism of higher sperm production in patients with a fruit/vegetable diet is related to dietary factors or reflects an epiphenomen.

Nutritionally deficient diets, lacking antioxidant vitamins and synergistic minerals, do not enable the quenching of reactive oxygen molecules. For example, Vitamin C and Vitamin E are essential antioxidants that protect the body's cells from damage due to oxidative stress and free radicals. Vitamin C is the most abundant antioxidant in the semen of fertile men, and it contributes to the maintenance of healthy sperm by protecting the sperm's DNA from free radical damage [140]. Vitamin E is a fat-soluble vitamin that helps protect the sperm's cell membrane from damage. Studies have shown that Vitamin E improves sperm motility and morphology. Vitamin C functions to regenerate Vitamin E, thus these vitamins may work together to improve sperm function [140–143]. Selenium is a mineral that also functions as an antioxidant and selenium supplements have been shown to increase sperm motility. A combination of selenium and Vitamin E has been shown to decrease damage due to free radicals and improve sperm motility in infertile men [144]. Diets deficient in these substances will then be unable to provide the benefits mentioned above.

Obese, overweight, and high body mass index (BMI) subjects may be at risk of infertility [145–147]. Men with BMI's greater than 25 are up to three times more at risk of infertility due to reduction in sperm count and increased DNA fragmentation. Many clarifications have been given to explain the link between obesity and decreased spermatogenesis. Firstly, excess adipose tissue leads to the conversion of more testosterone to estrogen. This subsequently results in the development of secondary hypogonadism through hypothalamic-pituitary-gonadal axis inhibition [148], thereby decreasing the levels of circulating testosterone and increasing the levels of estradiol [36, 37, 149–151]. This change in testosterone: estradiol ratio is often accompanied by reduced levels of LH and FSH [145]. More than likely, the decreased testosterone levels in the testis are responsible for impaired spermatogenesis [152].

Secondly, accumulation of suprapubic and inner thigh fat in severely obese men could lead to infertility via increased scrotal temperatures. Deposition of fat around the scrotal blood vessels can also cause impaired blood cooling and elevate testicular temperature [153]. Obese men also tend to be more sedentary which would exacerbate any temperature increases as discussed elsewhere under the Sect. 11.3.2.5.

Finally, obesity and several of its accompanying complications, namely, insulin resistance and dyslipidemia, are associated with systemic proinflammatory states and increased levels of oxidative stress [154, 155]. Oxidative stress causes sperm membrane lipid peroxidation, which results in the impairment of sperm motility, DNA damage, and impaired sperm-oocyte interaction [156, 157]. Conversely, adipose tissue releases proinflammatory adipokines that increase leukocyte production of ROS [158].

Both endocrine and exocrine (spermatogenesis) functions of the testis are believed to be influenced in direct proportion with the current trend of increased BMI and obesity in men throughout the world.

11.3.2.4 Psychological and Noise Stress

Mental stress is associated with lower levels of antioxidants, such as glutathione (GSH) and SOD, as well as higher levels of prooxidants [159]. This can create oxidative stress. Various studies have shown a correlation between stress and semen quality. One such study in particular reported that students have lower sperm counts and sperm quality during the highly stressful periods of exams [160]. Eskiocak et al. [161] were also able to link periods of psychological stress with a reduction in sperm quality, mediated by an increase in seminal plasma ROS generation and a reduction in antioxidant protection [161, 162]. It has also been established that stress can lead to increased levels of glucocorticoids and decreased levels of testosterone [163].

Similarly, Ruffoli et al. [164] demonstrated that chronic noise stress can cause accumulation of lipofuscin in the testis of mice. Moreover, it subsequently led to a decrease in testosterone production in these animals. It was previously established that corticosterone administration caused free radical production in the mitochondria of Leydig cells and that free radicals are known to stimulate lipofuscin formation [165, 166]. Ruffoli et al. [164] went on to conclude that exposure to above the normal levels of noise in the workplace or environment may be detrimental to testicular function.

11.3.2.5 Scrotal Heat Stress

The exteriorization of the male gonads into the scrotum is a uniquely mammalian feature. The most plausible explanation for such evolution is that optimal spermatogenesis requires a temperature (±34°C) markedly lower than core abdominal temperature (±37°C) [167, 168].

The concept that an elevation of testicular temperature results in impairment of spermatogenesis is widely accepted. For instance, rats whose testes were immersed into a luke warm water bath (43–45°C for 15–30 min) showed deterioration in spermatogenesis [169]. It was found that apoptosis of the pachytene spermatocytes and round spermatids were induced via the mitochondrial pathway [170–175].

Various mechanisms have evolved to allow for the testes to be kept 3–4°C below core body temperature. First, the testes descend into the very bottom of the scrotum – as far away from the body surface as possible. Second, the presence of a countercurrent heat exchanger in the form of the pampiniform plexus, as well as a vascular-rich corrugated scrotal surface (third mechanism) through which heat loss can occur, ensures further cooling of the testes.

The lower temperature leads to reduced rates of oxidative DNA damage and consequently fewer mutations in resulting sperm cells [168, 176]. Spermatozoa are stored in the epididymis often for many days or weeks. Storage occurs specifically in the cauda epididymis which is found in the coolest area of the scrotum, thereby reducing metabolic rates and oxidative damage of these spermatozoa [177].

Scrotal pathologies such as varicocele and cryptorchidism can increase testicular temperature excessively; however, lifestyle and occupation can also lead to chronically elevated scrotal temperatures that can contribute to the global trend in declining male reproductive parameters [167].

Occupational exposure to increased ambient temperatures (welders, bakers, stokers, foundry workers, furnace operators) has been shown to increase scrotal temperatures, decrease sperm density, motility and morphology, as well as significantly prolong time to pregnancy [178–180]. A few studies, however, reported no differences in sperm concentration and semen quality in men with similar occupations [181, 182]. Therefore, the influence of occupational heat exposure not yet allows for definitive conclusions [169].

Extended periods of sitting have also been correlated with increased scrotal temperatures [183, 184]. Hjollund reported a progressive increase in scrotal temperature in office workers in relation to sedentary time with sperm density being significantly decreased in men with more than 75% of their daytime scrotal temperature above 35°C [185, 186]. Various other studies support these findings. More generally speaking, sperm density is believed to decrease by 40% per 1°C increment of median daytime scrotal temperatures [186, 187]. The difference in scrotal temperatures between sitting in the office chair and sitting in a car was shown to be statistically insignificant [183]. Professional drivers such as lorry and taxi drivers have also been shown to experience reduced semen quality and increased time to pregnancy [178, 188–190].

Several studies have investigated the impact of tight vs. loose fitting underwear. On the whole, these studies are in agreement that the type of clothing can increase genital temperature [190–194]. A few studies found no significant differences [195, 196], but in general most of these studies were not well controlled. Recently, Jung et al. [197] analyzed the influence of the type of underpants under highly controlled conditions and reported that scrotal temperatures were significantly higher for tight fitting, less for loose fitting, and the least for no underwear.

Prolonged hot baths and saunas also increase scrotal temperature and have been implicated to impair spermatogenesis [192, 198–200]. Furthermore, obesity and the accompanying accumulation of adipose tissue within the groin region also result in raised testicular temperature. This has been linked to the generation of ROS and development of oxidative stress in the testis resulting in reduced sperm quality [201–203].

Febrile illnesses (e.g., influenza, Malaria) are another factor that can lead to increased scrotal temperatures. Several studies demonstrated a decrease in total sperm counts and semen quality even up to a few months after these episodes of fever [183, 204, 205].

Failure to cool the scrotum adequately therefore appears to be associated in the adult with impaired spermatogenesis.

11.3.2.6 Cell Phone and Ionizing Radiation

Stopczyk et al. [206] demonstrated that radiofrequency electromagnetic waves (RF-EMW), produced by cell phones, significantly depleted SOD-1 activity while increasing the concentration of malonyldialdehyde (MDA) after 1, 5, and 7 min of exposure in a suspension of human blood platelets. On the grounds of these results, the authors conclude that oxidative stress after exposure to microwaves may be the reason for many adverse changes in cells and could cause a number of systemic disturbances in the human body. Several animal studies also demonstrated that cell phone radiation can increase levels of MDA and decrease the levels of antioxidant enzymes, while other studies consistently reported that cell phone radiation leads to a decrease in male fertility. A few studies, however, showed conflicting results [207].

Various epidemiological studies proposed that cell phone usage may cause decreases in sperm count and other sperm parameters [208–212]. A study by Agarwal et al. [213] provided evidence that cell phone radiation can lead to generation of ROS. Results showed a significant increase in ROS production and a decrease in sperm motility, viability, and ROS-TAC score in exposed semen samples. A plausible explanation for the ROS production is stimulation of the spermatozoa's plasma membrane redox system (increase in the activity of spermatozoal NADH oxidase) by RF-EMW or the effect of EMW on leukocytes present in the neat semen. Recently, Friedman et al. [214] also suggested that RF-EMW stimulate plasma membrane NADH oxidase in mammalian cells and cause production of ROS. EMW-dependent decrease in melatonin, an antioxidant, can also predispose sperm to oxidative stress [215].

It is furthermore speculated that RF-EMW emitted from cell phones might also influence spermatogenesis via a thermal molecular effect [208]. Leydig cells are among the most susceptible cells to EMW and injury to these cells may affect spermatogenesis. A decrease in seminiferous tubular diameter and epithelium thickness was also observed after RF-EMW exposure [216].

Although many animal as well as in vitro studies have provided evidence that cell phone radiation may lead to a decrease in sperm parameters, considerable research is still required to confirm that cell phone usage impact spermatogenesis.

Chronic exposure to ionizing radiation can also cause decreased sperm quality coupled to endocrine disruption [217–219]. Results are mainly from animal studies, but prisoners volunteering for testicle X-ray irradiation as well as men exposed to radiation after the Chernobyl nuclear accident were also studied. In all cases, the doses of exposure seem to be the important determinant of the effect on spermatogenesis with higher dosages leading to even permanent sterility [47, 218, 220].

11.4 Environmental Insults, Epigenetics, and Spermatogenesis

The ability of environmental factors to promote a phenotype or disease state not only in the individual exposed, but also in subsequent progeny for successive generations is termed transgenerational inheritance. The majority of environmental factors such as nutrition or toxins do not promote genetic mutations or alterations in DNA sequence. However, these factors do have the capacity to alter the epigenome. Epimutations in the germline which become permanently programmed can allow transmission of epigenetic transgenerational phenotypes [221]. Skinner et al. [221] furthermore define epigenetics as molecular factors and processes around DNA that are mitotically stable and regulate genome activity independent of DNA sequence.

Epigenetic elements identified include DNA methylation and histone modifications [222, 223]. A special category of genes, called imprinted genes, are subjected to epigenetic programming and can be influenced by environmental exposure[224]. Epigenetic influences have been observed with environmental compounds (Fig. 11.1), nutritional factors (X45 X46), inorganic contaminants such as arsenic [225, 226], PAHs [227], endocrine disruptors such as BPA [228–230], phytoestrogens [231, 232], and chemicals used as fungicides and pesticides [233, 234].

The crucial period for epigenetic regulation and modification of the germline is during the period of primordial germ cell migration and gonadal sex determination. The permanent alteration in the epigenetic programming of the germline appears to be the mechanism involved in the transgenerational phenotype [233, 235]. The endocrine disruptor vinclozolin was used in one of the initial studies to demonstrate the ability of an environmental factor to modify epigenetic programming of the male germline. Embryonic exposure of rats through maternal administration led to adult onset of disease in the first through fourth subsequent generations [233]. This phenomenon was found to be caused by male germline changes in DNA methylation, resulting in heritable changes in transcription in tissues such as the testis [236]. It also correlated with reduced sperm number in the adult due to increases in apoptotic germ cell numbers in the testis of pubertal and adult animals [237].

Transient early life exposures in the affected individual, or transgenerational exposures if the germline is involved, are now included as causal factors for adult onset disease. Endocrine disruptors are one of the most prevalent groups of environmental compounds humans are exposed to daily. Although these compounds disrupt the endocrine system, it is the long-term response of molecular processes such as epigenetics that will promote downstream developmental-events and adult onset disease [1, 221]. Epigenetic events in the testis have just begun to be studied. New work on the function of specific histone modifications, chromatin modifiers, DNA methylation, and impact of the environment on spermotogenesis suggests that the setting of the epigenome is required for male reproductive health [1].

11.5 Conclusion

The increase in defective spermatogenesis, testicular cancer, cryptorchidism, and TDS during the past few decades is an immense cause of concern. As highlighted in this chapter, many environmental factors can impinge on human testicular function. Increased concern in many Western countries regarding the deleterious effects of environmental chemicals on male reproduction exists, but attention to this issue should now be given by developing countries as well.

Environmental chemicals and toxicants can have endocrine-disrupting properties, thereby affecting normal regulation of the hypothalamus-pituitary-gonadal axis and sperm production. Other effects of exposure can include development of oxidative stress, which in turn is also deleterious to sperm production. Similarly, a host of lifestyle and occupational factors can influence spermatogenesis as well.

As spermatogenesis exclusively occurs in the mature testis, adulthood exposure impacts directly sperm number and quality. On the contrary, perinatal exposure to environmental insults can have lasting and more severe effects on gamete production, even transgenerationally. These emphasize the importance of environmental impacts throughout the life course.

With the onset of assisted reproductive technologies, specifically intracytoplasmic sperm injection, a major proportion of infertile men is now afforded the opportunity and ability to procreate. The dilemma of this situation is that the fundamental and root cause of male fertility is not addressed, only the symptoms. Tragically, these advances in infertility treatments are also negating any advances in understanding the etiology and treatment of male infertility. It is therefore paramount that research on the reasons for male infertility, specifically with regard to the effects of environmental insults on spermatogenesis, be performed in order to solve for prevention and cure and not leaving it to future generations to try and resolve when it might already be too late.

References

1. Godmann M, Lambrot R, Kimmins S. The dynamic epigenetic program in male germ cells: its role in spermatogenesis, testis cancer, and its response to the environment. Microsc Res Tech. 2009;72(8):603–19.
2. Sharpe RM. Environmental/lifestyle effects on spermatogenesis. Philos Trans R Soc Lond. 2010; 365(1546):1697–712.
3. Toppari J, Larsen JC, Christiansen P, et al. Male reproductive health and environmental xenoestrogens. Environ Health Perspect. 1996;104 Suppl 4:741–803.
4. Irvine S, Cawood E, Richardson D, MacDonald E, Aitken J. Evidence of deteriorating semen quality in the United Kingdom: birth cohort study in 577 men in Scotland over 11 years. BMJ. 1996;312(7029): 467–71.
5. Andersen AG, Jensen TK, Carlsen E, et al. High frequency of sub-optimal semen quality in an unselected population of young men. Hum Reprod. 2000;15(2): 366–72.
6. Swan SH, Elkin EP, Fenster L. The question of declining sperm density revisited: an analysis of 101 studies published 1934-1996. Environ Health Perspect. 2000; 108(10):961–6.

7. Irvine DS. Declining sperm quality: a review of facts and hypotheses. Baillières Clin Obstet Gynaecol. 1997;11(4):655–71.
8. Carlsen E, Giwercman A, Keiding N, Skakkebaek NE. Evidence for decreasing quality of semen during past 50 years. BMJ. 1992;305(6854):609–13.
9. Agarwal A, Desai NR, Ruffoli R, Carpi A. Lifestyle and testicular dysfunction: a brief update. Biomed Pharmacother. 2008;62(8):550–3.
10. Droller MJ. Environment and the genitourinary tract. Otolaryngol Head Neck Surg. 1996;114(2):248–52.
11. Aitken RJ, Koopman P, Lewis SE. Seeds of concern. Nature. 2004;432(7013):48–52.
12. Bribiescas RG. Reproductive ecology and life history of the human male. Am J Phys Anthropol. 2001;Suppl 33:148–76.
13. Mann DR, Gould KG, Collins DC, Wallen K. Blockade of neonatal activation of the pituitary-testicular axis: effect on peripubertal luteinizing hormone and testosterone secretion and on testicular development in male monkeys. J Clin Endocrinol Metab. 1989;68(3):600–7.
14. Orth JM, Jester WF, Li LH, Laslett AL. Gonocyte-Sertoli cell interactions during development of the neonatal rodent testis. Curr Top Dev Biol. 2000;50:103–24.
15. Rajpert-De Meyts E. Developmental model for the pathogenesis of testicular carcinoma in situ: genetic and environmental aspects. Hum Reprod Update. 2006;12(3):303–23.
16. Mitchell RT, Cowan G, Morris KD, et al. Germ cell differentiation in the marmoset (*Callithrix jacchus*) during fetal and neonatal life closely parallels that in the human. Hum Reprod. 2008;23(12):2755–65.
17. Johnson L, Thompson Jr DL, Varner DD. Role of Sertoli cell number and function on regulation of spermatogenesis. Anim Reprod Sci. 2008;105(1–2):23–51.
18. McLachlan RI, Wreford NG, Robertson DM, de Kretser DM. Hormonal control of spermatogenesis. Trends Endocrinol Metab. 1995;6(3):95–101.
19. Johnson L. Spermatogenesis and aging in the human. J Androl. 1986;7(6):331–54.
20. Johnson L, Zane RS, Petty CS, Neaves WB. Quantification of the human Sertoli cell population: its distribution, relation to germ cell numbers, and age-related decline. Biol Reprod. 1984;31(4):785–95.
21. Andersson AM, Toppari J, Haavisto AM, et al. Longitudinal reproductive hormone profiles in infants: peak of inhibin B levels in infant boys exceeds levels in adult men. J Clin Endocrinol Metab. 1998;83(2):675–81.
22. Dym M, Raj HG. Response of adult rat Sertoli cells and Leydig cells to depletion of luteinizing hormone and testosterone. Biol Reprod. 1977;17(5):676–96.
23. Feig LA, Bellve AR, Erickson NH, Klagsbrun M. Sertoli cells contain a mitogenic polypeptide. Proc Natl Acad Sci USA. 1980;77(8):4774–8.
24. Jutte NH, Jansen R, Grootegoed JA, Rommerts FF, Clausen OP, van der Molen HJ. Regulation of survival of rat pachytene spermatocytes by lactate supply from Sertoli cells. J Reprod Fertil. 1982;65(2):431–8.
25. Jutte NH, Jansen R, Grootegoed JA, Rommerts FF, van der Molen HJ. FSH stimulation of the production of pyruvate and lactate by rat Sertoli cells may be involved in hormonal regulation of spermatogenesis. J Reprod Fertil. 1983;68(1):219–26.
26. Tres LL, Smith EP, Van Wyk JJ, Kierszenbaum AL. Immunoreactive sites and accumulation of somatomedin-C in rat Sertoli-spermatogenic cell co-cultures. Exp Cell Res. 1986;162(1):33–50.
27. Bellve AR, Zheng W. Growth factors as autocrine and paracrine modulators of male gonadal functions. J Reprod Fertil. 1989;85(2):771–93.
28. Johnson L, Varner DD, Thompson Jr DL. Effect of age and season on the establishment of spermatogenesis in the horse. J Reprod Fertil Suppl. 1991;44:87–97.
29. Sharpe RM, McKinnell C, Kivlin C, Fisher JS. Proliferation and functional maturation of Sertoli cells, and their relevance to disorders of testis function in adulthood. Reproduction. 2003;125(6):769–84.
30. Scott HM, Hutchison GR, Mahood IK, et al. Role of androgens in fetal testis development and dysgenesis. Endocrinology. 2007;148(5):2027–36.
31. Johnston H, Baker PJ, Abel M, et al. Regulation of Sertoli cell number and activity by follicle-stimulating hormone and androgen during postnatal development in the mouse. Endocrinology. 2004;145(1):318–29.
32. Cortes D, Muller J, Skakkebaek NE. Proliferation of Sertoli cells during development of the human testis assessed by stereological methods. Int J Androl. 1987;10(4):589–96.
33. Skakkebaek NE, Rajpert-De Meyts E, Main KM. Testicular dysgenesis syndrome: an increasingly common developmental disorder with environmental aspects. Hum Reprod. 2001;16(5):972–8.
34. Mocarelli P, Gerthoux PM, Patterson Jr DG, et al. Dioxin exposure, from infancy through puberty, produces endocrine disruption and affects human semen quality. Environ Health Perspect. 2008;116(1):70–7.
35. Storgaard L, Bonde JP, Ernst E, et al. Does smoking during pregnancy affect sons' sperm counts? Epidemiology. 2003;14(3):278–86.
36. Jensen TK, Jorgensen N, Punab M, et al. Association of in utero exposure to maternal smoking with reduced semen quality and testis size in adulthood: a cross-sectional study of 1, 770 young men from the general population in five European countries. Am J Epidemiol. 2004;159(1):49–58.
37. Jensen TK, Andersson AM, Jorgensen N, et al. Body mass index in relation to semen quality and reproductive hormones among 1, 558 Danish men. Fertil Steril. 2004;82(4):863–70.
38. Ramlau-Hansen CH, Thulstrup AM, Storgaard L, Toft G, Olsen J, Bonde JP. Is prenatal exposure to tobacco smoking a cause of poor semen quality? A follow-up study. Am J Epidemiol. 2007;165(12):1372–9.
39. Kizu R, Okamura K, Toriba A, et al. A role of aryl hydrocarbon receptor in the antiandrogenic effects of

polycyclic aromatic hydrocarbons in LNCaP human prostate carcinoma cells. Arch Toxicol. 2003;77(6): 335–43.

40. Barnes-Ellerbe S, Knudsen KE, Puga A. 2, 3, 7, 8-Tetrachlorodibenzo-p-dioxin blocks androgen-dependent cell proliferation of LNCaP cells through modulation of pRB phosphorylation. Mol Pharmacol. 2004;66(3):502–11.
41. Ramlau-Hansen CH, Nohr EA, Thulstrup AM, Bonde JP, Storgaard L, Olsen J. Is maternal obesity related to semen quality in the male offspring? A pilot study. Hum Reprod. 2007;22(10):2758–62.
42. Swan SH, Liu F, Overstreet JW, Brazil C, Skakkebaek NE. Semen quality of fertile US males in relation to their mothers' beef consumption during pregnancy. Hum Reprod. 2007;22(6):1497–502.
43. Sharpe RM. The 'oestrogen hypothesis' – where do we stand now? Int J Androl. 2003;26(1):2–15.
44. Hughes PI. How vulnerable is the developing testis to the external environment? Arch Dis Child. 2000; 83(4):281–2.
45. Partsch CJ, Aukamp M, Sippell WG. Scrotal temperature is increased in disposable plastic lined nappies. Arch Dis Child. 2000;83(4):364–8.
46. de Rooij DG, Russell LD. All you wanted to know about spermatogonia but were afraid to ask. J Androl. 2000;21(6):776–98.
47. Lahdetie J. Occupation- and exposure-related studies on human sperm. J Occup Environ Med. 1995;37(8): 922–30.
48. Sharpe RM. Lifestyle and environmental contribution to male infertility. Br Med Bull. 2000;56(3): 630–42.
49. Le HH, Carlson EM, Chua JP, Belcher SM. Bisphenol A is released from polycarbonate drinking bottles and mimics the neurotoxic actions of estrogen in developing cerebellar neurons. Toxicol Lett. 2008;176(2): 149–56.
50. Korasli D, Ziraman F, Ozyurt P, Cehreli SB. Microleakage of self-etch primer/adhesives in endodontically treated teeth. J Am Dent Assoc. 2007; 138(5):634–40.
51. Chitra KC, Latchoumycandane C, Mathur PP. Induction of oxidative stress by bisphenol A in the epididymal sperm of rats. Toxicology. 2003;185(1–2): 119–27.
52. Kabuto H, Amakawa M, Shishibori T. Exposure to bisphenol A during embryonic/fetal life and infancy increases oxidative injury and causes underdevelopment of the brain and testis in mice. Life Sci. 2004; 74(24):2931–40.
53. Obata T, Kubota S. Formation of hydroxy radicals by environmental estrogen-like chemicals in rat striatum. Neurosci Lett. 2000;296(1):41–4.
54. Gesler RM. Toxicology of di-2-ethylhexyl phthalate and other phthalic acid ester plasticizers. Environ Health Perspect. 1973;3:73–9.
55. Peakall DB. Phthalate esters: occurrence and biological effects. Residue Rev. 1975;54:1–41.
56. Ishihara M, Itoh M, Miyamoto K, et al. Spermatogenic disturbance induced by di-(2-ethylhexyl) phthalate is significantly prevented by treatment with antioxidant vitamins in the rat. Int J Androl. 2000;23(2):85–94.
57. Third National Report on Human Exposure to Environmental Chemicals. In: Center for Disease Control, 2005. http://www.cluin.org/download/contaminantfocus/pcb/third-report.pdf
58. Lee E, Ahn MY, Kim HJ, et al. Effect of di(n-butyl) phthalate on testicular oxidative damage and antioxidant enzymes in hyperthyroid rats. Environ Toxicol. 2007;22(3):245–55.
59. Kasahara E, Sato EF, Miyoshi M, et al. Role of oxidative stress in germ cell apoptosis induced by di (2-ethylhexyl)phthalate. Biochem J. 2002;365(Pt 3): 849–56.
60. Park JD, Habeebu SS, Klaassen CD. Testicular toxicity of di-(2-ethylhexyl)phthalate in young Sprague-Dawley rats. Toxicology. 2002;171(2–3):105–15.
61. Chitra KC, Mathur PP. Vitamin E prevents nonylphenol-induced oxidative stress in testis of rats. Indian J Exp Biol. 2004;42(2):220–3.
62. Hayashi K, Nakae A, Fukushima Y, et al. Contamination of rice by etofenprox, diethyl phthalate and alkylphenols: effects on first delivery and sperm count in mice. J Toxicol Sci. 2010;35(1):49–55.
63. Duty SM, Silva MJ, Barr DB, et al. Phthalate exposure and human semen parameters. Epidemiology. 2003;14(3):269–77.
64. Hauser R, Chen Z, Pothier L, Ryan L, Altshul L. The relationship between human semen parameters and environmental exposure to polychlorinated biphenyls and p, p'-DDE. Environ Health Perspect. 2003; 111(12):1505–11.
65. Hsu PC, Guo YL. Antioxidant nutrients and lead toxicity. Toxicology. 2002;180(1):33–44.
66. Acharya UR, Acharya S, Mishra M. Lead acetate induced cytotoxicity in male germinal cells of Swiss mice. Ind Health. 2003;41(3):291–4.
67. Xu DX, Shen HM, Zhu QX, et al. The associations among semen quality, oxidative DNA damage in human spermatozoa and concentrations of cadmium, lead and selenium in seminal plasma. Mutat Res. 2003;534(1–2):155–63.
68. Naha N, Chowdhury AR. Inorganic lead exposure in battery and paint factory: effect on human sperm structure and functional activity. J UOEH. 2006; 28(2):157–71.
69. Shiau CY, Wang JD, Chen PC. Decreased fecundity among male lead workers. Occup Environ Med. 2004;61(11):915–23.
70. Figa-Talamanca I, Traina ME, Urbani E. Occupational exposures to metals, solvents and pesticides: recent evidence on male reproductive effects and biological markers. Occup Med (Lond). 2001;51(3):174–88.
71. Ahamed M, Siddiqui MK. Low level lead exposure and oxidative stress: current opinions. Clin Chim Acta. 2007;383(1–2):57–64.
72. Benoff S, Hauser R, Marmar JL, Hurley IR, Napolitano B, Centola GM. Cadmium concentrations in blood and seminal plasma: correlations with sperm number and motility in three male populations (infertility

patients, artificial insemination donors, and unselected volunteers). Mol Med. 2009;15(7–8):248–62.
73. Gunnarsson D, Svensson M, Selstam G, Nordberg G. Pronounced induction of testicular PGF(2 alpha) and suppression of testosterone by cadmium-prevention by zinc. Toxicology. 2004;200(1):49–58.
74. Yang JM, Arnush M, Chen QY, Wu XD, Pang B, Jiang XZ. Cadmium-induced damage to primary cultures of rat Leydig cells. Reprod Toxicol. 2003; 17(5):553–60.
75. Benoff S, Auborn K, Marmar JL, Hurley IR. Link between low-dose environmentally relevant cadmium exposures and asthenozoospermia in a rat model. Fertil Steril. 2008;89(2 Suppl):e73–9.
76. Siu ER, Mruk DD, Porto CS, Cheng CY. Cadmium-induced testicular injury. Toxicol Appl Pharmacol. 2009;238(3):240–9.
77. Gennart JP, Buchet JP, Roels H, Ghyselen P, Ceulemans E, Lauwerys R. Fertility of male workers exposed to cadmium, lead, or manganese. Am J Epidemiol. 1992;135(11):1208–19.
78. Bonde JP. The risk of male subfecundity attributable to welding of metals. Studies of semen quality, infertility, fertility, adverse pregnancy outcome and childhood malignancy. Int J Androl. 1993;16 Suppl 1:1–29.
79. Jurasovic J, Cvitkovic P, Pizent A, Colak B, Telisman S. Semen quality and reproductive endocrine function with regard to blood cadmium in Croatian male subjects. Biometals. 2004;17(6):735–43.
80. Telisman S, Cvitkovic P, Jurasovic J, Pizent A, Gavella M, Rocic B. Semen quality and reproductive endocrine function in relation to biomarkers of lead, cadmium, zinc, and copper in men. Environ Health Perspect. 2000;108(1):45–53.
81. Chia SE, Xu B, Ong CN, Tsakok FM, Lee ST. Effect of cadmium and cigarette smoking on human semen quality. Int J Fertil Menopausal Stud. 1994;39(5):292–8.
82. Vitousek PM, Aber J, Howarth RW, et al. Human alteration of the global nitrogen cycle: sources and consequences. Ecol Appl. 1997;7:737–50.
83. Vitousek PM, Hattenschwiler S, Olander L, Allison S. Nitrogen and nature. Ambio. 2002;31(2):97–101.
84. Aber JD. Nitrogen cycling and nitrogen saturation in temperate forest ecosystems. Trends Ecol Evol. 1992; 7:220–3.
85. Wu TP, Huang BM, Tsai HC, Lui MC, Liu MY. Effects of nitric oxide on human spermatozoa activity, fertilization and mouse embryonic development. Arch Androl. 2004;50(3):173–9.
86. Jurewicz J, Hanke W, Radwan M, Bonde JP. Environmental factors and semen quality. Int J Occup Med Environ Health. 2009;22(4):305–29.
87. Wong WY, Zielhuis GA, Thomas CM, Merkus HM, Steegers-Theunissen RP. New evidence of the influence of exogenous and endogenous factors on sperm count in man. Eur J Obstet Gynecol Reprod Biol. 2003;110(1):49–54.
88. Oliva A, Spira A, Multigner L. Contribution of environmental factors to the risk of male infertility. Hum Reprod. 2001;16(8):1768–76.
89. Chitra KC, Sujatha R, Latchoumycandane C, Mathur PP. Effect of lindane on antioxidant enzymes in epididymis and epididymal sperm of adult rats. Asian J Androl. 2001;3(3):205–8.
90. Latchoumycandane C, Chitra KC, Mathur PP. 2, 3, 7, 8-Tetrachlorodibenzo-p-dioxin (TCDD) induces oxidative stress in the epididymis and epididymal sperm of adult rats. Arch Toxicol. 2003;77(5):280–4.
91. Latchoumycandane C, Mathur PP. Induction of oxidative stress in the rat testis after short-term exposure to the organochlorine pesticide methoxychlor. Arch Toxicol. 2002;76(12):692–8.
92. Vaithinathan S, Saradha B, Mathur PP. Transient inhibitory effect of methoxychlor on testicular steroidogenesis in rat: an in vivo study. Arch Toxicol. 2008;82(11):833–9.
93. Defamie N, Mograbi B, Roger C, et al. Disruption of gap junctional intercellular communication by lindane is associated with aberrant localization of connexin43 and zonula occludens-1 in 42GPA9 Sertoli cells. Carcinogenesis. 2001;22(9):1537–42.
94. Saradha B, Vaithinathan S, Mathur PP. Single exposure to low dose of lindane causes transient decrease in testicular steroidogenesis in adult male Wistar rats. Toxicology. 2008;244(2–3):190–7.
95. Selmanoglu G, Barlas N, Songur S, Kockaya EA. Carbendazim-induced haematological, biochemical and histopathological changes to the liver and kidney of male rats. Hum Exp Toxicol. 2001;20(12): 625–30.
96. Carter SD, Hess RA, Laskey JW. The fungicide methyl 2-benzimidazole carbamate causes infertility in male Sprague-Dawley rats. Biol Reprod. 1987; 37(3):709–17.
97. Akbarsha MA, Kadalmani B, Girija R, Faridha A, Hamid KS. Spermatotoxic effect of carbendazim. Indian J Exp Biol. 2001;39(9):921–4.
98. Rajeswary S, Kumaran B, Ilangovan R, et al. Modulation of antioxidant defense system by the environmental fungicide carbendazim in Leydig cells of rats. Reprod Toxicol. 2007;24(3–4): 371–80.
99. Kovacic P, Pozos RS. Cell signaling (mechanism and reproductive toxicity): redox chains, radicals, electrons, relays, conduit, electrochemistry, and other medical implications. Birth Defects Res C Embryo Today. 2006;78(4):333–44.
100. Edelfors S, Hass U, Hougaard KS. Changes in markers of oxidative stress and membrane properties in synaptosomes from rats exposed prenatally to toluene. Pharmacol Toxicol. 2002;90(1):26–31.
101. Nakai N, Murata M, Nagahama M, et al. Oxidative DNA damage induced by toluene is involved in its male reproductive toxicity. Free Radic Res. 2003; 37(1):69–76.
102. Xiao G, Pan C, Cai Y, Lin H, Fu Z. Effect of benzene, toluene, xylene on the semen quality of exposed workers. Chin Med J. 1999;112(8):709–12.
103. Chen Q, Vazquez EJ, Moghaddas S, Hoppel CL, Lesnefsky EJ. Production of reactive oxygen species

by mitochondria: central role of complex III. J Biol Chem. 2003;278(38):36027–31.
104. Adam-Vizi V. Production of reactive oxygen species in brain mitochondria: contribution by electron transport chain and non-electron transport chain sources. Antioxid Redox Signal. 2005;7(9–10):1140–9.
105. Vine MF, Tse CK, Hu P, Truong KY. Cigarette smoking and semen quality. Fertil Steril. 1996;65(4): 835–42.
106. Kunzle R, Mueller MD, Hanggi W, Birkhauser MH, Drescher H, Bersinger NA. Semen quality of male smokers and nonsmokers in infertile couples. Fertil Steril. 2003;79(2):287–91.
107. Saleh RA, Agarwal A, Sharma RK, Nelson DR, Thomas Jr AJ. Effect of cigarette smoking on levels of seminal oxidative stress in infertile men: a prospective study. Fertil Steril. 2002;78(3):491–9.
108. Ramlau-Hansen CH, Thulstrup AM, Aggerholm AS, Jensen MS, Toft G, Bonde JP. Is smoking a risk factor for decreased semen quality? A cross-sectional analysis. Hum Reprod. 2007;22(1):188–96.
109. Vine MF, Margolin BH, Morrison HI, Hulka BS. Cigarette smoking and sperm density: a meta-analysis. Fertil Steril. 1994;61(1):35–43.
110. Traber MG, van der Vliet A, Reznick AZ, Cross CE. Tobacco-related diseases. Is there a role for antioxidant micronutrient supplementation? Clin Chest Med. 2000;21(1):173–87, x.
111. Cross CE, Halliwell B, Borish ET, et al. Oxygen radicals and human disease. Ann Intern Med. 1987;107(4):526–45.
112. Richthoff J, Elzanaty S, Rylander L, Hagmar L, Giwercman A. Association between tobacco exposure and reproductive parameters in adolescent males. Int J Androl. 2008;31(1):31–9.
113. Mostafa T, Anis TH, El-Nashar A, Imam H, Othman IA. Varicocelectomy reduces reactive oxygen species levels and increases antioxidant activity of seminal plasma from infertile men with varicocele. Int J Androl. 2001;24(5):261–5.
114. Fraga CG, Motchnik PA, Wyrobek AJ, Rempel DM, Ames BN. Smoking and low antioxidant levels increase oxidative damage to sperm DNA. Mutat Res. 1996;351(2):199–203.
115. Maddocks S, Hargreave TB, Reddie K, Fraser HM, Kerr JB, Sharpe RM. Intratesticular hormone levels and the route of secretion of hormones from the testis of the rat, guinea pig, monkey and human. Int J Androl. 1993;16(4):272–8.
116. Piner J, Sutherland M, Millar M, Turner K, Newall D, Sharpe RM. Changes in vascular dynamics of the adult rat testis leading to transient accumulation of seminiferous tubule fluid after administration of a novel 5-hydroxytryptamine (5-HT) agonist. Reprod Toxicol. 2002;16(2):141–50.
117. Gaur DS, Talekar M, Pathak VP. Effect of cigarette smoking on semen quality of infertile men. Singapore Med J. 2007;48(2):119–23.
118. Marinelli D, Gaspari L, Pedotti P, Taioli E. Mini-review of studies on the effect of smoking and drinking habits on semen parameters. Int J Hyg Environ Health. 2004; 207(3):185–92.
119. Martini AC, Molina RI, Estofan D, Senestrari D, Fiol de Cuneo M, Ruiz RD. Effects of alcohol and cigarette consumption on human seminal quality. Fertil Steril. 2004;82(2):374–7.
120. Villalta J, Ballesca JL, Nicolas JM, Martinez de Osaba MJ, Antunez E, Pimentel C. Testicular function in asymptomatic chronic alcoholics: relation to ethanol intake. Alcohol Clin Exp Res. 1997;21(1): 128–33.
121. Boyden TW, Pamenter RW. Effects of ethanol on the male hypothalamic-pituitary-gonadal axis. Endocr Rev. Fall 1983;4(4):389–95.
122. Muthusami KR, Chinnaswamy P. Effect of chronic alcoholism on male fertility hormones and semen quality. Fertil Steril. 2005;84(4):919–24.
123. Goverde HJ, Dekker HS, Janssen HJ, Bastiaans BA, Rolland R, Zielhuis GA. Semen quality and frequency of smoking and alcohol consumption – an explorative study. Int J Fertil Menopausal Stud. 1995;40(3):135–8.
124. Maneesh M, Dutta S, Chakrabarti A, Vasudevan DM. Alcohol abuse-duration dependent decrease in plasma testosterone and antioxidants in males. Indian J Physiol Pharmacol. 2006;50(3):291–6.
125. Dahchour A, Lallemand F, Ward RJ, De Witte P. Production of reactive oxygen species following acute ethanol or acetaldehyde and its reduction by acamprosate in chronically alcoholized rats. Eur J Pharmacol. 2005;520(1–3):51–8.
126. Lieber CS. The discovery of the microsomal ethanol oxidizing system and its physiologic and pathologic role. Drug Metab Rev. 2004;36(3–4):511–29.
127. Agarwal A, Prabakaran SA. Mechanism, measurement, and prevention of oxidative stress in male reproductive physiology. Indian J Exp Biol. 2005;43(11):963–74.
128. Wiseman H, Halliwell B. Damage to DNA by reactive oxygen and nitrogen species: role in inflammatory disease and progression to cancer. Biochem J. 1996;313(Pt 1):17–29.
129. Wu D, Cederbaum AI. Alcohol, oxidative stress, and free radical damage. Alcohol Res Health. 2003;27(4):277–84.
130. Koch OR, Pani G, Borrello S, et al. Oxidative stress and antioxidant defenses in ethanol-induced cell injury. Mol Aspects Med. 2004;25(1–2):191–8.
131. Shalet SM. Effects of cancer chemotherapy on gonadal function of patients. Cancer Treat Rev. 1980;7(3):141–52.
132. Schlegel PN, Chang TS, Marshall FF. Antibiotics: potential hazards to male fertility. Fertil Steril. 1991;55(2):235–42.
133. Ericsson RJ, Baker VF. Binding of tetracycline to mammalian spermatozoa. Nature. 1967;214(5086): 403–4.
134. O'Morain C, Smethurst P, Dore CJ, Levi AJ. Reversible male infertility due to sulphasalazine: studies in man and rat. Gut. 1984;25(10):1078–84.

135. Hayashi T, Miyata A, Yamada T. The impact of commonly prescribed drugs on male fertility. Hum Fertil. 2008;11(3):191–6.
136. Sikka SC, Wang R. Endocrine disruptors and estrogenic effects on male reproductive axis. Asian J Androl. 2008;10(1):134–45.
137. Anderson RA, Baird DT. Male contraception. Endocr Rev. 2002;23(6):735–62.
138. Knuth UA, Maniera H, Nieschlag E. Anabolic steroids and semen parameters in bodybuilders. Fertil Steril. 1989;52(6):1041–7.
139. Du Plessis SS, Cabler S, McAlister DA, Sabanegh E, Agarwal A. The effect of obesity on sperm disorders and male infertility. Nat Rev Urol. 2010;7(3): 153–61.
140. Song GJ, Norkus EP, Lewis V. Relationship between seminal ascorbic acid and sperm DNA integrity in infertile men. Int J Androl. 2006;29(6):569–75.
141. Eskenazi B, Kidd SA, Marks AR, Sloter E, Block G, Wyrobek AJ. Antioxidant intake is associated with semen quality in healthy men. Hum Reprod. 2005;20(4):1006–12.
142. Therond P, Auger J, Legrand A, Jouannet P. alpha-Tocopherol in human spermatozoa and seminal plasma: relationships with motility, antioxidant enzymes and leukocytes. Mol Hum Reprod. 1996;2(10):739–44.
143. Fraga CG, Motchnik PA, Shigenaga MK, Helbock HJ, Jacob RA, Ames BN. Ascorbic acid protects against endogenous oxidative DNA damage in human sperm. Proc Natl Acad Sci U S A. 1991; 88(24):11003–6.
144. Hawkes WC, Turek PJ. Effects of dietary selenium on sperm motility in healthy men. J Androl. 2001; 22(5):764–72.
145. Hammoud AO, Gibson M, Peterson CM, Hamilton BD, Carrell DT. Obesity and male reproductive potential. J Androl. 2006;27(5):619–26.
146. Hammoud AO, Gibson M, Peterson CM, Meikle AW, Carrell DT. Impact of male obesity on infertility: a critical review of the current literature. Fertil Steril. 2008;90(4):897–904.
147. Nielsen TL, Hagen C, Wraae K, et al. Visceral and subcutaneous adipose tissue assessed by magnetic resonance imaging in relation to circulating androgens, sex hormone-binding globulin, and luteinizing hormone in young men. J Clin Endocrinol Metab. 2007;92(7):2696–705.
148. Fejes I, Koloszar S, Zavaczki Z, Daru J, Szollosi J, Pal A. Effect of body weight on testosterone/estradiol ratio in oligozoospermic patients. Arch Androl. 2006;52(2):97–102.
149. Kort HI, Massey JB, Elsner CW, et al. Impact of body mass index values on sperm quantity and quality. J Androl. 2006;27(3):450–2.
150. Nguyen RH, Wilcox AJ, Skjaerven R, Baird DD. Men's body mass index and infertility. Hum Reprod. 2007;22(9):2488–93.
151. Koloszar S, Fejes I, Zavaczki Z, Daru J, Szollosi J, Pal A. Effect of body weight on sperm concentration in normozoospermic males. Arch Androl. 2005; 51(4):299–304.
152. Cabler S, Agarwal A, Flint M, du Plessis SS. Obesity: modern man's fertility nemesis. Asian J Androl. 2010;12(4):480–9.
153. Shafik A, Olfat S. Scrotal lipomatosis. Br J Urol. 1981;53(1):50–4.
154. Dandona P, Aljada A, Chaudhuri A, Mohanty P, Garg R. Metabolic syndrome: a comprehensive perspective based on interactions between obesity, diabetes, and inflammation. Circulation. 2005;111(11): 1448–54.
155. Davi G, Falco A. Oxidant stress, inflammation and atherogenesis. Lupus. 2005;14(9):760–4.
156. Kodama H, Yamaguchi R, Fukuda J, Kasai H, Tanaka T. Increased oxidative deoxyribonucleic acid damage in the spermatozoa of infertile male patients. Fertil Steril. 1997;68(3):519–24.
157. Twigg J, Fulton N, Gomez E, Irvine DS, Aitken RJ. Analysis of the impact of intracellular reactive oxygen species generation on the structural and functional integrity of human spermatozoa: lipid peroxidation, DNA fragmentation and effectiveness of antioxidants. Hum Reprod. 1998;13(6): 1429–36.
158. Singer G, Granger DN. Inflammatory responses underlying the microvascular dysfunction associated with obesity and insulin resistance. Microcirculation. 2007;14(4–5):375–87.
159. Eskiocak S, Gozen AS, Kilic AS, Molla S. Association between mental stress & some antioxidant enzymes of seminal plasma. Indian J Med Res. 2005;122(6):491–6.
160. Eskiocak S, Gozen AS, Yapar SB, Tavas F, Kilic AS, Eskiocak M. Glutathione and free sulphydryl content of seminal plasma in healthy medical students during and after exam stress. Hum Reprod. 2005; 20(9):2595–600.
161. Eskiocak S, Gozen AS, Taskiran A, Kilic AS, Eskiocak M, Gulen S. Effect of psychological stress on the L-arginine-nitric oxide pathway and semen quality. Braz J Med Biol Res. 2006;39(5):581–8.
162. Tremellen K. Oxidative stress and male infertility – a clinical perspective. Hum Reprod Update. 2008; 14(3):243–58.
163. Monder C, Miroff Y, Marandici A, Hardy MP. 11 beta-Hydroxysteroid dehydrogenase alleviates glucocorticoid-mediated inhibition of steroidogenesis in rat Leydig cells. Endocrinology. 1994;134(3): 1199–204.
164. Ruffoli R, Carpi A, Giambelluca MA, Grasso L, Scavuzzo MC, Giannessi FF. Diazepam administration prevents testosterone decrease and lipofuscin accumulation in testis of mouse exposed to chronic noise stress. Andrologia. 2006;38(5):159–65.
165. Terman A, Brunk UT. Lipofuscin. Int J Biochem Cell Biol. 2004;36(8):1400–4.
166. Gao HB, Tong MH, Hu YQ, et al. Mechanisms of glucocorticoid-induced Leydig cell apoptosis. Mol Cell Endocrinol. 2003;199(1–2):153–63.

167. Ivell R. Lifestyle impact and the biology of the human scrotum. Reprod Biol Endocrinol. 2007; 5:15.
168. Werdelin L, Nilsonne A. The evolution of the scrotum and testicular descent in mammals: a phylogenetic view. J Theor Biol. 1999;196(1):61–72.
169. Jung A, Schuppe HC. Influence of genital heat stress on semen quality in humans. Andrologia. 2007;39(6): 203–15.
170. Lue YH, Hikim AP, Swerdloff RS, et al. Single exposure to heat induces stage-specific germ cell apoptosis in rats: role of intratesticular testosterone on stage specificity. Endocrinology. 1999;140(4):1709–17.
171. Lue YH, Lasley BL, Laughlin LS, et al. Mild testicular hyperthermia induces profound transitional spermatogenic suppression through increased germ cell apoptosis in adult cynomolgus monkeys (*Macaca fascicularis*). J Androl. 2002;23(6):799–805.
172. Yamamoto CM, Sinha Hikim AP, Huynh PN, et al. Redistribution of Bax is an early step in an apoptotic pathway leading to germ cell death in rats, triggered by mild testicular hyperthermia. Biol Reprod. 2000; 63(6):1683–90.
173. Vera Y, Rodriguez S, Castanares M, et al. Functional role of caspases in heat-induced testicular germ cell apoptosis. Biol Reprod. 2005;72(3):516–22.
174. Kandeel FR, Swerdloff RS. Role of temperature in regulation of spermatogenesis and the use of heating as a method for contraception. Fertil Steril. 1988; 49(1):1–23.
175. Zhang ZH, Jin X, Zhang XS, et al. Bcl-2 and Bax are involved in experimental cryptorchidism-induced testicular germ cell apoptosis in rhesus monkey. Contraception. 2003;68(4):297–301.
176. Short RV. The testis: the witness of the mating system, the site of mutation and the engine of desire. Acta Paediatr Suppl. 1997;422:3–7.
177. Bedford JM. Anatomical evidence for the epididymis as the prime mover in the evolution of the scrotum. Am J Anat. 1978;152(4):483–507.
178. Thonneau P, Ducot B, Bujan L, Mieusset R, Spira A. Effect of male occupational heat exposure on time to pregnancy. Int J Androl. 1997;20(5):274–8.
179. Thonneau P, Bujan L, Multigner L, Mieusset R. Occupational heat exposure and male fertility: a review. Hum Reprod. 1998;13(8):2122–5.
180. Bonde JP. Semen quality in welders exposed to radiant heat. Br J Ind Med. 1992;49(1):5–10.
181. Mur JM, Wild P, Rapp R, Vautrin JP, Coulon JP. Demographic evaluation of the fertility of aluminium industry workers: influence of exposure to heat and static magnetic fields. Hum Reprod. 1998;13(7): 2016–9.
182. Figa-Talamanca I, Dell'Orco V, Pupi A, et al. Fertility and semen quality of workers exposed to high temperatures in the ceramics industry. Reprod Toxicol. 1992;6(6):517–23.
183. Jung A, Schuppe HC, Schill WB. [Fever as etiology of temporary infertility in the man]. Hautarzt. 2001;52(12):1090–3.
184. Bujan L, Daudin M, Charlet JP, Thonneau P, Mieusset R. Increase in scrotal temperature in car drivers. Hum Reprod. 2000;15(6):1355–7.
185. Hjollund NH, Bonde JP, Jensen TK, Olsen J. Diurnal scrotal skin temperature and semen quality. The Danish First Pregnancy Planner Study Team. Int J Androl. 2000;23(5):309–18.
186. Hjollund NH, Storgaard L, Ernst E, Bonde JP, Olsen J. The relation between daily activities and scrotal temperature. Reprod Toxicol. 2002;16(3):209–14.
187. Magnusdottir EV, Thorsteinsson T, Thorsteinsdottir S, Heimisdottir M, Olafsdottir K. Persistent organochlorines, sedentary occupation, obesity and human male subfertility. Hum Reprod. 2005;20(1):208–15.
188. Sas M, Szollosi J. Impaired spermiogenesis as a common finding among professional drivers. Arch Androl. 1979;3(1):57–60.
189. Figa-Talamanca I, Cini C, Varricchio GC, et al. Effects of prolonged autovehicle driving on male reproduction function: a study among taxi drivers. Am J Ind Med. 1996;30(6):750–8.
190. Rock J, Robinson D. Effect of induced intrascrotal hyperthermia on testicular function in man. Am J Obstet Gynecol. 1965;93(6):793–801.
191. Yamaguchi M, Sakatoku J, Takihara H. The application of intrascrotal deep body temperature measurement for the noninvasive diagnosis of varicoceles. Fertil Steril. 1989;52(2):295–301.
192. Jockenhovel F, Grawe A, Nieschlag E. A portable digital data recorder for long-term monitoring of scrotal temperatures. Fertil Steril. 1990;54(4):694–700.
193. Parazzini F, Marchini M, Luchini L, Tozzi L, Mezzopane R, Fedele L. Tight underpants and trousers and risk of dyspermia. Int J Androl. 1995;18(3): 137–40.
194. Mieusset R, Bujan L. Testicular heating and its possible contributions to male infertility: a review. Int J Androl. 1995;18(4):169–84.
195. Zorgniotti A, Reiss H, Toth A, Sealfon A. Effect of clothing on scrotal temperature in normal men and patients with poor semen. Urology. 1982;19(2):176–8.
196. Munkelwitz R, Gilbert BR. Are boxer shorts really better? A critical analysis of the role of underwear type in male subfertility. J Urol. 1998;160(4): 1329–33.
197. Jung A, Leonhardt F, Schill WB, Schuppe HC. Influence of the type of undertrousers and physical activity on scrotal temperature. Hum Reprod. 2005;20(4):1022–7.
198. Procope BJ. Effect of repeated increase of body temperature on human sperm cells. Int J Fertil. 1965; 10(4):333–9.
199. Brown-Woodman PD, Post EJ, Gass GC, White IG. The effect of a single sauna exposure on spermatozoa. Arch Androl. 1984;12(1):9–15.
200. Setchell BP. The Parkes Lecture. Heat and the testis. J Reprod Fertil. 1998;114(2):179–94.
201. Banks S, King SA, Irvine DS, Saunders PT. Impact of a mild scrotal heat stress on DNA integrity in murine spermatozoa. Reproduction. 2005;129(4):505–14.

202. Ishii T, Matsuki S, Iuchi Y, et al. Accelerated impairment of spermatogenic cells in SOD1-knockout mice under heat stress. Free Radic Res. 2005;39(7):697–705.
203. Perez-Crespo M, Pintado B, Gutierrez-Adan A. Scrotal heat stress effects on sperm viability, sperm DNA integrity, and the offspring sex ratio in mice. Mol Reprod Dev. 2008;75(1):40–7.
204. Carlsen E, Andersson AM, Petersen JH, Skakkebaek NE. History of febrile illness and variation in semen quality. Hum Reprod. 2003;18(10):2089–92.
205. Evenson DP, Jost LK, Corzett M, Balhorn R. Characteristics of human sperm chromatin structure following an episode of influenza and high fever: a case study. J Androl. 2000;21(5):739–46.
206. Stopczyk D, Gnitecki W, Buczynski A, Kowalski W, Buczynska M, Kroc A. [Effect of electromagnetic field produced by mobile phones on the activity of superoxide dismutase (SOD-1) – in vitro researches]. Ann Acad Med Stetin. 2005;51 Suppl 1:125–8.
207. Dasdag S, Zulkuf Akdag M, Aksen F, et al. Whole body exposure of rats to microwaves emitted from a cell phone does not affect the testes. Bioelectromagnetics. 2003;24(3):182–8.
208. Deepinder F, Makker K, Agarwal A. Cell phones and male infertility: dissecting the relationship. Reprod Biomed Online. 2007;15(3):266–70.
209. Agarwal A, Deepinder F, Sharma RK, Ranga G, Li J. Effect of cell phone usage on semen analysis in men attending infertility clinic: an observational study. Fertil Steril. 2008;89(1):124–8.
210. Kilgallon SJ, Simmons LW. Image content influences men's semen quality. Biol Lett. 2005;1(3): 253–5.
211. Fejes I, Zavaczki Z, Szollosi J, et al. Is there a relationship between cell phone use and semen quality? Arch Androl. 2005;51(5):385–93.
212. Baste V, Riise T, Moen BE. Radiofrequency electromagnetic fields; male infertility and sex ratio of offspring. Eur J Epidemiol. 2008;23(5):369–77.
213. Agarwal A, Desai NR, Makker K, et al. Effects of radiofrequency electromagnetic waves (RF-EMW) from cellular phones on human ejaculated semen: an in vitro pilot study. Fertil Steril. 2009;92(4):1318–25.
214. Friedman J, Kraus S, Hauptman Y, Schiff Y, Seger R. Mechanism of short-term ERK activation by electromagnetic fields at mobile phone frequencies. Biochem J. 2007;405(3):559–68.
215. Burch JB, Reif JS, Yost MG, Keefe TJ, Pitrat CA. Nocturnal excretion of a urinary melatonin metabolite among electric utility workers. Scand J Work Environ Health. 1998;24(3):183–9.
216. Ozguner M, Koyu A, Cesur G, et al. Biological and morphological effects on the reproductive organ of rats after exposure to electromagnetic field. Saudi Med J. 2005;26(3):405–10.
217. Ash P. The influence of radiation on fertility in man. Br J Radiol. 1980;53(628):271–8.
218. Clifton DK, Bremner WJ. The effect of testicular x-irradiation on spermatogenesis in man. A comparison with the mouse. J Androl. 1983;4(6):387–92.
219. Popescu HI, Lancranjan I. Spermatogenesis alterations during protracted irradiation in man. Health Phys. 1975;28(5):567–73.
220. Cheburakov I, Cheburakova OP. [Disorders of spermatogenesis in people working at the clean-up of the Chernobyl nuclear power plant accident]. Radiats Biol Radioecol. 1993;33(6):771–4.
221. Skinner MK, Manikkam M, Guerrero-Bosagna C. Epigenetic transgenerational actions of environmental factors in disease etiology. Trends Endocrinol Metab. 2010;21(4):214–22.
222. Holliday R, Pugh JE. DNA modification mechanisms and gene activity during development. Science. 1975;187(4173):226–32.
223. Turner BM. Histone acetylation as an epigenetic determinant of long-term transcriptional competence. Cell Mol Life Sci. 1998;54(1):21–31.
224. Wu Q, Ohsako S, Ishimura R, Suzuki JS, Tohyama C. Exposure of mouse preimplantation embryos to 2, 3, 7, 8-tetrachlorodibenzo-p-dioxin (TCDD) alters the methylation status of imprinted genes H19 and Igf2. Biol Reprod. 2004;70(6):1790–7.
225. Waalkes MP, Liu J, Chen H, et al. Estrogen signaling in livers of male mice with hepatocellular carcinoma induced by exposure to arsenic in utero. J Natl Cancer Inst. 2004;96(6):466–74.
226. Singh KP, DuMond Jr JW. Genetic and epigenetic changes induced by chronic low dose exposure to arsenic of mouse testicular Leydig cells. Int J Oncol. 2007;30(1):253–60.
227. Perera F, Tang WY, Herbstman J, et al. Relation of DNA methylation of 5'-CpG island of ACSL3 to transplacental exposure to airborne polycyclic aromatic hydrocarbons and childhood asthma. PLoS One. 2009;4(2):e4488.
228. Yaoi T, Itoh K, Nakamura K, Ogi H, Fujiwara Y, Fushiki S. Genome-wide analysis of epigenomic alterations in fetal mouse forebrain after exposure to low doses of bisphenol A. Biochem Biophys Res Commun. 2008;376(3):563–7.
229. Dolinoy DC, Huang D, Jirtle RL. Maternal nutrient supplementation counteracts bisphenol A-induced DNA hypomethylation in early development. Proc Natl Acad Sci U S A. 2007;104(32):13056–61.
230. Ho SM, Tang WY, Belmonte de Frausto J, Prins GS. Developmental exposure to estradiol and bisphenol A increases susceptibility to prostate carcinogenesis and epigenetically regulates phosphodiesterase type 4 variant 4. Cancer Res. 2006;66(11):5624–32.
231. Guerrero-Bosagna CM, Sabat P, Valdovinos FS, Valladares LE, Clark SJ. Epigenetic and phenotypic changes result from a continuous pre and post natal dietary exposure to phytoestrogens in an experimental population of mice. BMC Physiol. 2008; 8:17.
232. Dolinoy DC, Weidman JR, Waterland RA, Jirtle RL. Maternal genistein alters coat color and protects Avy mouse offspring from obesity by modifying the fetal epigenome. Environ Health Perspect. 2006;114(4): 567–72.

233. Anway MD, Cupp AS, Uzumcu M, Skinner MK. Epigenetic transgenerational actions of endocrine disruptors and male fertility. Science. 2005; 308(5727):1466–9.
234. Andersen HR, Schmidt IM, Grandjean P, et al. Impaired reproductive development in sons of women occupationally exposed to pesticides during pregnancy. Environ Health Perspect. 2008;116(4): 566–72.
235. Jirtle RL, Skinner MK. Environmental epigenomics and disease susceptibility. Nat Rev. 2007;8(4):253–62.
236. Anway MD, Rekow SS, Skinner MK. Transgenerational epigenetic programming of the embryonic testis transcriptome. Genomics. 2008; 91(1):30–40.
237. Uzumcu M, Suzuki H, Skinner MK. Effect of the anti-androgenic endocrine disruptor vinclozolin on embryonic testis cord formation and postnatal testis development and function. Reprod Toxicol. 2004; 18(6):765–74.
238. Takeda K, Tsukue N, Yoshida S. Endocrine-disrupting activity of chemicals in diesel exhaust and diesel exhaust particles. Environ Sci. 2004;11(1): 33–45.
239. Kuriyama SN, Talsness CE, Grote K, Chahoud I. Developmental exposure to low dose PBDE 99: effects on male fertility and neurobehavior in rat offspring. Environ Health Perspect. 2005;113(2): 149–54.
240. Howdeshell KL, Wilson VS, Furr J, et al. A mixture of five phthalate esters inhibits fetal testicular testosterone production in the Sprague-Dawley rat in a cumulative, dose-additive manner. Toxicol Sci. 2008;105(1):153–65.
241. Danzo BJ. The effects of environmental hormones on reproduction. Cell Mol Life Sci. 1998;54(11): 1249–64.
242. Moutsatsou P. The spectrum of phytoestrogens in nature: our knowledge is expanding. Hormones (Athens). 2007;6(3):173–93.
243. Kabuto H, Hasuike S, Minagawa N, Shishibori T. Effects of bisphenol A on the metabolisms of active oxygen species in mouse tissues. Environ Res. 2003; 93(1):31–5.

Sperm DNA Damage: Causes and Guidelines for Current Clinical Practice

12

Aleksander Giwercman, Marcello Spanò, and Mona Bungum

Abstract

Infertility is a common health problem affecting approximately 15% of all couples. It is estimated that, in at least 50% of all cases, impairment of semen quality is a factor contributing to the problem of the couple. Furthermore, 10–15% of all infertility cases are "unexplained". Traditional sperm parameters – concentration, motility, morphology – were shown to have a poor predictive value, both in relation to fertility in vivo and in vitro. Thus, there is an urgent need of finding new sperm quality markers that can be used for the evaluation of the chance of a couple to conceive in a natural way, and also, if necessary, for the selection of the right assisted reproductive technique (ART). In this context, testing of sperm DNA integrity seems to be a potential candidate. The causes of sperm DNA damage are multi-factorial, including testicular and post-testicular, genetic and exposure-related mechanisms. For the assessment of sperm DNA damage, a number of different techniques is available. The results obtained by these methods are generally correlated, but, on the other hand, they seem to measure slightly different elements of sperm DNA integrity and they provide limited information on the nature of the lesions detected. So far, assessment of sperm DNA has proven to be the most powerful in predicting in vivo infertility, which means cases where the chance of pregnancy by natural conception or intrauterine insemination is close to zero. High percentage of sperms with DNA defects seems also to have a negative impact on the results of standard in vitro fertilisation (IVF), but not on that of intracytoplasmatic sperm injection (ICSI), even if the issue is debatable and under active scrutiny. Clinically applicable threshold values

A. Giwercman (✉)
Reproductive Medicine Center, Skåne University Hospital, Malmö, Sweden
and
Department of Clinical Sciences, Lund University, Malmö, Sweden
e-mail: aleksander.giwercman@med.lu.se

C. Racowsky et al. (eds.), *Biennial Review of Infertility: Volume 2*,
DOI 10.1007/978-1-4419-8456-2_12, © Springer Science+Business Media, LLC 2011

have been defined for one of the methods for assessment of sperm DNA integrity – the sperm chromatin structure assay (SCSA) – but not yet for the other techniques. There is a need for standardisation of technology for these assays in the same way as it has been achieved for SCSA. Thus, well-designed studies should be carried out in order to define the clinical role of these new measures of sperm quality. This is important from the diagnostic as well as therapeutic point of view, since a more nuanced characterisation of sperm DNA defects will not only lead to an improved choice of the ART methods, but may also help in developing cause-related therapy of male subfertility. From the biological point of view, it needs to be investigated whether sperm DNA damage transmitted to the embryo by use of IVF and ICSI can be hazardous to the offspring, taking into account the wealth of animal data demonstrating the link between sperm DNA damage and abnormalities in embryo development.

Keywords
Infertility • Sperm DNA • SCSA • TUNEL • Comet • Strand breaks • Insemination • Assisted reproductive technology • IVF • ICSI • Pregnancy

12.1 Case Story

Adam, 28 years old, has been referred for andrological examination due to involuntary childlessness. Together with Linda, 27 years, he has for 1 year tried to beget a child without succeeding. Linda has never been pregnant and Adam has no children and has never made any woman pregnant. They have intercourse 2–3 times per week. Gynaecological examination of Linda, including measurement of hormonal status and tubal patency, revealed no abnormalities. Adam's andrological history is unremarkable and the physical examination did not indicate any abnormality. He delivered two semen samples for examination both showing perfectly normal volume, sperm concentration, motility and morphology.

Since the infertility problem of the couple was characterised as "unexplained" and they were relatively young, the advice was to continue the attempt to achieve spontaneous pregnancy. One year later, the couple was again referred to the infertility clinic since Linda has not got pregnant. They were thereafter referred for intrauterine insemination (IUI). Three attempts of IUI were unsuccessful. Adam delivered one more semen sample and the examination revealed again perfectly normal volume, concentration, motility and morphology. As additional test, sperm chromatin structure assay (SCSA) was performed, showing a DNA fragmentation index (DFI) of 36%. The SCSA was repeated this time showing a DFI of 39%. The couple was wondering why they were unable to achieve pregnancy and how they should proceed.

12.2 The Need for New Tests for the Assessment of Semen Quality

The case story presented above shows some of the basic problems of today routine infertility work-up:

(a) The predictive value of standard semen analysis in relation to the chance of achieving spontaneous pregnancy is rather poor [1, 2].
(b) The same is true in relation to choice of the method of assisted reproduction technique (ART), which means that couples may

undergo treatment a priori having a very low chance of success.

Traditional semen analysis is based on the guidelines of the World Health Organization [3], the main parameters to be assessed being volume, sperm number, motility and morphology. According to the most recent WHO guidelines [4], the 15×10^6/mL is to be considered as the lower reference limit. However, a population-based study has shown that optimal male fertility potential is not achieved before the sperm concentration reaches the level of $40–50 \times 10^6$/mL [1, 2]. On the other hand, spontaneous pregnancies are possible with sperm concentration far below this lower reference limit [1]. The wide overlap between "fertile" and "non-fertile" is true not only for sperm concentration, but also for the other parameters, i.e. motility and morphology [2]. Thus, when evaluating the results of semen analysis, we quite often are unable to predict the chance of the couple to achieve a natural pregnancy.

The other emerging problem related to the classical semen parameters is the poor link between the pathogenesis and the result of semen investigation. Thus, oligo-astheno-teratozoospermia may be due to different types of testicular as well as post-testicular pathologies [5]. This limitation highly restricts our possibilities to dig into the causes of male-related subfertility, and thereby, for finding and testing cause-related new treatment modalities.

Finally, even when the decision of performing ART has been made, standard semen parameters are only of limited value to select the best option among the different techniques available as IUI, standard in vitro fertilisation (IVF) or intracytoplasmatic sperm injection (ICSI).

For these reasons, during the recent years, a lot of attention has been given to sperm DNA damage as an additional and useful marker of sperm function and as an alternative indicator of the mechanisms behind male subfertility [6, 7].

12.3 Human Sperm Chromatin

Due to the limited size of the head of the spermatozoa, a significantly more compact packaging of the genetic material than in the case of a somatic nucleus is needed. In fact, a mature sperm nucleus containing the haploid genome must adopt a volume 40 times less than that of a normal somatic nucleus [8]. In order to achieve such architectural compression, the nucleosomal organisation is dismantled in the last part of spermiogenesis, and histones are replaced by a new set of nuclear proteins, the protamines, more basic and much smaller than histones [9]. The fundamental packaging unit of mammalian sperm chromatin is a toroid containing 50–60 kb of DNA. Individual toroids represent DNA loop-domains highly condensed by protamines and fixed at the nuclear matrix. The toroids are further compacted by the intra- and inter-molecular disulfide cross-links, formed by oxidation of sulfhydryl groups of cysteine present in the protamines [9, 10]. Thus, each chromosome represents a garland of toroids, and all 23 chromosomes are clustered by centromeres into a compact chromocenter positioned well inside the nucleus with telomere ends united into dimers exposed to the nuclear periphery [11, 12]. This condensed, insoluble and highly organised nature of sperm chromatin acts to protect genetic integrity during transport of the paternal genome through the male and female reproductive tracts as the mature sperm is a repair-deficient cell. It also ensures that the paternal DNA is delivered in the form that sterically allows the proper fusion of two gametic genomes and enables the developing embryo to correctly express the genetic information [11, 13].

In many animal species, protamines comprise 95% of the spermatozoal nucleoproteins. However, in humans this percentage is usually only 85%. This may be one of the reasons why human sperm chromatin is less compacted and more frequently contains DNA strand breaks [14]. In comparison with other species [15], human sperm chromatin packaging is also exceptionally variable, both within and between men. Moreover, in contrast to the bull, cat, boar and ram, whose spermatozoa contain only one type of protamine (P1), human and mouse spermatozoa contain a second type of protamine (P2), which contains fewer cysteine groups [16]. Consequently, the diminished level of disulfide cross-linking could be one of the responsible factors underlying the looser human sperm chromatin packaging as compared to the sperm chromatin of other species containing P1 alone [17].

12.4 Origin of Human Sperm DNA Damage

The origin of human sperm DNA damage is heterogeneous involving, in a not mutually exclusive ways, both testicular and post-testicular mechanisms. The most common types of DNA damage include abasic sites, chemical modification of a base, inter- and intra-strand cross-links, and single or double DNA strand breaks. Both sperm nuclear and mitochondrial DNA can be damaged, but since the latter makes no contribution to the functionality of the male gamete, the attention will be given to impairment of the integrity of the nuclear genetic material. Testicular mechanisms include (a) alterations in chromatin modelling during the process of spermiogenesis and (b) abortive apoptosis, whereas post-testicular factors are mostly related to the action of (c) reactive oxygen species (ROS) and (d) activation of caspases and endonucleases [18, 19].

12.4.1 Chromatin Modelling During the Process of Spermiogenesis

The process of chromatin condensation and packing during the spermiogenetic steps includes the induction of DNA nicks to provide relief of torsional stress to aid chromatin arrangement during the displacement of histones by protamines. Type II DNA topoisomerase is the enzyme responsible of the induction and sealing of these nicks because of the endonuclease and ligase activity of the enzyme [20]. The intermediate breaks allow the DNA to be untangled or unwound, and at the end of these processes, the DNA is reconnected again. Any impairment of this process, occurring in round spermatids, will lead to long-term consequences such as an increased number of sperm DNA strand breaks and/or higher susceptibility to other assaults.

12.4.2 Abortive Apoptosis

Under the process of spermatogenesis, germ cells are under the control of Sertoli cells resulting in induction of apoptosis in 50–60% of the germ cells before they enter meiosis I [21]. For several reasons including (a) inability of spermatozoa to undergo "programmed cell death" due to lack of transcriptional and translational capacity; (b) reduced nucleosome content because of extensive protamination and thereof following inability to exhibit the characteristic DNA laddering seen in somatic cells; and (c) endonucleases activated in the cytoplasm or released from the mitochondria being prevented from physically accessing the DNA due to the physical architecture of the spermatozoa, the apoptotic process in male germ cells cannot be identical to that in other cell types. Therefore, ideally, the spermatozoa earmarked by the apoptotic markers of *Fas* type should be eliminated by being phagoctosed by the Sertoli cells. However, this process seems not to be completely efficient leading to some of the "abortive apoptosis" meaning that some of the cells escape the apoptosis and may, thereafter, appear in the ejaculate [20].

12.4.3 Reactive Oxygen Species

Oxidative stress is supposed to be the major contributory factor behind defective sperm function and is supposed to be due to an imbalance between the amount of ROS produced and the ability of the antioxidants to scavenge these. Spermatozoa seem to be susceptible to the attack of free radicals due to superabundance of polyunsaturated fatty acids, necessary for a proper fertilisation process. The sources of the oxidative stress leading to DNA damage in the germ cells include factors as loss of antioxidant protection, infection and/or intrinsic (spermatozoa), and extrinsic radical production [22].

Spermatozoa are relatively deficient of ROS-scavenging enzymes, for that reason the antioxidant protection being of a crucial importance for their DNA integrity. Epididymis secretes an array of antioxidant factors including vitamin C, uric acid, taurine and thioredoxin, superoxide dismutase and gluthatione peroxidise. Secretion of some of those factors is under androgenic control. Even the seminal plasma may provide some antioxidant protection; however, unlike the epididymis, sperm spend very little time in seminal plasma and the role of seminal antioxidants is not completely clarified. However, it has been shown that the degree of sperm DNA fragmentation in ejaculated spermatozoa can be higher than in those obtained from the testis and caput or corpus epididymis [22, 23].

Leukocytes, mainly neutrophils and macrophages, generate ROS and are important contributors to the general seminal level of ROS. Infection is the major cause of leukocytic infiltration into the male genital tract, and in a vast majority of cases, the spermatozoa get in contact with the leukocytes at ejaculation [23].

However, the origin of ROS which may be deleterious to the integrity of sperm DNA may not only be extrinsic but even intrinsic, the major source being sperm mitochondria [24]. The net result in terms of the degree of sperm DNA damage depends on the balance between extrinsic and intrinsic ROS production and the protective ability of the seminal fluid.

12.4.4 Activation of Caspases and Endonucleases

We should also mention that sperm DNA fragmentation can even be induced by activation of sperm's own caspases and endonucleases activated by oxygen radicals and physicochemical factors, including heat exposure. This also means that ROS may induce DNA strand breaks in the spermatozoa by exerting a direct effect, or indirectly, by inducing a cascade of events involving the above-mentioned enzymes [19].

The proposed mechanisms to explain the very origin of sperm DNA damage are obviously not mutually exclusive and, recently, a two-step hypothesis has been put forward where faulty spermatogenesis can lead to defective chromatin remodelling with the DNA more susceptible and vulnerable to a variety of stressors [22].

There are a variety of etiologic factors that have been associated with sperm DNA fragmentation and/or defective chromatin. Sperm DNA breaks have also been linked to exposure to cancer treatment, radiotherapy and chemotherapy [25], as well as to some environmental toxicants, e.g. PCBs, phthalates and air pollution [26, 27]. The exact mechanisms behind the effects of such exposures in relation to sperm DNA integrity are not known. However, these might include a direct effect on the DNA of the spermatozoa as well as indirect effect caused by changes in the endocrine milieu of the testis and/or epididymis and, thereby, lowered activity of the testosterone-dependent DNA enzyme topoisomerase as well as reduced epidymal production of antioxidants.

Both single- (SSB) and double-stranded (DSB) DNA breaks can occur. Generally, SSB is easier to repair and has a better prognosis than the DSB. SSB are usually due to unrepaired DNA nicks introduced during the spermiogenesis or as a consequence of the action of ROS. However, the latter may also lead to DSB, which also can be a consequence of abortive apoptosis and/or the action of caspases and endonucleases. DSBs are considered the nastiest DNA lesions that, if left unrepaired, would lead to gross structural alteration of the chromosome complement. Therefore, a sperm DSB is considered to be a most serious DNA lesion which has potential deleterious impact of the healthy development of the progeny [7].

Some recent review articles [18, 19] provide more finely detailed reviews of the possible mechanisms entangled behind sperm DNA damage. From the clinical point of view, it is important to stress that the cause of sperm DNA fragmentation may be multi-factorial and is partly unknown. Most of the available techniques for detection of sperm DNA damage provide limited information on the nature of the DNA lesions detected and none of them enables us to depict the exact aetiology and pathogenesis of impairment of sperm DNA, this diagnostic problem reducing our possibilities of giving a cause-related efficient therapy.

12.5 Methods for Assessment of Sperm DNA Damage

Several methods for assessment of sperm DNA damage are now available. Below some details of the most commonly applied techniques will be given.

12.5.1 TdT and TUNNEL

The terminal deoxynucleotidyl transferase (TdT)-mediated 2′-deoxyuridine 5′-triphosphate-nick end labelling (TUNEL) assay uses TdT, an enzyme able to catalyse, in the presence of DNA nicks, the addition of dUTPs that are secondarily labelled with a marker, generally fluorescent. TdT preferentially labels the blunt 3′-OH ends of double-stranded DNA breaks, but also works on the single-strand 3′-OH [28]. The assay detects the DNA breaks directly, which means without initial step of denaturation by introducing acid or alkaline pH. However, the peculiar sperm chromatin compaction may impede its effectiveness and limit the access of the enzyme to all 3′-OH break ends [29]. TUNEL tests can be based on microscopic evaluation of 2–500 cells, and if the labelling is fluorescent, flow cytometric analysis is also possible thus increasing statistical reliability (the number of scored cells can be 5–10,000), precision, and sensitivity of the measurements.

12.5.2 Comet

Comet assay [30] is a single cell gel electrophoresis of immobilised sperm, which involves their encapsulation in agarose, lysis (at different pH), and electrophoresis. When the electric field is applied, the DNA, which has an overall negative charge, is drawn towards the anode, which is positively charged. Undamaged DNA strands are too large and do not leave the nucleus, whereas the smaller the fragments, the farther they are free to move in a given period of time. Therefore, the amount of DNA that leaves the nucleus is a measure of the amount of DNA damage in the cell. The cells are stained with a fluorescent DNA-binding dye. The overall intensity of the fluorescence for the whole nucleoid and the fluorescence of the migrated DNA is measured by image analysis. The stronger the signal from the migrated DNA, the more damage there is present. The overall structure resembles a comet (hence "Comet assay") with a circular head corresponding to the undamaged DNA that remains in the nucleus and a tail of damaged DNA. The brighter and longer the tail, the higher the level of damage. Comet assay can be performed under neutral as well as alkaline conditions. By choosing different pH conditions for electrophoresis and the preceding incubation, different damage types and different levels of sensitivity can be assessed. Under neutral (pH 8–9) conditions, mainly DSB are detected, although some SSB due to the relaxation of supercoiled loops containing the breaks might also contribute to the observed comet [31]. Alternatively, under alkaline conditions, DSB and SSB (at pH 12.3) and additionally alkali labile sites (at pH ≥13) can be visualised resulting in increased DNA migration in the electrophoretic field [32]. Comet assay, requiring a much smaller number of cells (typically, only 100) for analysis than other tests, has been considered as particularly useful and suitable for measures of testicular and oligozoospermic sperm samples where cells are scarce [33].

12.5.3 Sperm Chromatin Structure Assay

SCSA is a flow cytometric test where sperm DNA breaks can be evaluated indirectly through DNA denaturability. The assay measures the susceptibility of sperm DNA to acid-induced DNA denaturation in situ (the low-pH solution potentially denatures only the DNA that is damaged), followed by staining with the fluorescence dye acridine orange [34–36] and quantifying the metachromatic shift of acridine orange fluorescence from green (native DNA) to red (denatured DNA) under a blue light excitation. By using a flow cytometer, 5–10,000 sperm can be analysed within a short time. Through a specific SCSA-software (SCSA-Soft®, SCSA, Brookings, ND), the ratio of red to total (green plus red) fluorescence is calculated for each sperm and the frequency distribution, called DFI, of all the accumulated measured sperm is generated, together with scattergrams formed by a proper combination of sperm fluorescent parameters. From these data, the percentage of spermatozoa with an abnormally high DNA stainability and the level of DNA fragmentation are calculated. The sperm fraction with the most intensive green colour is called high DNA stainable (HDS). It is still unclear precisely which mechanisms and types of DNA damage are lying behind DFI and HDS; however, it is believed that DFI are related to the percentage of sperm with both SSB and DSB and/or impairment of normal protamination. HDS is thought to represent immature spermatozoa. One of the benefits of SCSA is adhering to a standardised protocol that minimises inter-laboratory variation [37].

These three methods are to be considered as major tests applied for clinical evaluation of sperm DNA integrity. However, other potential techniques can be mentioned.

12.5.4 Acridine Orange Test

Acridine orange test (*AOT*) is based on exactly the same principle as the SCSA (see above). However, the evaluation of the proportion of cells with denaturated DNA is based on a microscopic examination of a smear. The main advantage is its simplicity and there is no need of expensive equipment. However, due to a low number of cells which are scored, unpredictable artifactual of acridine orange on a glass surface because of its critical equilibrium staining and the subjectivity in the assessment of the level of intra- and inter-laboratory variation are significantly higher than the case is for the SCSA assay. Such conditions could preclude use of AOT for reliable clinical diagnosis and prognosis of a semen sample.

12.5.5 Toluidine Blue Test

Toluidine blue (*TB*) *test* is also based on microscopic examination of smears stained with the thiazine dye toluidine blue. Like in SCSA and AOT, prior to staining, the DNA of the spermatozoa is denaturated by lowering the pH. The test measures the availability of the sperm chromatin DNA phosphate residues for staining with TB, which is dependent on both the protein state and DNA integrity. It has been reported [38, 39] that sperm nuclei with red fluorescence by AOT corresponded to those that stain dark-purple with TB, whereas sperm with green fluorescence correspond to those that stain light blue with TB. The number of dark-purple-stained cells as percentage of all cells is assessed by microscopic examination. The results of the TB test correlate well with the results of the SCSA and TUNEL assay [40] and the test could be amenable of clinical application also because of its relative simplicity and inexpensiveness.

12.5.6 Sperm Chromatin Dispersion

Sperm chromatin dispersion (*SCD*) test is based on the principle that sperm with fragmented DNA fails to produce the characteristic halo of dispersed DNA loops that are observed on sperm with non-fragmented DNA, when mixed with aqueous agarose following acid denaturation and removal of chromatin nuclear proteins [41]. This relatively simple procedure can be performed either with fluorescence or Diff-Quick staining, and consequently, the SCD can be assessed either by fluorescence microscopy or by bright field microscopy. Approximately 500 cells are, after initial denaturation and staining procedure, evaluated under the microscope and the halo size of each cell is evaluated by the relative parameter: area of the halo divided by that of the whole nucleoid. Since some sperm cells may have different nuclear sizes, this relative parameter avoids the distortion that would result if absolute sizes were considered. A complete kit (Halosperm, INDAS Biotech, Madrid, Spain) has been developed.

12.5.7 Oxidised Deoxynucleoside

Oxidised deoxynucleoside, 8-oxo-7,8-dihydro-2′deoxyguanosine (*8-oxodG*) level is considered to be a biomarker of oxidative stress in sperm which could also have negative effects on sperm function [42–44]. The levels of 8-oxodG and dG in nuclear sperm DNA are chemically determined by high pressure liquid chromatography (HPLC) after DNA extraction from nuclei isolated from the sample and digestion to the deoxynucleosides by means of nuclease P1 and alkaline phosphatase. The level of 8-oxodG is reported per 10^5 unoxidized dG. Recently, the formation of the 8-oxodG base lesion can also be measured using fluorescently labelled anti-8-oxodG antibodies and their abundance can be assessed by measuring the fluorescence level using flow cytometry [45].

12.5.8 Chromomycin A3 Staining

Chromomycin A3 (*CMA3*) *staining* is considered as a test assessing the packaging quality of the chromatin in spermatozoa and may allow indirect visualisation of protamine deficiency [46]. It is based on the ability of CMA3 to compete with the protamines for binding to the minor groove of DNA. The fraction of CMA3 positive cells is commonly assessed by scoring 200 cells under a fluorescence microscope.

Furthermore, two other tests do not directly detect sperm DNA strand breaks, but detect earlier stages of the apoptotic cascade which ultimately leads to DNA fragmentation.

12.5.9 Annexin V-Binding Ability Assay

Annexin V-binding ability assay is a method based on the ability of Annexin V to bind to phosphatidylserine (PS), a well-established early apoptosis marker [47]. Sperm suspension is washed and, thereafter, centrifuged. Annexin V labelled with fluorescein isothiocyanate (FITC) is added to the pellet and subsequently a smear is made and evaluated with a fluorescence microscope for assessment of the percentage of green-fluorescing sperm (Annexin V positive) cells.

12.5.10 Evaluation of Anti- or Pro-Apoptotic Proteins

Evaluation of anti- or pro-apoptotic proteins. Antibodies against anti- (e.g. Bcl-xL) and pro-apoptotic (e.g. caspase-3 and Fas) can be used for evaluation of the percentage of abortive apoptotic spermatozoa. Quantification can be done by use of microscopy or flow cytometry [48].

Although these tests differ, both as we consider the technical principle but also what they specifically are measuring, a number of investigations have shown a moderate association when same sample is assessed by use of two or more of these tests [40] (Table 12.1). However, the correlations coefficients between the results of different tests are usually of a magnitude not higher than 0.4–0.6. To a certain extent, all these tests may complement each other as each test could address a particular facet of the complex processes involved in sperm nuclear packaging, and consequently, in the formation and detection of sperm DNA breaks [49]. Finally, with the exception of SCSA, each test requires a definitive protocol propaedeutic to its standardisation.

12.6 Clinical Usefulness of Sperm DNA Tests

Animal studies incontestably show that sperm DNA damage does impair normal embryo development and a healthy progress of pregnancy. Whereas there is also no doubt that there is an association between the percentage of human sperms with DNA damage and the fertility potential of a couple, the question is what the clinical usefulness of testing for sperm DNA integrity is? The literature does not give any unequivocal answer regarding this issue, the conclusions varying from "very useful" to "not useful" or more often "more research is needed". Some of the confusion regarding the role of sperm DNA integrity testing in the clinical set-up is related to lack of standardisation in methodology applied for assessment of sperm DNA integrity (see above), but also limited power of many studies due to a low number of patients included. Furthermore,

Table 12.1 Correlation levels between results of different sperm DNA fragmentation assays from selected studies (with >50 men)

Techniques	General population or healthy donors, *n*	Subfertile men, *n*	Correlation coefficient	References
SCSA vs. Comet assay				
SCSA vs. Comet, neutral pH 8	80		N.S.	[116]
SCSA vs. Comet, alkaline pH 13	80		N.S.	[116]
SCSA vs. Comet, alkaline pH 12.1		55	0.31	[117]
SCSA vs. TUNEL assay				
SCSA vs. FlM-TUNEL	7	60	0.90	[118]
SCSA vs. FlM-TUNEL	25	55	0.50	[119]
SCSA vs. FCM-TUNEL	24	96	0.41	[112]
SCSA vs. FCM-TUNEL	666		0.56	Toft (personal communication)
SCSA vs. FCM-TUNEL		58	0.27	[117]
SCSA vs. AOT				
SCSA vs. AOT		185	N.S.	[120]
SCSA vs. AOT	7	60	N.S.	[118]
SCSA vs. SCD	7	60	0.87–0.98	[118]
SCSA vs. toluidine blue	63	79	0.47	[59]
FCM- vs. FlM-TUNEL assay				
FCM-TUNEL vs. FlM-TUNEL		66	0.72	[121]
FCM-TUNEL vs. FlM-TUNEL		68	0.94	[122]
TUNEL assay vs. Comet assay				
FCM-TUNEL vs. Comet (alkaline pH 10)	42	21	0.56	[123]
FCM-TUNEL vs. Comet (alkaline pH 12.1)		58	N.S.	[117]
TUNEL assay vs. CMA3				
FlM-TUNEL vs. CMA3		61	0.76	[62]
FlM-TUNEL vs. CMA3		132	0.53	[124]
FCM TUNEL vs. CMA3	39	28	0.83–0.96	[24]
TUNEL assay vs. SCD				
M-TUNEL vs. SCD	30	60	0.6–0.9	[125]
FlM-TUNEL vs. SCD	7	60	0.9	[118, 126]
SCD vs. CMA3		78	$r=0.29$	[126]
8-oxodG vs. TUNEL assay		94	0.25 (0.77)[a]	[24]

Levels of correlation: ≤0.15 not correlated, 0.15–0.39 poorly, 0.4–0.45 moderately

AOT acridine orange test; *CMA3* chromomycin A3; *SCD* sperm chromatin dispersion test; *SCSA* sperm chromatin structure assay; *TUNEL* terminal deoxynucleotidyl transferase dUTP nick end labelling; *M-TUNEL* TUNEL assay, bright field microscopy; *FlM-TUNEL* TUNEL assay, fluorescence microscopy; *FCM-TUNEL* TUNEL assay, flow cytometry; *N.S.* not statistically significant

[a] Calculated for Percoll high density separated semen fraction

the majority of reports focusing on ART do not discriminate between different methods (IUI; IVF; ICSI) applied for achieving pregnancy. From a clinical point of view, the following questions seem relevant to ask:

1. Is sperm DNA integrity testing a good predictor of the chance of achieving spontaneous pregnancy?
2. Can it be used for selection of most appropriate method of ART?

3. How robust are the tests in terms of intra-individual variation?

Below, we will try to give answer to these questions with focus on summarising of the existing knowledge rather than an extensive review of the literature.

12.6.1 Sperm DNA Integrity and Chance of Spontaneous Pregnancy

Very few studies have addressed the issue of sperm DNA integrity in relation to fertility in the general population. The two major reports within this area, one carried out in USA (the Georgetown study, 165 couples) and the other carried out in Europe (the Danish first pregnancy planners study, 215 couples), have been based on the use of SCSA. Both demonstrated that in couples from the general population, the chance of spontaneous pregnancy, measured by the time-to-pregnancy (TTP), decreases when DFI exceeded 20–30% [50, 51]. If the DFI was more than 30%, TTP tended to become infinite and the chances of spontaneous pregnancies were quite negligible. Stratifying the population into two groups, below and above a DFI threshold at 30%, the probability of pregnancy for the group with DFI <30% was statistically significantly higher than that for the group with DFI >30%. These two in vivo studies showed that the pregnancy rates are significantly higher for the group with DFI below the thresholds of 30% [52]. However, whereas DFI above 30% was highly predictive of low chance of spontaneous pregnancy, in a significant proportion of cases with DFI<30% the couples were unable to conceive. Thus, these data indicated that sperm DNA integrity testing, or at least SCSA, is a better marker of "infertility" than of "fertility" in vivo.

In the above-mentioned population of Danish first pregnancy planners [50], the likelihood of pregnancy occurring in a single menstrual cycle was inversely associated with the level of 8-oxodG [53]. These data suggest that sperm DNA oxidative damage influences fecundity, corroborating the result of the previous SCSA analysis and reinforcing the notion that oxidative DNA damage can play a major role in the genesis of DNA breaks [18].

These results based on couples from general population have been confirmed in a more recent study of 127 men from infertile couples where female factors contributing to the infertility problem were excluded and 137 men with proven fertility. Using SCSA as the method for assessing sperm DNA and the group of men with DFI <10% as reference group, the risk of being infertile was increased when DFI >20% (OR 5.1) in men with normal standard semen parameters, whereas if one of the WHO parameters were abnormal, the OR for infertility was increased already at DFI above 10% (OR 16) [54].

The above-mentioned study not only indicated that SCSA can be used in prediction of the chance of spontaneous pregnancy, independently of the standard sperm parameters (Table 12.2), but since DFI above 20% was found in 40% of men with otherwise normal standard parameters [54], it seems that in almost half of the cases of so-called "unexplained" infertility, sperm DNA defects are at least a contributing factor to the problem.

Interestingly, a cut-off fraction around 20% of defective sperm discriminating between normal healthy donors and male factor infertile men has been found by two studies using the TUNEL assay evaluated by flow cytometry [28, 55].

Also, other SCSA-based studies have shown higher DFI in men from infertile couples as compared to fertile men or to donors [56, 57]. This is also true for reports based on use of other techniques as Comet assay [58], TUNEL [55], TB [59], 8-oxodG [60], AO [61], SCD [41] and CMA3 [62]. However, although the vast majority of published data of such difference was found, this is not true for all of them [63]. Furthermore, generally, perhaps due to a significantly less degree of standardisation, the "threshold" values for infertility differ significantly, from study to study, when other techniques than SCSA have been applied for assessment of sperm DNA integrity [63].

When evaluating infertile men (Table 12.3), it has generally been noted that dyspermic men have also a higher fraction of chromatin defective sperm, supporting the intuitive notion that, in the presence of spermatogenic defects leading to oligoasthenoteratozoospermia, the chance of an increased chromatin damage is also more probable. This has been noted in a variety of studies

Table 12.2 Correlation levels between sperm DNA fragmentation and the WHO parameters of concentration, motility, and morphology from selected studies (with >150 men)

Technique	General population or healthy donors, *n*	Subfertile men, *n*	Concentration	Morphology	Motility	References
SCSA						
SCSA	277		–0.31	–0.38		[100]
SCSA	215		–0.23	–0.25		[50]
SCSA	278		–0.12			[127]
SCSA	171		–0.26		–0.43 (–0.53[a])	[37]
SCSA	278		–0.12		–0.25 (–0.38[a])	[37]
SCSA		201	–0.22	–0.46	–0.56	[120]
SCSA		249		–0.36	–0.41	[70]
SCSA	707		N.S.	–0.17	–0.23	[94]
SCSA		374		N.S.		[69]
SCSA	209		N.S.	–0.22	–0.19	[106]
SCSA		2,586	–0.22	–0.40	–0.61	[128]
SCSA		279	–0.41	–0.35	–0.50	[57]
SCSA		175	Negative	Negative	Negative	[128]
M-TUNEL		332		–0.2	–0.2	[129]
Fl M-TUNEL		150	N.S.	Negative	Negative	[91]
Fl M-TUNEL		262	N.S.	–0.44	–0.60	[130]
Fl M-TUNEL		167			N.S.	[131]
Fl M-TUNEL		167			0.12	[131]
FCM-TUNEL		298	–0.18	–0.34	–0.12	[92]
FCM-TUNEL		1,633	N.S.	N.S.	N.S.[a]	[122]
Comet assay (neutral)		257	–1.42	–0.05	–0.43	[132]
SCD		622	–0.13	–0.32	–0.28	[133]
AOT						
AOT		187	–0.58	–0.48	–0.42	[134]
AOT		185	N.S.	0.18	N.S.	[120]
AOT		234			0.21	[131]
AOT		234			0.20	[131]
Aniline blue	75	90	N.S.	N.S.	N.S.	[90]

Levels of correlation: ≤0.15 not correlated, 0.15–0.39 poorly, 0.4–0.45 moderately

AOT acridine orange test; *SCD* sperm chromatin dispersion test; *SCSA* sperm chromatin structure assay; *TUNEL* terminal deoxynucleotidyl transferase dUTP nick end labelling; *M-TUNEL* TUNEL assay, bright field microscopy; *FlM-TUNEL* TUNEL assay, fluorescence microscopy; *FCM-TUNEL* TUNEL assay, flow cytometry; *N.S.* not statistically significant

[a] Evaluated by computer-assisted sperm analysis (CASA)

using the Comet assay [64], the TUNEL assay [65, 66], CMA3 and in situ nick translation [67], SCSA [56, 68–71], the SCD test [72], and toluidine blue staining [40].

A higher fraction of sperm with DNA fragmentation emerged also in men with abnormal protamine 1/protamione 2 ratio, implying a protective role of protamines against sperm DNA damage [73].

12.6.2 Sperm DNA Integrity Testing and ART

ART are widely used in cases when the chance of spontaneous pregnancy is considered as non-existing or very low. If the infertility problem of the couple is unexplained or the impairment of semen quality is considered as "mild", the IUI may be the first choice treatment. If the

Table 12.3 Selected studies (with >100 individuals) reporting prevalence of DNA defective sperm in infertile men as compared to normal controls

Technique	Controls, *n*	Subfertile men, *n*	Notes	References
SCSA	165	115	DFI significantly higher in infertility men (24.4%) than in controls (13.7 ± 7.2%)	[51]
SCSA	13	88	DFI significantly higher in infertile men (23.1 ± 1.7%) than in controls (10.8 ± 1.6%)	[56]
SCSA	16	92	DFI significantly higher in infertile men (28%) than in controls (15%)	[71]
SCSA	13	101	DFI significantly higher in infertile men (22.0 ± 1.5%) than in controls (10.8 ± 1.8%)	[135]
SCSA	100	200	DFI significantly higher in infertile men (20.2–23.8%) than in controls (5.2–6.6%)	[136]
SCSA	22	279	DFI significantly higher in infertile men (range 3.8–90.8%) than in controls (range 6.43–25.74%)	[57]
SCSA	137	127	DFI significantly higher in infertile men (23%) than in controls (12%)	[54]
M-TUNEL	20	236	Fraction of TUNEL positive sperm significantly lower in controls (0.3 ± 0.4%) than in infertile men	[82]
FlM-TUNEL	23	87	Fraction of TUNEL positive sperm significantly lower in controls (2.5 ± 1.2%) than in infertile men (11.3 ± 4.9%)	[137]
FlM-TUNEL	49	61	Fraction of TUNEL positive sperm significantly lower in controls (6.2 ± 1.8%) than in infertile men (30.0 ± 7.1%)	[62]
FCM-TUNEL	47	66	Fraction of TUNEL positive sperm significantly lower in controls (13.1 ± 7.3%) than in infertile men (40.9 ± 14.3%) Cut-off at 20%	[28]
FCM-TUNEL	25	194	Fraction of TUNEL positive sperm significantly lower in controls (11.9 ± 6.8%) than in infertile men (29.5 ± 18.7%) Cut-off at 19.25%	[55]
CMA3	49	61	Fraction of CMA3 positive sperm significantly higher in infertile men (31.5 ± 7.1%) than in controls (6.3 ± 1.8%)	[62]
Aniline blue	75	90	Fraction of condensed sperm significantly higher in control (78.0 ± 19.0%) than in infertile men (55.0 ± 12.0%)	[90]
Toluidine blue	63	79	Controls have a significant higher fraction on normal toluidine blue light cells than infertile men (51 ± 21 vs. 32 ± 20%) and significantly less abnormal toluidine blue dark cells (24 ± 13 vs. 47 ± 24%) Cut-off for infertility 45% toluidine blue dark cells	[59]
8-oxodG	54	60	Levels of 8-oxodG significantly higher in infertile men than in controls (10.0 vs. 4.8/10^5 deoxyguanosines)	[60]

CMA3 chromomycin A3; *DFI* DNA fragmentation index, evaluated by SCSA; *SCSA* sperm chromatin structure assay; *TUNEL* terminal deoxynucleotidyl transferase dUTP nick end labelling; *M-TUNEL* TUNEL assay, bright field microscopy; *FlM-TUNEL* TUNEL assay, fluorescence microscopy; *FCM-TUNEL* TUNEL assay, flow cytometry; *8-oxodG* 8-hydroxydeoxyguanosine level evaluated by high-performance liquid chromatography

IUI treatment is unsuccessful or there is a serious female pathology, as, for example, occlusion of the fallopian tubes, those couples may go directly for IVF. In cases of poor semen quality and/or unsuccessful standard IVF, ICSI becomes the method of choice.

Although the panorama of ART includes a number of potentially powerful techniques, the results are still somewhat disappointing and two third or more of the treatment do not lead to a child birth. One of the reasons behind this problem is the low predictive value of standard sperm parameters in relation to ART, which become quite meaningless in the case of ICSI. Therefore, better markers are needed in order to avoid ART treatment with an a priori low chance of success, but also to give the most simple and least invasive type of therapy.

It should be also kept in mind that the reproductive end points in relation to ART may differ according to whether the fertilisation is achieved in vivo or in vitro. The latter scenario allows for evaluation of not only pregnancy or birth rate, but also of parameters as fertilisation, embryo quality and early miscarriage.

12.6.2.1 Intrauterine Insemination

Numerous studies have shown association between level of indices of sperm DNA damage and IUI pregnancy rate. The pioneering report by Duran et al. [74] has shown in 154 couples lack of pregnancy when DFI, as measured by the TUNEL assay on prepared semen, was above 12%. Similar findings have been reported by Saleh et al. [75] who performed a small study where 12 of 19 couples had a DFI value as measured by SCSA above 28% and none of these couples achieved a pregnancy. Boe-Hansen and colleagues used the SCSA in a study on 48 IUI-couples. Only two of the couples had a DFI value above 30%, and none of them obtained a pregnancy [69]. In our own report based on 387 IUI cycles, DFI as assessed by SCSA was shown to be a predictor of fertility independent of other sperm parameters [76]. While the proportion of children born per cycle was 19.0% when the DFI value was below 30%, those with a DFI value above 30% only had a take-home-baby rate of 1.5%. The chance of IUI pregnancy was unaffected by the variation of DFI within the range 0–20%, but started to decrease when the value exceeded the 20% level. This result is well in accordance with the other SCSA data based on in vivo conception, those based on general population or couples with unexplained infertility (see above). In contrast, no correlation was found between SCD results and pregnancy outcome in 100 Spanish IUI-patients [77].

12.6.2.2 IVF and ICSI

Earlier studies based on quite limited numbers of couples indicated that DFI above 27% as measured by SCSA could be used as a cut-off value for infertility, not only in vivo but even in vitro. It was reported that in couples with a DFI >27%, no pregnancy could be obtained, regardless of the type of ART applied [78, 79]. However, in 2004 three independent SCSA reports demonstrated that a DFI level above 27% was indeed compatible with pregnancy and delivery after both IVF and ICSI [70, 80, 81] meaning that use of ART compensates for poor sperm chromatin quality.

Our own study [76] based on 388 IVF and 223 ICSI cycles has shown no statistically significant difference between the outcomes of ICSI and ICSI when DFI of 30% was used as a threshold. However, in the DFI >30% group, the results of ICSI were significantly better than those of IVF, no such difference being seen for lower levels of sperm DNA damage. When comparing ICSI to IVF (reference), the odds ratios (ORs) for biochemical pregnancy (BP), clinical pregnancy (CP) and delivery (D) were 3.0 (95% CI: 1.4–6.2), 2.3 (5% CI: 1.1–4.6) and 2.2 (95% CI: 1.0–4.5), respectively.

These data are in agreement with other previous smaller reports using TUNEL or Comet assays, showing that sperm DNA damage is more predictive in IVF and much less so in ICSI [82, 83]. Also a very recent study of Simon et al. [84], using Comet assay, has shown that the difference in percentage of sperms with impairment of DNA integrity, when comparing successful and unsuccessful treatment, is much more clear for IVF than for ICSI. In contrast, one single study reported that DFI threshold values were not valid for prediction of IVF outcome [85]. However, this study did not discriminate between standard IVF and ICSI.

Whereas several studies have shown some association between the ART outcome and DFI, the other parameter measured by SCSA, HDS, has not yet been shown of any clinical significance.

The data regarding the relationship between sperm DNA fragmentation and fertilisation rates after IVF and ICSI are conflicting. Ahmadi and Ng in a mouse model demonstrated that despite DNA damage, a spermatozoa was able to fertilise an oocyte [86]. Also, human studies have shown that the fertilisation rate is the same for men with high number of sperm with damaged DNA as for those with a low proportion of such cells, when using SCSA [76, 79, 87] or other sperm DNA integrity assays [88–90]. On the other hand, the presence of damaged sperm DNA was shown to have a significant inverse relationship with fertilisation in other studies [82, 91, 92].

Although fertilisation may be independent of sperm DNA integrity, it has been suggested that the post-fertilisation development of the pre-embryo can be impaired by such incomplete or aberrant sperm DNA repair by the oocyte leading to implantation failure, early miscarriages or in the worst cases diseases in the offspring [6, 22]. The human data regarding pre-embryo development in relation to sperm DNA damage is also conflicting. While some authors have reported similar cleavage stage embryo developmental rates between high and low DFI groups as measured by SCSA [79, 80], others have shown that sperm DNA damage is negatively correlated with embryo quality after IVF and ICSI [92, 93]. Two studies have also reported that men with high levels of DNA fragmentation are at increased risk of low blastocyst formation compared to men with a low DFI [94, 95].

12.6.3 Intra-Individual Variation in Sperm DNA Integrity

One of the limitations in use of standard semen parameters in the daily clinical routine is the considerable intra-individual variation with respect to sperm concentration, motility and morphology [96–98]. Even DFI, as measured by use of SCSA, seems to be a subject of such variation. Thus, for this parameter, CVs of 21–29% have been found [99–101]. In this subgroup, a switch of DFI to a higher level may have implications for the selection of the ART treatment, since the DFI of 30% was found to represent a clinically relevant cut-off level [76].

Comparison between TUNEL and SCSA indicated a less variation over the data collection period for the latter method with a DFI within-subject CVs of 47.4 and 22.3%, respectively [102].

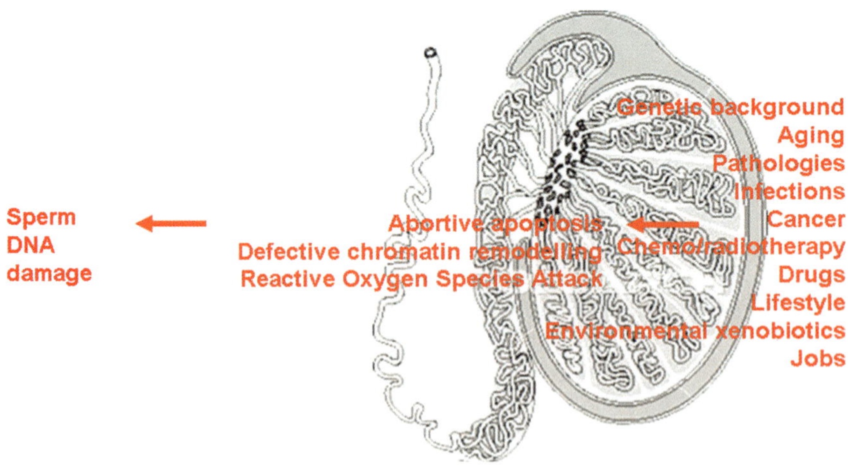

Fig. 12.1 A two-step hypothesis of origin of human sperm DNA damage according to Aitken and De Iuliis [18]. The figure does also visualise where in the male reproductive system the damage occurs

In another TUNEL study, the CV sperm DFI ranged from 12.9 to 43.9%, whereas parallel measurements on cell counts showed within-donor CVs ranging from 16.7 up to 63.2% [103].

Although even DFI seems to be a subject of some intra-individual variation, the question is whether it is of any clinical significance? Our own data (Oleszczuk, personal communication) have shown that among 616 men referred due to infertility, 85% remained in the same category of DFI; ≤30% or >30% when comparing first and second SCSA test. This implies that only in 15% a repeated analysis implied a reclassification of the SCSA-based prediction of fertility potential of the patient.

The biological background for the intra-individual variation in DFI is not completely known, although some lifestyle-related factors may be of an importance (Fig. 12.1).

12.7 The Effects of Lifestyle and Environmental Factors

Several lifestyle- and environment-related factors have been linked to increase in percentage of sperms with impairment of DNA integrity. A number of studies have shown positive association between the length of the abstinence period and both SCSA DFI [100], although the correlations found were usually weak to moderate. Although it might be expected that cigarette smoking implies an impairment of sperm DNA integrity, the data in the literature are quite controversial with some of the largest studies not showing such effect [104, 105]. So far there is lack of information regarding other lifestyle factors as consumption of alcohol, caffeine or recreational drugs.

Among environmental factors, the most consistent association between exposure and DFI has been found for polychlorinated biphenyls (PCBs) and phthalates, although some reports have indicated impairment of sperm DNA integrity related to air pollution, styrene, lead, pesticide and dichlorodiphenyldichloroethylene (*p,p′*-DDE – a metabolite of DDT) exposure [26, 27, 106].

Interestingly, for PCBs, an ethnic difference in susceptibility to the effect of the exposure has been seen. Thus, high PCB levels in serum were associated with increase in DFI in Caucasian, but not in Inuit men [27]. Whether this difference is due to genetic diversity or to other lifestyle factors, for example, food intake, is not known. Knowledge to the link between lifestyle/environment and sperm DNA integrity is interesting from a biological point of view; the clinical implications are so far limited. These data are summarised in Table 12.4.

Furthermore, some studies evidenced that the association between sperm chromatin damage and environmental exposure emerged if absent or resulted exacerbated if already present only in selected subpopulations characterised by a particular gene polymorphism, thus implying that a suspected gene–environment interplay can be at work [107–109].

12.8 Sperm DNA Integrity and Cancer

Males treated for cancer represent a potential source of worry in relation to sperm DNA integrity. It could be expected that cancer therapy – both irradiation and cytotoxic drugs – might introduce sperm DNA defects, which could be transmitted to the offspring, mainly if IVF or ICSI are used as methods of conception.

The available data indicate that both adult and childhood cancer per se can lead to a slight increase in DFI [110, 111]. Cancer treatment may add to the impairment of sperm DNA integrity, and this effect, even if transiently, seems to be most pronounced for the irradiation treatment [25], whereas it is limited or not seen at all in men given chemotherapy [112]. Sperm cryopreservation has, in some studies, been shown to imply an increase in percentage of sperms with abnormal DFI [113], although even these findings have been questioned by others [110]. Epidemiological data show that in vitro conceived children of men treated for cancer have no increased risk of congenital malformations as compared to those IVF/ICSI children not having a father with a history of malignancy.

Table 12.4 Epidemiologic studies of ambient chemical exposures and sperm DNA damage

Noxia	Subjects	Indicator of exposure	Technique	Association	References
Polycyclic aromatic hydrocarbons (PAH)					
	42 Taiwan coke-oven workers	Urinary 1-hydroxypyrene levels	SCSA	Positive	[138]
	273 Chinese fertile and 620 infertile men	Urinary 1-hydroxypyrene levels	TUNEL assay (FCM)	Positive	[139]
Air pollution					
	266 Young Czech	Ambient air pollution monitoring	SCSA	Positive	[140]
	36 Young Czech	Ambient air pollution monitoring	SCSA	Positive	[26, 108]
Plastics					
Styrene					
	21 Danish farmers unexposed 23 Danish reinforced plastic workers	Urinary mandelic acid levels	SCSA	Positive	[141]
Styrene (mandelic acid urinary concentration)	46 Italian plastics workers 27 Unexposed controls	Urinary mandelic acid levels	Comet assay (alkaline)	Positive	[142]
Phthalates					
	168 US men from infertile couples	Phthalate metabolites urinary concentration	Comet assay (neutral)	Positive	[143]
	379 US men from infertile couples	Phthalate metabolites urinary concentration	Comet assay (neutral)	Positive	[105]
	234 Young Swedish from general population	Phthalate metabolites urinary concentration	SCSA	N.S.	[144]
	300 Indian men (200 infertile, 100 fertile) from infertility clinics		SCSA	Positive	[136]
Acrylonitrile	30 Chinese acrylonitrile exposed workers 30 Non-exposed controls	Ambient air monitoring of acrylonitrile in the workplace	Comet assay (alkaline)	Positive	[145]
Persistant organic pollutants (POPs)					
DDT					
	212 US men from infertile couples	Serum *p,p'*-DDE levels	Comet assay (neutral)	N.S.	[146]
	176 Swedish fishermen	Serum *p,p'*-DDE levels	SCSA	N.S.	[104]
	514 European and 193 Inuit men from general population	Serum *p,p'*-DDE levels	SCSA	N.S.	[27]
	452 European and 200 Inuit men from general population	Serum *p,p'*-DDE levels	TUNEL assay (FCM)	N.S.	[48]
	116 Mexican residents in malaria areas	Serum *p,p'*-DDE levels	Aniline blue	Positive	[147]
	209 South Africans living in malaria areas	Serum *p,p'*-DDE levels	SCSA	Positive	[106]
PCBs					
	212 US men from infertile couples	Serum concentration of congeners PCB 118, PCB 138, PCB 153	Comet assay (neutral)	N.S.	[146]
	176 Swedish fishermen	Serum concentration of PCB congener 153	SCSA	Positive	[104]

(continued)

Table 12.4 (continued)

Noxia	Subjects	Indicator of exposure	Technique	Association	References
	514 European and 193 Inuit men from general population	Serum concentration of PCB congener 153	SCSA	Positive (in Europeans only)	[27]
	452 European and 200 Inuit men from general population	Serum concentration of PCB congener 153	TUNEL assay (FCM)	Positive (in Europeans only)	[48]
Hexachlorobenzene (HCB)	212 US men from infertile couples	Serum concentration of HCB	Comet assay (neutral)	N.S.	[146]
Pesticides					
	169 Danish pesticide spraying farmers 82 Danish not spraying farmers	Interview	SCSA	N.S.	[148]
	33 Mexican agricultural workers	Urinary concentration of diethylthiophosphate (DETP)	SCSA	Positive	[149]
	21 Chinese pesticide factory workers 23 Internal controls 19 External controls	Ambient air monitoring of fenvalerate in the workplace	Comet assay (alkaline) and TUNEL assay (FCM)	Positive	[123]
	260 US men from infertile couples	Urinary metabolite concentrations of chlorpyrifos (3,5,6-trichloro-2-pyridinol) and carbaryl (1-naphthol)	Comet assay (neutral)	Positive	[150]
	207 US men from infertile couples	Urinary concentration of pyrethroid metabolites 3-phenoxybenzoic acid and *cis*- and *trans*-3-(2, 2-dichlorovinyl)-2,2-dimethylcyclopropane carboxylic acid	Comet assay (neutral)	Positive	[151]
	54 Mexican agricultural workers	Interview	ISNT assay	Positive	[107]
	16 Chinese pesticide factory workers 30 internal and external controls	Ambient air monitoring of carbaryl in the workplace	TUNEL assay (FCM)	Positive	[152]
Metals – lead					
	362 European Pb-exposed workers 141 Non-exposed men	Blood Pb concentration	SCSA	Positive	[153]
	68 Mexican fertile men	Pb concentration in seminal fluid, spermatozoa, and blood	NCD	Positive	[154]
	80 Taiwan battery plant workers	Blood Pb concentration	SCSA	Positive	[155]

DDE p,p′ dichlorodiphenyldichloroethylene; *DDT 1,1,1* trichloro-2,2-bis(chlorodiphenyl)ethane; *FCM* flow cytometry; *ISNT* in situ nick translation assay; *NCD* nuclear chromatin decondensation test; *PCBs* polychlorinated biphenyls; *SCSA* sperm chromatin structure assay; *TUNEL* terminal deoxynucleotidyl transferase-mediated dUTP nick end labelling; *N.S.* not statistically significant

12.9 Clinical Recommendations

Whereas the testing of sperm DNA integrity has proved to be an important tool both in reproductive and in environmental research, its role in the daily clinical practice is still widely debated. Thus, the Practice Committee of the American Society for Reproductive Medicine [114] concluded: "Sperm DNA damage is more common in infertile men and may contribute to poor reproductive performance. However, current methods for evaluating sperm DNA integrity do not reliable predict treatment outcomes, and no treatment for abnormal DNA integrity has proven clinical value". Furthermore, "At present, the results of sperm DNA integrity testing alone do not predict pregnancy rates achieved with intercourse, IUI, IVF and ICSI".

On the other hand, in an Editorial in Molecular Human Reproduction, Barratt [115] claims that "... there is an urgent need to develop new assessments of male reproductive potential and testing of DNA and its packaging in the human spermatozoa is likely to be a very important tool in the armamentarium. Importantly, there are already considerable data to support the clinical use of DNA damage assays".

There are several reasons for the confusion regarding the clinical usefulness of sperm DNA integrity testing:

(a) The vast majority of studies are based on small patient cohorts and are, therefore, underpowered.
(b) Furthermore, most available reports focus on difference between fertile and infertile subjects in percentage of sperms with DNA damage rather than on predictive value of these tests in a clinical set-up.
(c) Uniform criteria for selection of patients for these studies are lacking. Thus, in many studies, no consideration is taken to the possible contribution of the female partner. Furthermore, in order to reach higher number of patients, couples receiving different types of ART are pooled together. As indicated above, sperm DNA testing seems to be the most powerful predictor for in vivo fertility, and among the two in vitro methods, more related to the outcome of IVF than that of ICSI.
(d) In several "meta analyses" and review papers, no discrimination is made between the results obtained by different methods for sperm DNA testing, SCSA, Comet assay and TUNEL.

So far, clinical threshold values have only been established for the SCSA, perhaps because the methodology has been highly standardised, which is witnessed by very low intra- and inter-laboratory variation [99]. When evaluating the clinical applicability of this method, the poor predictive value of standard semen parameters should also be taken into consideration. Furthermore, although the SCSA is based on use of expensive equipment – flow cytometer – the analysis can be centralised. We, therefore, consider the use of SCSA testing as clinically valuable in following cases:

1. Unexplained infertility and normal standard semen parameters combined with mild or treatable female subfertility.
   (a) DFI above 20% can, at least partly, explain the infertility problem of the couple.
   (b) If the DFI is above 30%, the couple can go directly to IVF/ICSI.
   (c) If the DFI is below 30% (at least two samples), treatment of the female in order to improve the chance of the couple to achieve spontaneous pregnancy can be tried.
2. Mild impairment of semen quality (e.g. only one of the standard parameters: concentration, motility or morphology below the reference range) and relatively short (<2 years) history of infertility.
   (a) DFI below 10% and the female partner without any pathology and below the age of 35 years: achieving spontaneous pregnancy can be tried (for 1/2–1 year).
   (b) DFI below 10% and the female partner with treatable subfertility: treatment of the female in order to improve the chance of the couple to achieve spontaneous pregnancy can be tried.
3. A couple referred for IUI and fulfilling criteria – including standard semen analysis – for this treatment.
   (a) DFI above 25–30% (in two samples): the couple should go directly for IVF/ICSI.

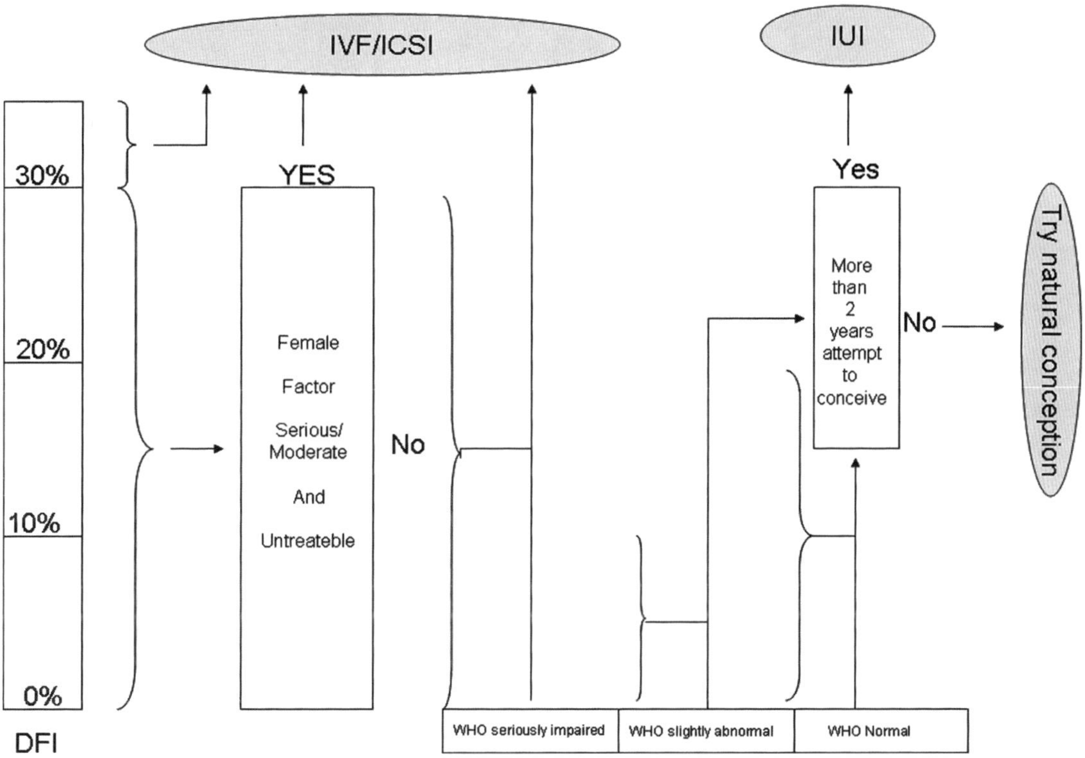

Fig. 12.2 Schematic flow chart illustrating clinical guidelines for use of SCSA DNA fragmentation index (DFI) analysis

4. A couple referred for standard IVF and fulfilling criteria – including standard semen analysis – for this treatment.
   (a) DFI above 30% (in two samples): ICSI should be considered.
5. These recommendations are summarised in Fig. 12.2.
6. So far, it seems that the SCSA analysis of sperm DNA integrity, to be clinically useful, should be performed on raw and not on prepared semen.

12.10 Future Perspectives

The clinical role of different methods for testing sperm DNA integrity needs to be established. Standardisation of the methodology, mainly for techniques other than SCSA, is needed and so are clinical studies based on sufficiently large and well-defined patient cohorts. This will, hopefully, lead to defining relevant threshold values for different clinical situations and treatment modalities. Since the techniques for measuring sperm DNA damage are not completely overlapping, it cannot be excluded that highest predictive value can be obtained by use of a panel of well-characterised and standardised methods.

From the biological point of view, we still need more information about the mechanisms behind sperm DNA damage and an improved methodology to discriminate between the underlying pathologies. This will enable us to develop targeted, cause-related therapies, so far an almost non-existing option within the field of male subfertility.

Furthermore, we need to learn more about the implications of sperm DNA damage, not only in relation to the fertility, but also as considers possible transmission of wrong genetic information to the offspring. This knowledge seems of particular interest in the current era of ICSI, which is bypassing the natural biological mechanisms preventing a defective sperm in fertilising an egg.

References

1. Bonde JPE, Ernst E, Jensen TK, et al. Relation between semen quality and fertility: a population-based study of 430 first-pregnancy planners. Lancet. 1998;352:1172–7.
2. Guzick DS, Overstreet JW, Factor-Litvak P, et al. Sperm morphology, motility, and concentration in fertile and infertile men. N Engl J Med. 2001; 345(19):1388–93.
3. WHO. WHO laboratory manual for the examination of human semen and sperm-cervical mucus interaction. Cambridge: Cambridge University Press; 1999.
4. WHO. WHO laboratory manual for the examination and processing of human semen. 5th ed. Geneva: World Health Organization; 1999.
5. Skakkebaek NE, Giwercman A, de Kretser D. Pathogenesis and management of male infertility. Lancet. 1994;343(8911):1473–9.
6. Agarwal A, Said TM. Role of sperm chromatin abnormalities and DNA damage in male infertility. Hum Reprod Update. 2003;9(4):331–45.
7. Erenpreiss J, Spano M, Erenpreisa J, Bungum M, Giwercman A. Sperm chromatin structure and male fertility: biological and clinical aspects. Asian J Androl. 2006;8(1):11–29.
8. Ward WS, Coffey DS. DNA packaging and organization in mammalian spermatozoa: comparison with somatic cells. Biol Reprod. 1991;44:569–74.
9. Fuentes-Mascorro G, Serrano H, Rosado A. Sperm chromatin. Arch Androl. 2000;45(3):215–25.
10. Ward WS. Deoxyribonucleic acid loop domain tertiary structure in mammalian spermatozoa. Biol Reprod. 1993;48(6):1193–201.
11. Solov'eva L, Svetlova M, Bodinski D, Zalensky AO. Nature of telomere dimers and chromosome looping in human spermatozoa. Chromosome Res. 2004; 12(8):817–23.
12. Zalensky AO, Allen MJ, Kobayashi A, Zalenskaya IA, Balhorn R, Bradbury EM. Well-defined genome architecture in the human sperm nucleus. Chromosoma. 1995;103(9):577–90.
13. Ward WS, Zalensky AO. The unique, complex organization of the transcriptionally silent sperm chromatin. Crit Rev Eukaryot Gene Expr. 1996; 6(2–3):139–47.
14. Bench GS, Friz AM, Corzett MH, Morse DH, Balhorn R. DNA and total protamine masses in individual sperm from fertile mammalian subjects. Cytometry. 1996;23(4):263–71.
15. Lewis JD, Song Y, de Jong ME, Bagha SM, Ausio J. A walk though vertebrate and invertebrate protamines. Chromosoma. 2003;111(8):473–82.
16. Corzett M, Mazrimas J, Balhorn R. Protamine 1: protamine 2 stoichiometry in the sperm of eutherian mammals. Mol Reprod Dev. 2002;61(4):519–27.
17. Jager S. Sperm nuclear stability and male infertility. Arch Androl. 1990;25(3):253–9.
18. Aitken RJ, De Iuliis GN. On the possible origins of DNA damage in human spermatozoa. Mol Hum Reprod. 2010;16(1):3–13.
19. Sakkas D, Alvarez JG. Sperm DNA fragmentation: mechanisms of origin, impact on reproductive outcome, and analysis. Fertil Steril. 2010;93(4):1027–36.
20. Sakkas D, Mariethoz E, Manicardi G, Bizzaro D, Bianchi PG, Bianchi U. Origin of DNA damage in ejaculated human spermatozoa. Rev Reprod. 1999;4(1):31–7.
21. Billig H, Furuta I, Rivier C, Tapanainen J, Parvinen M, Hsueh AJW. Apoptosis in testis germ cells: developmental changes in gonadotropin dependence and localization to selective tubule stages. Endocrinology. 1995;136:5–12.
22. Aitken RJ, Baker MA. Oxidative stress and male reproductive biology. Reprod Fertil Dev. 2004;16(5):581–8.
23. Aitken RJ, West KM. Analysis of the relationship between reactive oxygen species production and leucocyte infiltration in fractions of human semen separated on Percoll gradients. Int J Androl. 1990;13(6):433–51.
24. De Iuliis GN, Thomson LK, Mitchell LA, et al. DNA damage in human spermatozoa is highly correlated with the efficiency of chromatin remodeling and the formation of 8-hydroxy-2′-deoxyguanosine, a marker of oxidative stress. Biol Reprod. 2009;81(3):517–24.
25. Stahl O, Eberhard J, Jepson K, et al. The impact of testicular carcinoma and its treatment on sperm DNA integrity. Cancer. 2004;100(6):1137–44.
26. Rubes J, Selevan SG, Evenson DP, et al. Episodic air pollution is associated with increased DNA fragmentation in human sperm without other changes in semen quality. Hum Reprod. 2005;20(10):2776–83.
27. Spano M, Toft G, Hagmar L, et al. Exposure to PCB and p, p′-DDE in European and Inuit populations: impact on human sperm chromatin integrity. Hum Reprod. 2005;20(12):3488–99.
28. Sergerie M, Laforest G, Bujan L, Bissonnette F, Bleau G. Sperm DNA fragmentation: threshold value in male fertility. Hum Reprod. 2005;20(12):3446–51.
29. Mitchell LA, De Iuliis GN, Aitken RJ. The TUNEL assay consistently underestimates DNA damage in human spermatozoa and is influenced by DNA compaction and cell vitality: development of an improved methodology. Int J Androl. 2010;34(1):2–13.
30. Ostling O, Johanson KJ. Microelectrophoretic study of radiation-induced DNA damages in individual mammalian cells. Biochem Biophys Res Commun. 1984;123(1):291–8.
31. Collins AR. The comet assay for DNA damage and repair: principles, applications, and limitations. Mol Biotechnol. 2004;26(3):249–61.
32. Fairbairn DW, Olive PL, O'Neill KL. The comet assay: a comprehensive review. Mutat Res. 1995;339(1):37–59.
33. Lewis SE, O'Connell M, Stevenson M, Thompson-Cree L, McClure N. An algorithm to predict pregnancy in assisted reproduction. Hum Reprod. 2004;19(6):1385–94.

34. Evenson DP, Larson KL, Jost LK. Sperm chromatin structure assay: its clinical use for detecting sperm DNA fragmentation in male infertility and comparisons with other techniques. J Androl. 2002;23(1):25–43.
35. Evenson D, Jost L. Sperm chromatin structure assay is useful for fertility assessment. Methods Cell Sci. 2000;22(2–3):169–89.
36. Evenson DP. Flow cytometric analysis of male germ cell quality. Meth Cell Biol. 1990;33:401–10.
37. Giwercman A, Richthoff J, Hjollund H, et al. Correlation between sperm motility and sperm chromatin structure assay parameters. Fertil Steril. 2003;80(6):1404–12.
38. Erenpreisa J, Erenpreiss J, Freivalds T, et al. Toluidine blue test for sperm DNA integrity and elaboration of image cytometry algorithm. Cytom A. 2003;52(1):19–27.
39. Erenpreiss J, Bars J, Lipatnikova V, Erenpreisa J, Zalkalns J. Comparative study of cytochemical tests for sperm chromatin integrity. J Androl. 2001;22(1): 45–53.
40. Erenpreiss J, Jepson K, Giwercman A, Tsarev I, Erenpreisa J, Spano M. Toluidine blue cytometry test for sperm DNA conformation: comparison with the flow cytometric sperm chromatin structure and TUNEL assays. Hum Reprod. 2004;19(10):2277–82.
41. Fernandez JL, Muriel L, Rivero MT, Goyanes V, Vazquez R, Alvarez JG. The sperm chromatin dispersion test: a simple method for the determination of sperm DNA fragmentation. J Androl. 2003;24(1): 59–66.
42. Shen H, Ong C. Detection of oxidative DNA damage in human sperm and its association with sperm function and male infertility. Free Radic Biol Med. 2000;28(4):529–36.
43. Ni ZY, Liu YQ, Shen HM, Chia SE, Ong CN. Does the increase of 8-hydroxydeoxyguanosine lead to poor sperm quality? Mutat Res. 1997;381(1):77–82.
44. Chen CS, Chao HT, Pan RL, Wei YH. Hydroxyl radical-induced decline in motility and increase in lipid peroxidation and DNA modification in human sperm. Biochem Mol Biol Int. 1997;43(2):291–303.
45. De Iuliis GN, Newey RJ, King BV, Aitken RJ. Mobile phone radiation induces reactive oxygen species production and DNA damage in human spermatozoa in vitro. PLoS ONE. 2009;4(7):e6446.
46. Sakkas D, Urner F, Bizzaro D, et al. Sperm nuclear DNA damage and altered chromatin structure: effect on fertilization and embryo development. Hum Reprod. 1998;13 Suppl 4:11–9.
47. Gillan L, Evans G, Maxwell WM. Flow cytometric evaluation of sperm parameters in relation to fertility potential. Theriogenology. 2005;63(2):445–57.
48. Stronati A, Manicardi GC, Cecati M, et al. Relationships between sperm DNA fragmentation, sperm apoptotic markers and serum levels of CB-153 and p,p′-DDE in European and Inuit populations. Reproduction. 2006;132(6):949–58.
49. Perreault SD, Aitken RJ, Baker HW, et al. Integrating new tests of sperm genetic integrity into semen analysis: breakout group discussion. Adv Exp Med Biol. 2003;518:253–68.
50. Spano M, Bonde JP, Hjollund HI, Kolstad HA, Cordelli E, Leter G. Sperm chromatin damage impairs human fertility. The Danish First Pregnancy Planner Study Team. Fertil Steril. 2000;73(1):43–50.
51. Evenson DP, Jost LK, Marshall D, et al. Utility of the sperm chromatin structure assay as a diagnostic and prognostic tool in the human fertility clinic. Hum Reprod. 1999;14:1039–49.
52. Evenson DP, Wixon R. Data analysis of two in vivo fertility studies using Sperm Chromatin Structure Assay-derived DNA fragmentation index vs pregnancy outcome. Fertil Steril. 2008;90(4):1229–31.
53. Loft S, Kold-Jensen T, Hjollund NH, et al. Oxidative DNA damage in human sperm influences time to pregnancy. Hum Reprod. 2003;18(6):1265–72.
54. Giwercman A, Lindstedt L, Larsson M, et al. Sperm chromatin structure assay as an independent predictor of fertility in vivo: a case-control study. Int J Androl. 2009;33(1):e221–7.
55. Sharma RK, Sabanegh E, Mahfouz R, Gupta S, Thiyagarajan A, Agarwal A. TUNEL as a test for sperm DNA damage in the evaluation of male infertility. Urology. 2010;76(6):1380–6.
56. Zini A, Fischer MA, Sharir S, Shayegan B, Phang D, Jarvi K. Prevalence of abnormal sperm DNA denaturation in fertile and infertile men. Urology. 2002;60(6):1069–72.
57. Smit M, Romijn JC, Wildhagen MF, Weber RF, Dohle GR. Sperm chromatin structure is associated with the quality of spermatogenesis in infertile patients. Fertil Steril. 2009;94(5):1748–52.
58. Lewis SE, Agbaje IM. Using the alkaline comet assay in prognostic tests for male infertility and assisted reproductive technology outcomes. Mutagenesis. 2008;23(3):163–70.
59. Tsarev I, Bungum M, Giwercman A, et al. Evaluation of male fertility potential by toluidine blue test for sperm chromatin structure assessment. Hum Reprod. 2009;24(7):1569–74.
60. Shen HM, Chia SE, Ong CN. Evaluation of oxidative DNA damage in human sperm and its association with male infertility. J Androl. 1999;20(6):718–23.
61. Tejada RI, Mitchell JC, Norman A, Marik JJ, Friedman S. A test for the practical evaluation of male fertility by acridine orange (AO) fluorescence. Fertil Steril. 1984;42(1):87–91.
62. Plastira K, Msaouel P, Angelopoulou R, et al. The effects of age on DNA fragmentation, chromatin packaging and conventional semen parameters in spermatozoa of oligoasthenoteratozoospermic patients. J Assist Reprod Genet. 2007;24(10):437–43.
63. Zini A, Sigman M. Are tests of sperm DNA damage clinically useful? Pros and cons. J Androl. 2009; 30(3):219–29.
64. Sakkas D, Moffatt O, Manicardi GC, Mariethoz E, Tarozzi N, Bizzaro D. Nature of DNA damage in ejaculated human spermatozoa and the possible involvement of apoptosis. Biol Reprod. 2002;66:1061–7.

65. Liu CH, Tsao HM, Cheng TC, et al. DNA fragmentation, mitochondrial dysfunction and chromosomal aneuploidy in the spermatozoa of oligoasthenoteratozoospermic males. J Assist Reprod Genet. 2004; 21(4):119–26.
66. Host E, Lindenberg S, Kahn J, Christensen F. DNA strand breaks in human sperm cells: a comparison between men with normal and oligozoospermic sperm samples. Acta Obstet Gynecol Scand. 1999;78(4):336–9.
67. Tomlinson M, Turner J, Powell G, Sakkas D. One-step disposable chambers for sperm concentration and motility assessment: how do they compare with the World Health Organization's recommended methods? Hum Reprod. 2001;16(1):121–4.
68. Erenpreiss J, Elzanaty S, Giwercman A. Sperm DNA damage in men from infertile couples. Asian J Androl. 2008;10(5):786–90.
69. Boe-Hansen GB, Fedder J, Ersboll AK, Christensen P. The sperm chromatin structure assay as a diagnostic tool in the human fertility clinic. Hum Reprod. 2006;21(6):1576–82.
70. Virro MR, Larson-Cook KL, Evenson DP. Sperm chromatin structure assay (scsa(R)) parameters are related to fertilization, blastocyst development, and ongoing pregnancy in in vitro fertilization and intracytoplasmic sperm injection cycles. Fertil Steril. 2004;81:1289–95.
71. Saleh RA, Agarwal A, Nelson DR, et al. Increased sperm nuclear DNA damage in normozoospermic infertile men: a prospective study. Fertil Steril. 2002;78(2):313–8.
72. Fernandez JL, Muriel L, Goyanes V, et al. Simple determination of human sperm DNA fragmentation with an improved sperm chromatin dispersion test. Fertil Steril. 2005;84(4):833–42.
73. Aoki VW, Moskovtsev SI, Willis J, Liu L, Mullen JB, Carrell DT. DNA integrity is compromised in protamine-deficient human sperm. J Androl. 2005;26(6):741–8.
74. Duran EH, Morshedi M, Taylor S, Oehninger S. Sperm DNA quality predicts intrauterine insemination outcome: a prospective cohort study. Hum Reprod. 2002;17(12):3122–8.
75. Saleh RA, Agarwal A, Sharma RK, Said TM, Sikka SC, Thomas Jr AJ. Evaluation of nuclear DNA damage in spermatozoa from infertile men with varicocele. Fertil Steril. 2003;80(6):1431–6.
76. Bungum M, Humaidan P, Axmon A, et al. Sperm DNA integrity assessment in prediction of assisted reproduction technology outcome. Hum Reprod. 2007;22(1):174–9.
77. Muriel L, Meseguer M, Fernandez JL, et al. Value of the sperm chromatin dispersion test in predicting pregnancy outcome in intrauterine insemination: a blind prospective study. Hum Reprod. 2006;21(3): 738–44.
78. Larson-Cook KL, Brannian JD, Hansen KA, Kasperson KM, Aamold ET, Evenson DP. Relationship between the outcomes of assisted reproductive techniques and sperm DNA fragmentation as measured by the sperm chromatin structure assay. Fertil Steril. 2003;80(4):895–902.
79. Larson KL, DeJonge CJ, Barnes AM, Jost LK, Evenson DP. Sperm chromatin structure assay parameters as predictors of failed pregnancy following assisted reproductive techniques. Hum Reprod. 2000;15(8):1717–22.
80. Gandini L, Lombardo F, Paoli D, et al. Full-term pregnancies achieved with ICSI despite high levels of sperm chromatin damage. Hum Reprod. 2004;19(6):1409–17.
81. Bungum M, Humaidan P, Spano M, Jepson K, Bungum L, Giwercman A. The predictive value of sperm chromatin structure assay (SCSA) parameters for the outcome of intrauterine insemination, IVF and ICSI. Hum Reprod. 2004;19(6):1401–8.
82. Host E, Lindenberg S, Smidt-Jensen S. The role of DNA strand breaks in human spermatozoa used for IVF and ICSI. Acta Obstet Gynecol Scand. 2000;79(7):559–63.
83. Hammadeh ME, Stieber M, Haidl G, Schmidt W. Association between sperm cell chromatin condensation, morphology based on strict criteria, and fertilization, cleavage and pregnancy rates in an IVF program. Andrologia. 1998;30(1):29–35.
84. Simon L, Brunborg G, Stevenson M, Lutton D, McManus J, Lewis SE. Clinical significance of sperm DNA damage in assisted reproduction outcome. Hum Reprod. 2010;25(7):1594–608.
85. Payne JF, Raburn DJ, Couchman GM, Price TM, Jamison MG, Walmer DK. Redefining the relationship between sperm deoxyribonucleic acid fragmentation as measured by the sperm chromatin structure assay and outcomes of assisted reproductive techniques. Fertil Steril. 2005;84(2):356–64.
86. Ahmadi A, Ng SC. Fertilizing capacity of DNA damaged spermatozoa. J Exp Zool. 1999;286:696–704.
87. Twigg JP, Irvine DS, Aitken RJ. Oxidative damage to DNA in human spermatozoa does not preclude pronucleus formation at intracytoplasmic sperm injection. Hum Reprod. 1998;13(7):1864–71.
88. Sakkas D, Urner F, Bianchi PG, et al. Sperm chromatin anomalies can influence decondensation after intracytoplasmic sperm injection. Hum Reprod. 1996;11(4): 837–43.
89. Tomlinson MJ, Moffatt O, Manicardi GC, Bizzaro D, Afnan M, Sakkas D. Interrelationships between seminal parameters and sperm nuclear DNA damage before and after density gradient centrifugation: implications for assisted conception. Hum Reprod. 2001;16(10):2160–5.
90. Hammadeh ME, Al-Hasani S, Gauss C, et al. Predictive value of chromatin decondensation in vitro on fertilization rate after intracytoplasmic sperm injection (ICSI). Int J Androl. 2001;24(5):311–6.
91. Lopes S, Sun JG, Jurisicova A, Meriano J, Casper RF. Sperm deoxyribonucleic acid fragmentation is

increased in poor-quality semen samples and correlates with failed fertilization in intracytoplasmic sperm injection. Fertil Steril. 1998;69(3):528–32.
92. Sun JG et al. Detection of deoxyribomucleic acid fragmentation in human sperm: correlation with fertilization in vitro. Biol Reprod. 1997;56:602–7.
93. Morris ID, Ilott S, Dixon L, Brison DR. The spectrum of DNA damage in human sperm assessed by single cell gel electrophoresis (Comet assay) and its relationship to fertilization and embryo development. Hum Reprod. 2002;17(4):990–8.
94. Spano M, Seli E, Bizzaro D, Manicardi GC, Sakkas D. The significance of sperm nuclear DNA strand breaks on reproductive outcome. Curr Opin Obstet Gynecol. 2005;17(3):255–60.
95. Seli E, Gardner DK, Schoolcraft WB, Moffatt O, Sakkas D. Extent of nuclear DNA damage in ejaculated spermatozoa impacts on blastocyst development after in vitro fertilization. Fertil Steril. 2004;82(2):378–83.
96. Keel BA. Within- and between-subject variation in semen parameters in infertile men and normal semen donors. Fertil Steril. 2006;85(1):128–34.
97. Neuwinger J, Behre HM, Nieschlag E. External quality control in the andrology laboratory: an experimental multicenter trial. Fertil Steril. 1990;54(2):308–14.
98. Cooper TG, Neuwinger J, Bahrs S, Nieschlag E. Internal quality control of semen analysis. Fertil Steril. 1992;58(1):172–8.
99. Erenpreiss J, Bungum M, Spano M, Elzanaty S, Orbidans J, Giwercman A. Intra-individual variation in sperm chromatin structure assay parameters in men from infertile couples: clinical implications. Hum Reprod. 2006;21(8):2061–4.
100. Spano M, Kolstad AH, Larsen SB, et al. The applicability of the flow cytometric sperm chromatin structure assay as diagnostic and prognostic tool in then human fertility clinic. Hum Reprod. 1998;13:2495–505.
101. Evenson DP, Jost LK, Baer RK, Turner TW, Schrader SM. Individuality of DNA denaturation patterns in human sperm as measured by the sperm chromatin structure assay. Reprod Toxicol. 1991;5(2):115–25.
102. Sergerie M, Mieusset R, Daudin M, Thonneau P, Bujan L. Ten-year variation in semen parameters and sperm deoxyribonucleic acid integrity in a healthy fertile man. Fertil Steril. 2006;86(5):1513.e11–8.
103. Sergerie M, Laforest G, Boulanger K, Bissonnette F, Bleau G. Longitudinal study of sperm DNA fragmentation as measured by terminal uridine nick end-labelling assay. Hum Reprod. 2005;20(7):1921–7.
104. Rignell-Hydbom A, Rylander L, Giwercman A, et al. Exposure to PCBs and p, p′-DDE and human sperm chromatin integrity. Environ Health Perspect. 2005;113(2):175–9.
105. Hauser R, Meeker JD, Singh NP, et al. DNA damage in human sperm is related to urinary levels of phthalate monoester and oxidative metabolites. Hum Reprod. 2007;22(3):688–95.
106. de Jager C, Aneck-Hahn NH, Bornman MS, et al. Sperm chromatin integrity in DDT-exposed young men living in a malaria area in the Limpopo Province, South Africa. Hum Reprod. 2009;24(10):2429–38.
107. Perez-Herrera N, Polanco-Minaya H, Salazar-Arredondo E, et al. PON1Q192R genetic polymorphism modifies organophosphorous pesticide effects on semen quality and DNA integrity in agricultural workers from southern Mexico. Toxicol Appl Pharmacol. 2008;230(2):261–8.
108. Rubes J, Selevan SG, Sram RJ, Evenson DP, Perreault SD. GSTM1 genotype influences the susceptibility of men to sperm DNA damage associated with exposure to air pollution. Mutat Res. 2007;625(1–2):20–8.
109. Giwercman A, Rylander L, Rignell-Hydbom A, et al. Androgen receptor gene CAG repeat length as a modifier of the association between persistent organohalogen pollutant exposure markers and semen characteristics. Pharmacogenet Genomics. 2007;17(6):391–401.
110. Stahl O, Eberhard J, Cavallin-Stahl E, et al. Sperm DNA integrity in cancer patients: the effect of disease and treatment. Int J Androl. 2008;32(6):695–703.
111. Romerius P, Stahl O, Moell C, et al. Sperm DNA integrity in men treated for childhood cancer. Clin Cancer Res. 2010;16(15):3843–50.
112. Stahl O, Eberhard J, Jepson K, et al. Sperm DNA integrity in testicular cancer patients. Hum Reprod. 2006;21(12):3199–205.
113. Gandini L, Lombardo F, Lenzi A, Spano M, Dondero F. Cryopreservation and sperm DNA integrity. Cell Tissue Bank. 2006;7(2):91–8.
114. Practice Committee of American Society for Reproductive Medicine. The clinical utility of sperm DNA integrity testing. Fertil Steril. 2008;90(5 Suppl):S178–80.
115. Barratt CL, Aitken RJ, Bjorndahl L, et al. Sperm DNA: organization, protection and vulnerability: from basic science to clinical applications – a position report. Hum Reprod. 2010;25(4):824–38.
116. Schmid TE, Eskenazi B, Baumgartner A, et al. The effects of male age on sperm DNA damage in healthy non-smokers. Hum Reprod. 2007;22(1):180–7.
117. O'Flaherty C, Vaisheva F, Hales BF, Chan P, Robaire B. Characterization of sperm chromatin quality in testicular cancer and Hodgkin's lymphoma patients prior to chemotherapy. Hum Reprod. 2008;23(5):1044–52.
118. Chohan KR, Griffin JT, Lafromboise M, De Jonge CJ, Carrell DT. Comparison of chromatin assays for DNA fragmentation evaluation in human sperm. J Androl. 2006;27(1):53–9.
119. Smith R, Kaune H, Parodi D, et al. Increased sperm DNA damage in patients with varicocele: relationship with seminal oxidative stress. Hum Reprod. 2006;21(4):986–93.
120. Apedaile AE, Garrett C, Liu DY, Clarke GN, Johnston SA, Baker HW. Flow cytometry and microscopic acridine orange test: relationship with standard semen analysis. Reprod Biomed Online. 2004;8(4):398–407.

121. Dominguez-Fandos D, Camejo MI, Ballesca JL, Oliva R. Human sperm DNA fragmentation: correlation of TUNEL results as assessed by flow cytometry and optical microscopy. Cytom A. 2007;71(12):1011–8.
122. Cohen-Bacrie P, Belloc S, Menezo YJ, Clement P, Hamidi J, Benkhalifa M. Correlation between DNA damage and sperm parameters: a prospective study of 1, 633 patients. Fertil Steril. 2009;91(5):1801–5.
123. Bian Q, Xu LC, Wang SL, et al. Study on the relation between occupational fenvalerate exposure and spermatozoa DNA damage of pesticide factory workers. Occup Environ Med. 2004;61(12):999–1005.
124. Tarozzi N, Nadalini M, Stronati A, et al. Anomalies in sperm chromatin packaging: implications for assisted reproduction techniques. Reprod Biomed Online. 2009;18(4):486–95.
125. Zhang LH, Qiu Y, Wang KH, Wang Q, Tao G, Wang LG. Measurement of sperm DNA fragmentation using bright-field microscopy: comparison between sperm chromatin dispersion test and terminal uridine nick-end labeling assay. Fertil Steril. 2010;94(3): 1027–32.
126. Tavalaee M, Razavi S, Nasr-Esfahani MH. Influence of sperm chromatin anomalies on assisted reproductive technology outcome. Fertil Steril. 2009;91(4): 1119–26.
127. Richthoff J, Spano M, Giwercman YL, et al. The impact of testicular and accessory sex gland function on sperm chromatin integrity as assessed by sperm chromatin structure assay (SCSA). Hum Reprod. 2002;17:3162–9.
128. Hammiche F, Laven J, Boxmeer J, Dohle G, Steegers E, Steegers-Theunissen R. Semen quality decline among men below 60 years of age undergoing IVF or ICSI treatment. J Androl. 2010;32(1):70–6.
129. Benchaib M, Lornage J, Mazoyer C, Lejeune H, Salle B, Francois Guerin J. Sperm deoxyribonucleic acid fragmentation as a prognostic indicator of assisted reproductive technology outcome. Fertil Steril. 2007;87(1):93–100.
130. Henkel R, Kierspel E, Hajimohammad M, et al. DNA fragmentation of spermatozoa and assisted reproduction technology. Reprod Biomed Online. 2003;7(4):477–84.
131. Henkel R, Hajimohammad M, Stalf T, et al. Influence of deoxyribonucleic acid damage on fertilization and pregnancy. Fertil Steril. 2004;81(4):965–72.
132. Trisini AT, Singh NP, Duty SM, Hauser R. Relationship between human semen parameters and deoxyribonucleic acid damage assessed by the neutral comet assay. Fertil Steril. 2004;82(6):1623–32.
133. de la Calle JF Velez, Muller A, Walschaerts M, et al. Sperm deoxyribonucleic acid fragmentation as assessed by the sperm chromatin dispersion test in assisted reproductive technology programs: results of a large prospective multicenter study. Fertil Steril. 2008;90(5):1792–9.
134. Erenpreiss J, Hlevicka S, Zalkalns J, Erenpreisa J. Effect of leukocytospermia on sperm DNA integrity: a negative effect in abnormal semen samples. J Androl. 2002;23(5):717–23.
135. Fischer MA, Willis J, Zini A. Human sperm DNA integrity: correlation with sperm cytoplasmic droplets. Urology. 2003;61(1):207–11.
136. Pant N, Shukla M, Kumar Patel D, et al. Correlation of phthalate exposures with semen quality. Toxicol Appl Pharmacol. 2008;231(1):112–6.
137. Gandini L, Lombardo F, Paoli D, et al. Study of apoptotic DNA fragmentation in human spermatozoa. Hum Reprod. 2000;15:830–9.
138. Hsu PC, Chen IY, Pan CH, et al. Sperm DNA damage correlates with polycyclic aromatic hydrocarbons biomarker in coke-oven workers. Int Arch Occup Environ Health. 2006;79(5):349–56.
139. Ji G, Gu A, Zhu P, et al. Joint effects of XRCC1 polymorphisms and polycyclic aromatic hydrocarbons exposure on sperm DNA damage and male infertility. Toxicol Sci. 2010;116(1):92–8.
140. Selevan SG, Borkovec L, Slott VL, et al. Semen quality and reproductive health of young Czech men exposed to seasonal air pollution. Environ Health Perspect. 2000;108(9):887–94.
141. Kolstad HA, Bonde JP, Spano M, et al. Change in semen quality and sperm chromatin structure following occupational styrene exposure. ASCLEPIOS. Int Arch Occup Environ Health. 1999;72(3): 135–41.
142. Migliore L, Naccarati A, Zanello A, Scarpato R, Bramanti L, Mariani M. Assessment of sperm DNA integrity in workers exposed to styrene. Hum Reprod. 2002;17(11):2912–8.
143. Duty SM, Singh NP, Silva MJ, et al. The relationship between environmental exposures to phthalates and DNA damage in human sperm using the neutral comet assay. Environ Health Perspect. 2003;111(9):1164–9.
144. Jonsson BA, Richthoff J, Rylander L, Giwercman A, Hagmar L. Urinary phthalate metabolites and biomarkers of reproductive function in young men. Epidemiology. 2005;16(4):487–93.
145. Xu DX, Zhu QX, Zheng LK, et al. Exposure to acrylonitrile induced DNA strand breakage and sex chromosome aneuploidy in human spermatozoa. Mutat Res. 2003;537(1):93–100.
146. Hauser R, Singh NP, Chen Z, Pothier L, Altshul L. Lack of an association between environmental exposure to polychlorinated biphenyls and p, p′-DDE and DNA damage in human sperm measured using the neutral comet assay. Hum Reprod. 2003;18(12):2525–33.
147. De Jager C, Farias P, Barraza-Villarreal A, et al. Reduced seminal parameters associated with environmental DDT exposure and p,p′-DDE concentrations in men in Chiapas, Mexico: a cross-sectional study. J Androl. 2006;27(1):16–27.
148. Larsen SB, Giwercman A, Spano M, Bonde JP. A longitudinal study of semen quality in pesticide spraying Danish farmers. The ASCLEPIOS Study Group. Reproduct Toxicol. 1998;12(6):581–9.

149. Sanchez-Pena LC, Reyes BE, Lopez-Carrillo L, et al. Organophosphorous pesticide exposure alters sperm chromatin structure in Mexican agricultural workers. Toxicol Appl Pharmacol. 2004;196(1):108–13.
150. Meeker JD, Singh NP, Ryan L, et al. Urinary levels of insecticide metabolites and DNA damage in human sperm. Hum Reprod. 2004;19(11):2573–80.
151. Meeker JD, Barr DB, Hauser R. Human semen quality and sperm DNA damage in relation to urinary metabolites of pyrethroid insecticides. Hum Reprod. 2008;23(8):1932–40.
152. Xia Y, Cheng S, Bian Q, et al. Genotoxic effects on spermatozoa of carbaryl-exposed workers. Toxicol Sci. 2005;85(1):615–23.
153. Bonde JP, Joffe M, Apostoli P, et al. Sperm count and chromatin structure in men exposed to inorganic lead: lowest adverse effect levels. Occup Environ Med. 2002;59(4):234–42.
154. Hernandez-Ochoa I, Garcia-Vargas G, Lopez-Carrillo L, et al. Low lead environmental exposure alters semen quality and sperm chromatin condensation in northern Mexico. Reprod Toxicol. 2005;20(2):221–8.
155. Hsu PC, Chang HY, Guo YL, Liu YC, Shih TS. Effect of smoking on blood lead levels in workers and role of reactive oxygen species in lead-induced sperm chromatin DNA damage. Fertil Steril. 2009;91(4):1096–103.

13 The Emerging Role of the Sperm Epigenome and its Potential Role in Development

Sue Hammoud and Douglas T. Carrell

Abstract

The sperm genome has traditionally been thought to lack chromatin structure significant to affect embryonic development, since during spermatogenesis nucleosomes are widely replaced by protamines, which are believed to silence the genome, and the sperm DNA was known to be hypermethylated in comparison to the egg. The notion of an irrelevant sperm epigenome has been widely challenged due to many recent reports that suggest that sperm chromatin is actually poised similar to an embryonic stem cell, a finding that has been reported in the germline of many organisms. The significance of the mature sperm cellular epigenome is unknown; however, one may foresee two potential roles: either a role in developing embryo or a reminiscent memory of the spermatogonial stem cell with no significance beyond ensuring proper sperm differentiation and maturation. If these marks do help guide the embryo, then perturbations to the epigenome may have implications on embryo quality, likelihood of maintaining a pregnancy, or disease onset later in life.

Keywords

Epigenetics • Histone • Protamine • Imprinting • Methylation • Embryo quality

13.1 Introduction: The Significance of the Cellular Epigenome

Epigenetic modifications on the DNA sequence (DNA methylation) or on chromatin-associated proteins (i.e., histones) play an important role in the regulation of gene expression and are essential for normal mammalian development. DNA methylation usually occurs at CpG dinucleotides and is commonly associated with gene silencing [1, 2].

D.T. Carrell (✉)
Andrology and IVF Laboratories, Departments of Surgery (Urology), Obstetrics and Gynecology and Physiology, University of Utah School of Medicine, Salt Lake City, UT, USA
e-mail: douglas.carrell@hsc.utah.edu

C. Racowsky et al. (eds.), *Biennial Review of Infertility: Volume 2*,
DOI 10.1007/978-1-4419-8456-2_13,

Non-CpG methylation at gene bodies, repetitive DNA, and pericentromeric regions was initially described in plants [3, 4], but has recently been reported in mammalian embryonic stem cells [5] and unicellular/multicellular organisms [6, 7]. However, its significance is unknown. On the other hand, posttranslational modifications such as acetylation, methylation, and phosphorylation on the core nucleosomes, H2A, H2B, H3, and H4, promote gene activation or repression. The combination of DNA methylation and histone modifications refers to the cellular epigenome.

The cellular epigenome enables a dynamic and plastic cellular environment that facilitates the adaptation to cellular stress and environmental cues by modulating chromatin structure [8, 9], without altering the genomic content, to induce changes in gene expression. Altering the cellular transcriptome is a multifaceted process that requires first the recruitment of specific transcription factors and chromatin-modifying enzymes to amend the histone code and/or DNA methylation profile to allow gene promoters to become more or less accessible for transcriptional machinery. The role of the cellular epigenome has been increasingly highlighted and has been implicated in many cellular and developmental processes such as reprogramming (preimplantation embryos and primordial germ cell (PGC)), cellular differentiation, imprinting, X-chromosome inactivation, and genomic stability.

Alterations in epigenetic profiles have been seen in many complex diseases such as cancer [10–12], obesity [13], and infertility [14–19]. Considerable attention in recent years has been devoted towards understanding the nature and the extent of the relationship between infertility and epigenetic alterations [20–22]. These investigations were prompted by the emerging data from animal in-vitro fertilization (IVF) studies that showed an increased incidence of the large offspring syndrome (LOS) [14, 23]. LOS in animals is reminiscent to Beckwith–Wiedmann syndrome (BWS) in humans, both resulting from imprinting abnormalities [20, 24, 25]. Many have suggested that the increased frequency of imprinting abnormalities in IVF patients in animals may be due to oocyte stimulation, gamete manipulation, and/or embryo culture. However, more recent data in humans suggest that the gametes of subfertile patients are epigenetically altered [15–19]. These findings bolstered the concerns of the health outcome of offspring conceived by IVF and raise the question whether epigenetic abnormalities can be inherited.

The notion of transgenerational epigenetic inheritance in mammals has been raised on numerous occasions; however, the two waves of genome-wide epigenetic reprogramming occurring during embryogenesis and gametogenesis [26–28] may limit its likelihood. Although embryonic reprogramming may potentially explain the rare penetrance of epigenetic diseases, some reports in mice have shown that the IAP elements (retrotransposan) upstream of the Agouti locus escape reprogramming [29, 30]. The data from mice suggest that a few gene classes may escape reprogramming and the epigenome may not be completely erased and reestablished from a clean slate. Without a clear understanding of the extent of reprogramming, the safety and the risk assessment for transgenerational epigenetic inheritance for IVF patients is uncertain.

13.2 Chromatin Remodeling During Spermatogenesis

During postmeiotic maturation of male haploid germ cells, chromatin undergoes dramatic reorganization, including the exchange of canonical histones for protamines (Fig. 13.1) [31]. This change in chromatin composition facilitates the compaction of the paternal genome and protects the genomic content from DNA damaging agents during transit [32]. Several recent studies have shown that along with histone acetylation, histone ubiquination (upstream of H4) plays an essential role in the global histone replacement in spermatids. H2A/H2B ubiquination induces H4K16 acetylation (H4k16ac) [33, 34], which is known to be a key step in the remodeling of chromatin to more open conformation [35, 36]. In addition to an elevated H4k16ac signal at the time of histone to protamine transition, there was a general wave of H3 and H4 hyperacetylation [37]. Since acetylation adds negative charge to the nucleosome, it has been postulated that H3/H4

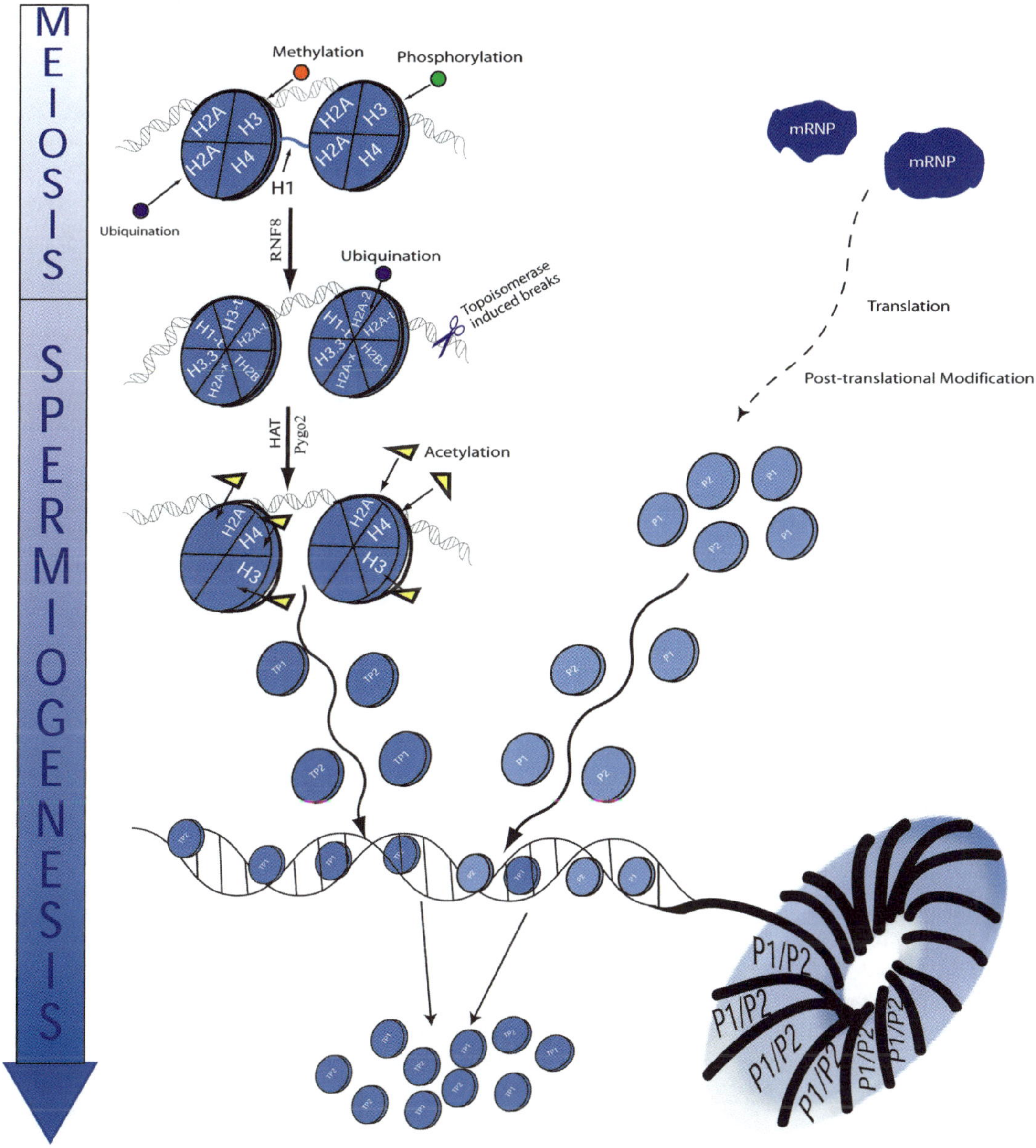

Fig. 13.1 Diagram highlighting the key and very well-described histone modification events that facilitate the transition of somatic histones to protamines. Somatic histones undergo site-specific methylation, phosphorylation, and ubiquitination. H2A ubiquination is set by ring finger protine 8, which later promotes H4 hyperacetylation. Hyperacetylation of H3/H4 relaxes the DNA coil to facilitate replacement of the testis-specific histones by the transition proteins. Transition proteins are subsequently replaced by protamines 1 and 2, processed from a pool of RNP particles, undergo maturation before and during binding to the DNA and replacement of the transition proteins. *RING8* ring finger 8 protein; *HAT* histone acetyltransferase; *Pygo2* pygopus homolog 2 (HAT) (figure modified from Carrell et al. [63])

hyperacetylation loosens histone-DNA interaction and enables the displacement of histone and replacement with transition proteins [38–40]. These studies suggest that changes in chromatin composition are intricately governed by the many waves of histone modifications that appear to ensure proper chromatin remodeling and packaging.

Changes in histone ubiquination and acetylation patterns have significant ramifications on spermatogenesis and reproductive potential. H2A in sperm is carried out by ring finger 8 (RNF8) and has been shown to have an important role in sex chromosome inactivation during meiotic prophase and in postmeiotic phases during the global histone replacement. However, RNF8$^{-/-}$ mice are proficient in meiotic sex chromosome inactivation and fail to replace histones with protamines, and the majority of the sperm cells undergo apoptosis [34]. To test the fertilization ability of the very few sperm cells that escaped apoptosis, IVF or intracytoplasmic sperm injection (ICSI) was used and showed that all microdrop samples resulted in no fertilization [34]. However, 5/28 fertilized oocytes reached the blastocyt stage with ICSI [34]. These data suggest that histone replacement is critical for normal sperm maturation, escaping testicular and epididymal apoptosis, and reproductive efficiency.

In addition to H2A ubiquination, histone acetylation (H3 and H4) is essential for the histone to protamine transition. Enzymes involved in H4 hyperacetylation in the round spermatid are unknown; nonetheless, two potential candidates expressed in the elongating spermatid at the time have shown to exhibit potent H4 acetylase activity may be: testis-specific chromodomain protein (CDY) and HAT (monocytic leukemia) 4 (MYST4) [41, 42]. Similar to the RNF8$^{-/-}$ phenotype, mice treated with general histone deacetylase (HDAC) inhibitors resulted in significantly reduced sperm counts and male infertility [43, 44]. On the other hand, H3 acetylation in the elongating spermatid was shown to be Pygopus 2 (Pygo 2)-dependent and loss of Pygo 2 function leads to spermatogenesis arrest and infertility. The mechanism through which H3/H4ac elicits this chromatin exchange is unknown; however, a few studies have suggested the involvement of BRDT, a testis-specific protein. BRDT associates with acetylated H4 nucleosomes [45–47] and mutating one of bromodomains (BD1) results in male sterility. Furthermore, ectopic expression of BRDT in somatic cells after treating cells with trichostatin A (a hyperacetylating agent) triggers a reorganization of chromatin [45–47].

Histone hyperacetylation is thought to promote the incorporation of transition proteins, but is subsequently replaced by protamines, which signal the end of sperm chromatin reorganization. Protamines are highly basic sperm-specific nuclear proteins that permit higher order of DNA packaging [48, 49]. Humans and mice express two protamine proteins, protamine 1 (P1) and protamine 2 (P2), both of which are expressed in relatively equal quantities [50]. The P1–P2 ratio in human sperm donors of known fertility lies close to 1 [51], ranging from 0.8 to 1.2 [32, 52], and deviations from this ratio is inversely correlated with the amount of histones retained [53, 54]. Patients with either a low or high P1/P2 ratio had significantly reduced semen parameter (lower sperm concentration, motility, and morphology), as compared to patients with normal P1/P2 ratios [52]. These patients also have increased sperm DNA damage and reduced fertilization ability. The reduced fertilization resulting from the sperm abnormalities can be overcome by the use of ICSI; however, implantation and pregnancy rates were significantly reduced [52, 55–58]. In mice, P1–P2 knockout or happloinsufficency resulted in similar findings to humans [59], which strongly suggests that protamine displacement may be an important trigger for ensuring proper embryonic development, most likely through a secondary mechanism, such as epigenetic mechanisms.

Alterations in chromatin remodeling at any point during the histone to protamine transition results in severe male subfertility and poor embryo outcome following IVF [59–61]. The reduction in reproductive efficiency resulting from improper sperm chromatin packaging prompts the question what is the true significance of chromatin reorganization: (a) protect the paternal genome and prevent apoptosis, (b) complete spermatogenesis, as has traditionally been thought, or (c) other possible reasons for the remodeling [32, 62, 63]. It has been proposed that the presence of protamines in the mature sperm and their replacement at the time of fertilization may be important for reprogramming the paternal pronucleus. Two potential mechanisms through which this may be mediated are: first, the DNA breaks resulting from protamine displacement may elicit the recruitment of the DNA repair-mediated DNA demethylases (GADD45, AID, MBD4) recently described in plants, mouse, and zebrafish (described in detail below). Second, the short stretches of naked DNA (after protamine ejection and prior to histone incorporation) may enable the recruitment of demethylases to the paternal genome and enhance reprogramming efficiency. Both mechanisms are speculative and a better understanding of the significance of the protamine transition and its role in development is essential.

Although sperm undergoes dramatic chromatin changes, the exchange process is incomplete, retaining approximately 5–15% of the genome packaged in nucleosomes [64–66]. The retained nucleosomes are comprised of canonical histone H2A, H3, and H4, but bear a testes-specific histone H2B with an unknown specialized function, along with very low levels of canonical H2B [65, 67]. Histone retention raises an intriguing question of whether the retained nucleosomes in the sperm nucleus may simply be due to inefficient protamine replacement, leading to a low random genome-wide distribution with no function in the embryo, or whether the retained nucleosomes, along with their attendant epigenetic modifications, can be enriched at particular genes/loci of significance to the developing embryo.

Prior to the availability of genome-wide array and modern sequencing technologies, two groups examined by qPCR the sperm chromatin composition at a few key loci required in embryogenesis and both reported significant enrichment of histones at the developmental loci [66, 68]. This suggested that histone retention maybe programmatically retained; however, these preliminary observations were not confirmed genome-wide until recently by three independent labs [69–71]. All three groups showed that histones were retained at developmental transcription factors, imprinted genes, cell cycle, and spermatogenesis gene promoters [69–71]. The spermatogenesis and cell cycle gene promoters retained high H3k4me, a mark of gene activation (Fig. 13.2) [72], whereas developmental transcription factor gene promoters were bivalently marked as seen in embryonic stem cells meaning that they retained both marks of activation and silencing (H3K4me and H3k27me), respectively (Fig. 13.2) [69–72]. Furthermore, histone retention at imprinted loci

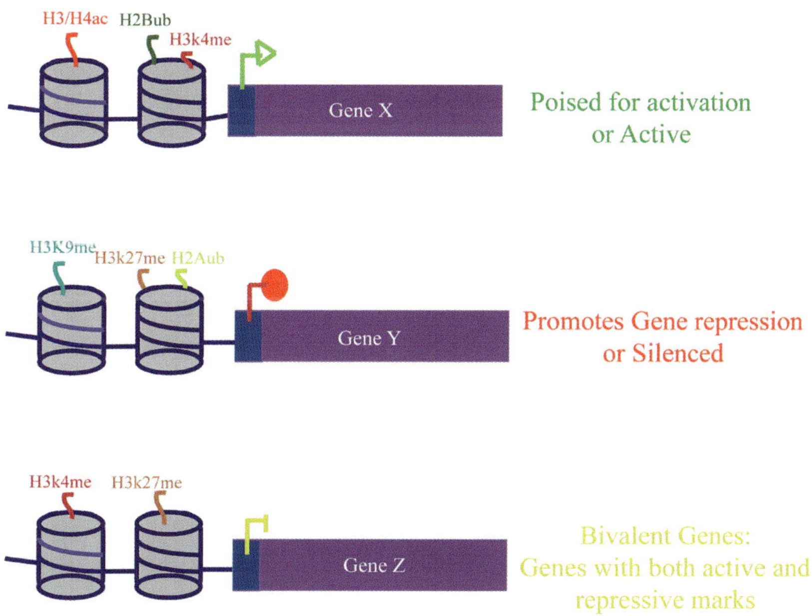

Fig. 13.2 Chromatin modifications determine gene state. Histone modifications promote either gene activation (i.e., spermatogenesis and cell cycle genes) or repression (i.e., organogenesis gene promoters); however, in embryonic stem cells and sperm, a subset of genes is commonly associated with both active and inactive marks (bivalent domains at developmental transcription factors and signaling factors). *ac* acetylation; *me* methylation; *ub* ubiquitination (figure obtained from Carrell and Hammoud [72])

was intriguing and showed differential profiles depending on whether the gene was maternally (lacked H3k4me) or paternally expressed (high H3k4me) [70]. Paternally expressed imprinted genes retained high levels of H3k4me, whereas maternally imprinted genes lacked H3k4me and a few loci tested by qPCR enriched for H3k9me.

This differential poising at spermatogenesis and cell cycle versus developmental transcription factors were not only unique to humans, but have been recently seen in mouse which retain less histone (~1%) and zebrafish sperm (complete histone genome) [69, 73]. This conservation in histone marking raises the question of whether the retained nucleosomal regions are important for early embryonic development or are only residual marks from the spermatogonial stem cell. Although a definitive answer for mammals is unknown, but in early zebrafish embryos H3k4me and H3k27me marks were erased and later reestablished after fertilization [73]. This suggests two possibilities either the histone marking in the paternal genome is not instructive to the early embryo or the levels of H3k4me and H3k27me were very low beyond antibody detection limits. In contrast, Brykczynska et al. reported in his discussion that paternal histones in mouse and human embryos are retained in the embryo [69]. Whether these differences in findings are attributed to species variation or due to the difference in the onset of zygotic transcription, 2–8 cell stage (mouse and human) vs. 500 cell stage (zebrafish) is unclear. For humans, if an epigenetic role is ascribed to the retained nucleosomes, there are obvious and profound implications for sperm with abnormal histone retention and protamine levels in humans, and for the use of such sperm, or any immature sperm, to achieve a pregnancy with the use of assisted reproductive technologies.

13.3 DNA Methylation and its Role in the Germline

DNA methylation in mammals primarily involves the modification of cytosine in a CpG context by a family of related DNA methyltransferases (DNMTs). This covalent mark is "read" by a family of methyl-binding domain proteins (MBDs) that associate with chromatin-modifying enzymes, including HDACs and histone methyltransferases (HMTs), that silence Pol II transcription [74–76]. Although the vast majority of DNA methylation resides on repetitive elements, the methylation of CpG sites in promoters can lead to gene silencing [77].

Genome-wide methylation studies in sperm have shown that the sperm epigenome differs markedly from that of somatic cells, but is very similar to ES cells and embryonic germ (EG) cells [78–81]. An examination of human gene promoters by several labs has revealed several important conclusions. First, promoters with "weak" CpG islands appear to be differentially methylated in sperm and somatic tissue or acquire methylation upon differentiation [70, 78–81]. Second, the target gene promoters of pluripotentcy network (e.g., OCT4, SOX2, NANOG, KLF4, and FOXD3 proteins) [82, 83] are hypomethylated in sperm, but acquire methylation upon differentiation to ensure cellular commitment, whereas several key members of the pluripotency/self-renewal network, OCT4, NANOG, and FOXD3 themselves, acquire methylation throughout spermatogenesis, consistent with recent studies in mice [78, 84]. To summarize, developmental and signaling gene promoters in mature sperm retain modified nucleosomes and are DNA hypomethylated, which suggests that the sperm chromatin are poised for activation, and this poising may enable transcriptional competence/activation of developmental regulators if needed in early embryonic development.

13.4 Imprinting and Alterations at Imprinted Genes Have Been Associated with Infertility

Genomic imprinting causes some genes to be monoallelically expressed and contributes to parental genome asymmetry. Approximately 100 imprinted genes have been identified, many of which are important for prenatal growth, placental development, and function and have been implicated in certain diseases [85]. Imprints are erased and reestablished in the germ line and maintained into embryogenesis [26, 86, 87]. One of the interesting features of the organization of imprinted genes is that most of them occur in clusters with long range cis-acting imprinting centers (ICs) [86]. These ICs carry allele-specific methylation marks, which subsequently influence epigenetic modifications of additional cis-acting regulators important for allele-specific, tissue-specific, or temporal-specific regulation of imprinted genes [88, 89].

Imprinted genes are classified as primary imprinted genes (such as H19/KCNQ1OT, etc.), which acquire their imprinted status in the germ line, whereas secondary imprinted genes are only imprinted for a short period of time during development (such as GTL2 IGDMR and CDKN1C) and then regain biallelic expression. Imprinting in the female germ line is primarily achieved using DNA methylation, whereas imprinting in males is primarily mediated through noncoding RNAs; however, two genes are known to be DNA methylated H19/Rasgraf.

A relationship between genomic imprinting and infertility first stemmed from early work of IVF in animal models. Offspring conceived by assisted reproductive technologies in animals had an increased incidence of LOS [23]. In humans, a meta-analysis showed that children born from assisted reproductive technology (ART) have a fourfold increased incidence of BWS compared with children conceived naturally [90–93].

Many speculations have been made suggesting that hormone stimulation, gamete manipulation, or embryo culture may alter oocyte/embryo imprinting. The effects of culture on embryo quality, embryo transcriptome and epigenetics, and long-term behavioral effects have been previously described [20, 94–96]. However, recently these findings have been confirmed by a very elegantly designed study using the agouti viable yellow (A^{vy}) allele in mice, which is one of the best-characterized alleles that display a labile epigenetic state [97–99]. This study shows that embryos cultured in commercially available embryo culture induced persistent epigenetic changes that altered coat color in mouse IVF offspring as compared to natural mating [99]. These findings are concerning and require a better understanding of the effects of existent or acquired epimutations on embryo quality, IVF success rate, or the true risk for transmission to counsel patients accordingly. However, more recently, it has been shown that IVF culture media may not be solely responsible for these changes, but also preexistent methylation alterations patterns are common in the gametes of infertile men [14–19]. These observations beg the question of whether methylation defects as well as other epigenetic defects (such as histone localization or modifications in the mature sperm) may affect embryo development, growth of ART offspring, and may last for future generations.

Evidence for germline epigenetic inheritance in humans has come almost exclusively from epidemiological studies. The strongest evidence for germline epigenetic inheritance in humans comes from the work of Horsthemke and colleagues [100]. They have shown that the presence of epimutations and not genetic mutations, at the SNRPN–SNURF, was inherited from the paternal grandmother [100]. More recently, a few reports have shown that a gain in methylation on the paternal alleles of LIT1 or MEST in sperm is maintained in the baby and associated with transient neonatal diabetes [101] or Silver–Russell syndrome [102]. Inheritance of epimutations from imprinted genes is intriguing since imprinted genes have tandem repeats in their gene promoters and repeats may be incompletely erased. Second, in mice the best known examples of transgenerational inheritance were described at two metastable epialleles known as the agouti viable yellow (A^{vy}) allele (coat color ranges from agouti to yellow) and the axin-fused ($Axin^{Fu}$) allele (normal to severe tail kinks). In both cases, isogenic animals displayed variable expressivity and phenotype variegation which correlated with the differential level of methylation acquired at the IAP retrotransposon inserted at each of the loci [101–105]. To date, epigenetic inheritance in mice and humans has been limited to a certain gene classes; genes that contain repeat elements in their promoter regions. One hypothesis can be that epigenetic inheritance is limited to repeat elements as they may escape reprogramming. However, epigenetic inheritance at a nonimprinted gene was suggested by Suter et al. and Chang et al., which showed that epimutations at the promoters of DNA repair genes, MLH1 and MSH2, were seen in some cases of familial colorectal cancer in successive generations [106, 107]. This study raises an interesting possibility that epigenetic marks may be maintained in families and are not efficiently cleared in the genome-wide reprogramming that takes place between generations. Future studies are needed to determine the perdurance of these marks.

13.5 Genome-Wide Reprogramming in Preimplantation Embryos and Primordial Germ Cells

Epigenetic reprogramming via demethylation of DNA occurs at two points in mammalian development. First, in early preimplantation embryos where the vast majority of the genome is demethylated, although some genes, including imprinted genes, escape this wave of DNA demethylation [29]. The second and more complete reprogramming happens in PGCs during which imprinted genes are erased and reestablished. The two waves reprogramming, first in the early embryo and a second in PGCs, may be needed to restore totipotency and limit the potential for transgenerational inheritance of epimutations [26, 108–115].

Genome-wide reprogramming can be mediated via two potential mechanisms: active demethylation, first described in plants, or passive demethylation. In plants, the active DNA demethylation process is important for plant gene imprinting and for general housekeeping functions to counteract the spreading of methylation from repetitive sequences to genes [116–121]. Loss of plant demethylases didn't result in significant changes in methylation on a genome-wide scale, but many genomic sites were hypermethylated [3, 119]. Surprisingly, the accumulation of methylation at many of the gene promoters did not alter gene expression [119, 122].

Mammals, on the other hand, lack orthologues for any of the characterized demethylases in plants or bacteria, but many of the recent findings suggest that the active DNA demethylation in mammals is achieved (embryo and PGCs), at least in part, by the base excision repair machinery [123–134]. First, 5-me C is deaminated by AID or Apobec, then followed by the T:G base excision repair by glycosylases such as TDG/MBD4 creating an abasic site, which is then filled by DNA polymerase and DNA ligase [134–136]. This multistep process results in a hypomethylated genome. The use of AID and other factors as a potential mechanism for active DNA demethylation was shown to be important for reprogramming mouse PGC and enhancing the efficiency of somatic cell reprogramming. Recent reports suggest that active DNA demethylation may be a more commonly used phenomena in mammalian cells than previously thought; it is seen at gene specific promoters (interleukin genes and estrogen responsive gene promoters) undergoing transcriptional cycling [128, 133, 137]. Demethylation at these gene promoters correlated with the recruitment of Dnmt3a, Dnmt3b, TDG, and other BER enzymes [128, 133, 137]. Evidence for such interaction between DNMTs (as deaminases), glycosylases, and BER was previously reported [138–140]. This raises the question whether there may be two active DNA demethylase complexes, one specified for a robust genome-wide demethtylation which includes AID (AID a mutagen – restricted to developmental time-points) and the other being a gene/class-specific reprogramming (involves DNMTs since they have weak deaminase activity, therefore their effect can be contained).

In contrast to the active demethylation process, the passive DNA demethylation occurs when maintenance methyltransferases are inactive during cell cycle following DNA replication and division, as seen in the female pronucleus shortly after fertilization or in early stages of germ cell migration. Recent data examining allele-specific methylation status of H19 and SNRPN in both migratory and postmigratory PGC (e9.5–e11.5) suggest that erasure process may begin before the arrival to the gonad (e9.5)

[141]. During migration, the majority of the cells analyzed were hypermethylated at the paternal H19 locus, but a very small subset of the alleles (~19%) get demethylated (<50% methylated) and the methylation continued to gradually decrease until e11.5 [141]. Consistent with the report above, Sato et al. 2003 showed that IGF2r DMR2 starts demethylation at e9.5 in some migrating PGC, before the cells colonize the genital ridge, but the progression of demethylation is augmented after entering the genital ridge [142]. These findings suggest that PGC reprogramming may begin as a passive demethylation process (because of cell doubling) followed by an active demethylation mechanism [143–145].

A better understanding of the mechanism responsible for erasing cellular memory and epigenetic information provides a better understanding for how epigenetic errors arise and potential reversal. Most importantly, reprogramming is essential for the success and efficiency regenerative medicine-based therapies such as stem cell transplantation, transdifferentiation, and gamete regeneration for azoospermic men, premature ovarian failure, or for fertility preservation for cancer patients who have undergone radiation or chemotherapy.

13.6 Conclusions and Future Directions

The sperm chromatin state is highly dynamic and retains important chromatin attributes, although the vast majority of the genome is packaged in protamines. The chromatin landscape of the mature sperm resembles that of an embryonic stem, in that developmental transcription factor gene promoters are DNA hypomethylated and bivalent (retain both activation and repression marks). The significance of this poising is yet unclear, but raises many questions: do these poised genes in sperm play an important role in early embryo development, how extensive is embryonic reprogramming, and is reprogramming essential since the sperm and maybe the egg genome is poised similar to an embryonic stem cell.

If epigenetic information can be inherited from the sperm and the oocyte to regulate gene expression in an appropriate manner, then this raises concern for the growing body of evidence that suggests that the ART procedure and/or infertility may provide an additional layer of complexity to the pregnancy and may elicit epigenetic changes in IVF offspring. Underlying support for these speculations comes from the work published from the CDC in 2002, which suggested that children conceived by IVF had an increased risk for preterm birth, low birth weight, congenital anomalies, preeclampsia, and perinatal mortality even in singleton pregnancies [146–148]. Low birth weight in naturally conceived babies has been connected to heart disease and metabolic syndrome later in life; whether these risks apply to low birth weight IVF babies too is unknown. Several groups have postulated that these abnormalities may be epigenetic in nature. Unfortunately, morphological assessment of gametes at the time of fertilization and grading embryos at the time of transfer is incapable of detecting epigenetic errors. Therefore, future studies are needed to determine whether the underlying epigenetic alterations in the gametes of infertile couple rather than the IVF technique or both are responsible for these complications seen in IVF babies.

References

1. Robertson KD, Wolffe AP. DNA methylation in health and disease. Nat Rev Genet. 2000;1(1):11–9.
2. Robertson KD, Ait-Si-Ali S, Yokochi T, Wade PA, Jones PL, Wolffe AP. DNMT1 forms a complex with Rb, E2F1 and HDAC1 and represses transcription from E2F-responsive promoters. Nat Genet. 2000; 25(3):338–42.
3. Lister R, O'Malley RC, Tonti-Filippini J, et al. Highly integrated single-base resolution maps of the epigenome in Arabidopsis. Cell. 2008;133(3):523–36.
4. Cokus SJ, Feng S, Zhang X, et al. Shotgun bisulphite sequencing of the Arabidopsis genome reveals DNA methylation patterning. Nature. 2008;452(7184): 215–9.
5. Lister R, Pelizzola M, Dowen RH, et al. Human DNA methylomes at base resolution show widespread epigenomic differences. Nature. 2009;462(7271):315–22.

6. Feng S, Cokus SJ, Zhang X, et al. Conservation and divergence of methylation patterning in plants and animals. Proc Natl Acad Sci USA. 2010;107(19):8689–94.
7. Zemach A, McDaniel IE, Silva P, Zilberman D. Genome-wide evolutionary analysis of eukaryotic DNA methylation. Science. 2010;328(5980):916–9.
8. Margueron R, Trojer P, Reinberg D. The key to development: interpreting the histone code? Curr Opin Genet Dev. 2005;15(2):163–76.
9. Jenuwein T, Allis CD. Translating the histone code. Science. 2001;293(5532):1074–80.
10. Ehrlich M. DNA methylation in cancer: too much, but also too little. Oncogene. 2002;21(35):5400–13.
11. Feinberg AP, Ohlsson R, Henikoff S. The epigenetic progenitor origin of human cancer. Nat Rev Genet. 2006;7(1):21–33.
12. Sharma S, Kelly TK, Jones PA. Epigenetics in cancer. Carcinogenesis. 2010;31(1):27–36.
13. Lomba A, Milagro FI, Garcia-Diaz DF, Marti A, Campion J, Martinez JA. Obesity induced by a pair-fed high fat sucrose diet: methylation and expression pattern of genes related to energy homeostasis. Lipids Health Dis. 2010;9(1):60.
14. Boissonnas CC, Abdalaoui HE, Haelewyn V, et al. Specific epigenetic alterations of IGF2-H19 locus in spermatozoa from infertile men. Eur J Hum Genet. 2010;18(1):73–80.
15. Hammoud SS, Purwar J, Pflueger C, Cairns BR, Carrell DT. Alterations in sperm DNA methylation patterns at imprinted loci in two classes of infertility. Fertil Steril. 2009;94(5):1728–33.
16. Kobayashi H, Sato A, Otsu E, et al. Aberrant DNA methylation of imprinted loci in sperm from oligospermic patients. Hum Mol Genet. 2007;16(21):2542–51.
17. Marques CJ, Carvalho F, Sousa M, Barros A. Genomic imprinting in disruptive spermatogenesis. Lancet. 2004;363(9422):1700–2.
18. Marques CJ, Costa P, Vaz B, et al. Abnormal methylation of imprinted genes in human sperm is associated with oligozoospermia. Mol Hum Reprod. 2008;14(2):67–74.
19. Marques CJ, Francisco T, Sousa S, Carvalho F, Barros A, Sousa M. Methylation defects of imprinted genes in human testicular spermatozoa. Fertil Steril. 2010;94(2):585–94.
20. Manipalviratn S, DeCherney A, Segars J. Imprinting disorders and assisted reproductive technology. Fertil Steril. 2009;91(2):305–15.
21. Owen CM, Segars Jr JH. Imprinting disorders and assisted reproductive technology. Semin Reprod Med. 2009;27(5):417–28.
22. Lawrence LT, Moley KH. Epigenetics and assisted reproductive technologies: human imprinting syndromes. Semin Reprod Med. 2008;26(2):143–52.
23. Young LE, Sinclair KD, Wilmut I. Large offspring syndrome in cattle and sheep. Rev Reprod. 1998;3(3):155–63.
24. Bliek J, Verde G, Callaway J, et al. Hypomethylation at multiple maternally methylated imprinted regions including PLAGL1 and GNAS loci in Beckwith–Wiedemann syndrome. Eur J Hum Genet. 2009;17(5):611–9.
25. Weksberg R, Shuman C, Beckwith JB. Beckwith–Wiedemann syndrome. Eur J Hum Genet. 2010;18(1):8–14.
26. Reik W, Dean W, Walter J. Epigenetic reprogramming in mammalian development. Science. 2001;293(5532):1089–93.
27. Reik W, Santos F, Mitsuya K, Morgan H, Dean W. Epigenetic asymmetry in the mammalian zygote and early embryo: relationship to lineage commitment? Philos Trans R Soc Lond B Biol Sci. 2003;358(1436):1403–9. discussion 1409.
28. Reik W, Santos F, Dean W. Mammalian epigenomics: reprogramming the genome for development and therapy. Theriogenology. 2003;59(1):21–32.
29. Olek A, Walter J. The pre-implantation ontogeny of the H19 methylation imprint. Nat Genet. 1997;17(3):275–6.
30. Lane N, Dean W, Erhardt S, et al. Resistance of IAPs to methylation reprogramming may provide a mechanism for epigenetic inheritance in the mouse. Genesis. 2003;35(2):88–93.
31. Seki Y, Hayashi K, Itoh K, Mizugaki M, Saitou M, Matsui Y. Extensive and orderly reprogramming of genome-wide chromatin modifications associated with specification and early development of germ cells in mice. Dev Biol. 2005;278:440–5.
32. Oliva R. Protamines and male infertility. Hum Reprod Update. 2006;12:417–35.
33. Lu LY, Wu J, Ye L, Gavrilina GB, Saunders TL, Yu X. RNF8-dependent histone modifications regulate nucleosome removal during spermatogenesis. Dev Cell. 2010;18(3):371–84.
34. Li L, Halaby MJ, Hakem A, et al. Rnf8 deficiency impairs class switch recombination, spermatogenesis, and genomic integrity and predisposes for cancer. J Exp Med. 2010;207(5):983–97.
35. Shogren-Knaak M, Ishii H, Sun JM, Pazin MJ, Davie JR, Peterson CL. Histone H4-K16 acetylation controls chromatin structure and protein interactions. Science. 2006;311(5762):844–7.
36. Dion MF, Altschuler SJ, Wu LF, Rando OJ. Genomic characterization reveals a simple histone H4 acetylation code. Proc Natl Acad Sci USA. 2005;102(15):5501–6.
37. Meistrich ML, Trostle-Weige PK, Lin R, Bhatnagar YM, Allis CD. Highly acetylated H4 is associated with histone displacement in rat spermatids. Mol Reprod Dev. 1992;31(3):170–81.
38. Nair M, Nagamori I, Sun P, et al. Nuclear regulator Pygo2 controls spermiogenesis and histone H3 acetylation. Dev Biol. 2008;320(2):446–55.
39. Hazzouri M, Pivot-Pajot C, Faure A, et al. Regulated hyperacetylation of core histones during mouse spermatogenesis: involvement of histone deacetylases. Eur J Cell Biol. 2000;79:950–60.

40. Sonnack V, Failing K, Bergmann M, Steger K. Expression of hyperacetylated histone H4 during normal and impaired human spermatogenesis. Andrologia. 2002;34(6):384–90.
41. McGraw S, Morin G, Vigneault C, Leclerc P, Sirard MA. Investigation of MYST4 histone acetyltransferase and its involvement in mammalian gametogenesis. BMC Dev Biol. 2007;7:123.
42. Lahn BT, Tang ZL, Zhou J, et al. Previously uncharacterized histone acetyltransferases implicated in mammalian spermatogenesis. Proc Natl Acad Sci USA. 2002;99(13):8707–12.
43. Fenic I, Sonnack V, Failing K, Bergmann M, Steger K. In vivo effects of histone-deacetylase inhibitor trichostatin-A on murine spermatogenesis. J Androl. 2004;25(5):811–8.
44. Fenic I, Hossain HM, Sonnack V, et al. In vivo application of histone deacetylase inhibitor trichostatin-a impairs murine male meiosis. J Androl. 2008;29(2):172–85.
45. Pivot-Pajot C, Caron C, Govin J, Vion A, Rousseaux S, Khochbin S. Acetylation-dependent chromatin reorganization by BRDT, a testis-specific bromodomain-containing protein. Mol Cell Biol. 2003;23(15):5354–65.
46. Shang E, Nickerson HD, Wen D, Wang X, Wolgemuth DJ. The first bromodomain of Brdt, a testis-specific member of the BET sub-family of double-bromodomain-containing proteins, is essential for male germ cell differentiation. Development. 2007;134(19):3507–15.
47. Moriniere J, Rousseaux S, Steuerwald U, et al. Cooperative binding of two acetylation marks on a histone tail by a single bromodomain. Nature. 2009;461(7264):664–8.
48. Krawetz SA, Dixon GH. Sequence similarities of the protamine genes: implications for regulation and evolution. J Mol Evol. 1988;27(4):291–7.
49. Balhorn R, The protamine family of sperm nuclear proteins. Genome Biol. 2007;8(9):227.
50. Corzett M, Mazrimas J, Balhorn R. Protamine 1: protamine 2 stoichiometry in the sperm of eutherian mammals. Mol Reprod Dev. 2002;61(4):519–27.
51. Carrell DT, Liu L. Altered protamine 2 expression is uncommon in donors of known fertility, but common among men with poor fertilizing capacity, and may reflect other abnormalities of spermiogenesis. J Androl. 2001;22(4):604–10.
52. Aoki VW, Liu L, Carrell DT. Identification and evaluation of a novel sperm protamine abnormality in a population of infertile males. Hum Reprod. 2005; 20(5):1298–306.
53. Zhang X, San Gabriel M, Zini A. Sperm nuclear histone to protamine ratio in fertile and infertile men: evidence of heterogeneous subpopulations of spermatozoa in the ejaculate. J Androl. 2006;27(3):414–20.
54. Zini A, Gabriel MS, Zhang X. The histone to protamine ratio in human spermatozoa: comparative study of whole and processed semen. Fertil Steril. 2007;87(1):217–9.
55. Aoki VW, Moskovtsev SI, Willis J, Liu L, Mullen JB, Carrell DT. DNA integrity is compromised in protamine-deficient human sperm. J Androl. 2005; 26(6):741–8.
56. Aoki VW, Liu L, Jones KP, et al. Sperm protamine 1/ protamine 2 ratios are related to in vitro fertilization pregnancy rates and predictive of fertilization ability. Fertil Steril. 2006;86(5):1408–15.
57. de Yebra L, Ballesca JL, Vanrell JA, Corzett M, Balhorn R, Oliva R. Detection of P2 precursors in the sperm cells of infertile patients who have reduced protamine P2 levels. Fertil Steril. 1998; 69(4):755–9.
58. Chevaillier P, Mauro N, Feneux D, Jouannet P, David G. Anomalous protein complement of sperm nuclei in some infertile men. Lancet. 1987;2(8562):806–7.
59. Cho C, Willis WD, Goulding EH, et al. Haploinsufficiency of protamine-1 or -2 causes infertility in mice. Nat Genet. 2001;28(1):82–6.
60. Zhao M, Shirley CR, Hayashi S, et al. Transition nuclear proteins are required for normal chromatin condensation and functional sperm development. Genesis. 2004;38(4):200–13.
61. Shirley CR, Hayashi S, Mounsey S, Yanagimachi R, Meistrich ML. Abnormalities and reduced reproductive potential of sperm from Tnp1- and Tnp2-null double mutant mice. Biol Reprod. 2004;71(4):1220–9.
62. Carrell DT, Emery BR, Hammoud S. Altered protamine expression and diminished spermatogenesis: what is the link? Hum Reprod Update. 2007;13(3):313–27.
63. Carrell DT, Emery BR, Hammoud S. The aetiology of sperm protamine abnormalities and their potential impact on the sperm epigenome. Int J Androl. 2008;31(6):537–45.
64. Gatewood JM, Cook GR, Balhorn R, Bradbury EM, Schmid CW. Sequence-specific packaging of DNA in human sperm chromatin. Science. 1987;236(4804): 962–4.
65. Gatewood JM, Cook GR, Balhorn R, Schmid CW, Bradbury EM. Isolation of four core histones from human sperm chromatin representing a minor subset of somatic histones. J Biol Chem. 1990;265(33):20662–6.
66. Wykes SM, Krawetz SA. The structural organization of sperm chromatin. J Biol Chem. 2003;278(32): 29471–7.
67. Kimmins S, Sassone-Corsi P. Chromatin remodelling and epigenetic features of germ cells. Nature. 2005;434(7033):583–9.
68. Gardiner-Garden M, Ballesteros M, Gordon M, Tam PP. Histone- and protamine-DNA association: conservation of different patterns within the beta-globin domain in human sperm. Mol Cell Biol. 1998; 18(6):3350–6.
69. Brykczynska U, Hisano M, Erkek S, et al. Repressive and active histone methylation mark distinct promoters in human and mouse spermatozoa. Nat Struct Mol Biol. 2010;17(6):679–87.
70. Hammoud SS, Nix DA, Zhang H, Purwar J, Carrell DT, Cairns BR. Distinctive chromatin in human sperm

packages genes for embryo development. Nature. 2009;460(7254):473–8.
71. Arpanahi A, Brinkworth M, Iles D, et al. Endonuclease-sensitive regions of human spermatozoal chromatin are highly enriched in promoter and CTCF binding sequences. Genome Res. 2009;19(8):1338–49.
72. Carrell DT, Hammoud SS. The human sperm epigenome and its potential role in embryonic development. Mol Hum Reprod. 2010;16(1):37–47.
73. Vastenhouw NL, Zhang Y, Woods IG, et al. Chromatin signature of embryonic pluripotency is established during genome activation. Nature. 2010;464(7290):922–6.
74. Bird A, Macleod D. Reading the DNA methylation signal. Cold Spring Harb Symp Quant Biol. 2004;69:113–8.
75. Fuks F, Burgers WA, Brehm A, Hughes-Davies L, Kouzarides T. DNA methyltransferase Dnmt1 associates with histone deacetylase activity. Nat Genet. 2000;24(1):88–91.
76. Rountree MR, Bachman KE, Baylin SB. DNMT1 binds HDAC2 and a new co-repressor, DMAP1, to form a complex at replication foci. Nat Genet. 2000;25(3):269–77.
77. Eden S, Cedar H. Role of DNA methylation in the regulation of transcription. Curr Opin Genet Dev. 1994;4(2):255–9.
78. Farthing CR, Ficz G, Ng RK, et al. Global mapping of DNA methylation in mouse promoters reveals epigenetic reprogramming of pluripotency genes. PLoS Genet. 2008;4(6):e1000116.
79. Weber M, Hellmann I, Stadler MB, et al. Distribution, silencing potential and evolutionary impact of promoter DNA methylation in the human genome. Nat Genet. 2007;39(4):457–66.
80. Oakes CC, La Salle S, Smiraglia DJ, Robaire B, Trasler JM. A unique configuration of genome-wide DNA methylation patterns in the testis. Proc Natl Acad Sci USA. 2007;104(1):228–33.
81. Eckhardt F, Lewin J, Cortese R, et al. DNA methylation profiling of human chromosomes 6, 20 and 22. Nat Genet. 2006;38(12):1378–85.
82. Mohn F, Weber M, Rebhan M, et al. Lineage-specific polycomb targets and de novo DNA methylation define restriction and potential of neuronal progenitors. Mol Cell. 2008;30(6):755–66.
83. Boyer LA, Lee TI, Cole MF, et al. Core transcriptional regulatory circuitry in human embryonic stem cells. Cell. 2005;122(6):947–56.
84. Down TA, Rakyan VK, Turner DJ, et al. A Bayesian deconvolution strategy for immunoprecipitation-based DNA methylome analysis. Nat Biotechnol. 2008;26(7):779–85.
85. Ferguson-Smith AC, Surani MA. Imprinting and the epigenetic asymmetry between parental genomes. Science. 2001;293(5532):1086–9.
86. Reik W, Walter J. Genomic imprinting: parental influence on the genome. Nat Rev Genet. 2001;2(1):21–32.
87. Allen ND, Norris ML, Surani MA. Epigenetic control of transgene expression and imprinting by genotype-specific modifiers. Cell. 1990;61(5):853–61.
88. Ferguson-Smith AC. Genetic imprinting: silencing elements have their say. Curr Biol. 2000;10(23):R872–5.
89. Paulsen M, Ferguson-Smith AC. DNA methylation in genomic imprinting, development, and disease. J Pathol. 2001;195(1):97–110.
90. Gosden R, Trasler J, Lucifero D, Faddy M. Rare congenital disorders, imprinted genes, and assisted reproductive technology. Lancet. 2003;361(9373):1975–7.
91. DeBaun MR, Niemitz EL, Feinberg AP. Association of in vitro fertilization with Beckwith–Wiedemann syndrome and epigenetic alterations of LIT1 and H19. Am J Hum Genet. 2003;72(1):156–60.
92. Niemitz EL, DeBaun MR, Fallon J, et al. Microdeletion of LIT1 in familial Beckwith–Wiedemann syndrome. Am J Hum Genet. 2004;75(5):844–9.
93. Cox GF, Burger J, Lip V, et al. Intracytoplasmic sperm injection may increase the risk of imprinting defects. Am J Hum Genet. 2002;71(1):162–4.
94. Fernandez-Gonzalez R, Moreira P, Bilbao A, et al. Long-term effect of in vitro culture of mouse embryos with serum on mRNA expression of imprinting genes, development, and behavior. Proc Natl Acad Sci USA. 2004;101(16):5880–5.
95. Lazzari G, Wrenzycki C, Herrmann D, et al. Cellular and molecular deviations in bovine in vitro-produced embryos are related to the large offspring syndrome. Biol Reprod. 2002;67(3):767–75.
96. Lonergan P, Rizos D, Gutierrez-Adan A, Fair T, Boland MP. Effect of culture environment on embryo quality and gene expression – experience from animal studies. Reprod Biomed Online. 2003;7(6):657–63.
97. Morgan HD, Sutherland HG, Martin DI, Whitelaw E. Epigenetic inheritance at the agouti locus in the mouse. Nat Genet. 1999;23(3):314–8.
98. Rakyan VK, Down TA, Thorne NP, et al. An integrated resource for genome-wide identification and analysis of human tissue-specific differentially methylated regions (tDMRs). Genome Res. 2008;18(9):1518–29.
99. Morgan HD, Jin XL, Li A, Whitelaw E, O'Neill C. The culture of zygotes to the blastocyst stage changes the postnatal expression of an epigenetically labile allele, agouti viable yellow, in mice. Biol Reprod. 2008;79(4):618–23.
100. Buiting K, Gross S, Lich C, Gillessen-Kaesbach G, El-Maarri O, Horsthemke B. Epimutations in Prader-Willi and Angelman syndromes: a molecular study of 136 patients with an imprinting defect. Am J Hum Genet. 2003;72(3):571–7.
101. Arima T, Kamikihara T, Hayashida T, et al. ZAC, LIT1 (KCNQ1OT1) and p57KIP2 (CDKN1C) are in an imprinted gene network that may play a role in Beckwith–Wiedemann syndrome. Nucleic Acids Res. 2005;33(8):2650–60.

102. Kagami M, Nagai T, Fukami M, Yamazawa K, Ogata T. Silver-Russell syndrome in a girl born after in vitro fertilization: partial hypermethylation at the differentially methylated region of PEG1/MEST. J Assist Reprod Genet. 2007;24(4):131–6.
103. Rakyan V, Whitelaw E. Transgenerational epigenetic inheritance. Curr Biol. 2003;13(1):R6.
104. Rakyan VK, Chong S, Champ ME, et al. Transgenerational inheritance of epigenetic states at the murine Axin(Fu) allele occurs after maternal and paternal transmission. Proc Natl Acad Sci USA. 2003;100(5):2538–43.
105. Blewitt ME, Vickaryous NK, Paldi A, Koseki H, Whitelaw E. Dynamic reprogramming of DNA methylation at an epigenetically sensitive allele in mice. PLoS Genet. 2006;2(4):e49.
106. Chan TL, Yuen ST, Kong CK, et al. Heritable germline epimutation of MSH2 in a family with hereditary nonpolyposis colorectal cancer. Nat Genet. 2006;38(10):1178–83.
107. Suter CM, Martin DI, Ward RL. Germline epimutation of MLH1 in individuals with multiple cancers. Nat Genet. 2004;36(5):497–501.
108. Yamazaki Y, Mann MR, Lee SS, et al. Reprogramming of primordial germ cells begins before migration into the genital ridge, making these cells inadequate donors for reproductive cloning. Proc Natl Acad Sci USA. 2003;100(21):12207–12.
109. Lee J, Inoue K, Ono R, et al. Erasing genomic imprinting memory in mouse clone embryos produced from day 11.5 primordial germ cells. Development. 2002;129(8):1807–17.
110. Hajkova P, Ancelin K, Waldmann T, et al. Chromatin dynamics during epigenetic reprogramming in the mouse germ line. Nature. 2008; 452(7189):877–81.
111. Hajkova P, Erhardt S, Lane N, et al. Epigenetic reprogramming in mouse primordial germ cells. Mech Dev. 2002;117(1–2):15–23.
112. Dean W, Santos F, Stojkovic M, et al. Conservation of methylation reprogramming in mammalian development: aberrant reprogramming in cloned embryos. Proc Natl Acad Sci USA. 2001;98(24):13734–8.
113. Mayer W, Niveleau A, Walter J, Fundele R, Haaf T. Demethylation of the zygotic paternal genome. Nature. 2000;403(6769):501–2.
114. Oswald J, Engemann S, Lane N, et al. Active demethylation of the paternal genome in the mouse zygote. Curr Biol. 2000;10(8):475–8.
115. Sasaki H, Matsui Y. Epigenetic events in mammalian germ-cell development: reprogramming and beyond. Nat Rev Genet. 2008;9(2):129–40.
116. Choi Y, Gehring M, Johnson L, et al. DEMETER, a DNA glycosylase domain protein, is required for endosperm gene imprinting and seed viability in *Arabidopsis*. Cell. 2002;110(1):33–42.
117. Kinoshita T, Miura A, Choi Y, et al. One-way control of FWA imprinting in *Arabidopsis* endosperm by DNA methylation. Science. 2004;303(5657): 521–3.
118. Jullien PE, Kinoshita T, Ohad N, Berger F. Maintenance of DNA methylation during the Arabidopsis life cycle is essential for parental imprinting. Plant Cell. 2006;18(6):1360–72.
119. Penterman J, Zilberman D, Huh JH, Ballinger T, Henikoff S, Fischer RL. DNA demethylation in the Arabidopsis genome. Proc Natl Acad Sci USA. 2007;104(16):6752–7.
120. Hsieh TF, Ibarra CA, Silva P, et al. Genome-wide demethylation of Arabidopsis endosperm. Science. 2009;324(5933):1451–4.
121. Gehring M, Reik W, Henikoff S. DNA demethylation by DNA repair. Trends Genet. 2009;25(2):82–90.
122. Zhu J, Kapoor A, Sridhar VV, Agius F, Zhu JK. The DNA glycosylase/lyase ROS1 functions in pruning DNA methylation patterns in *Arabidopsis*. Curr Biol. 2007;17(1):54–9.
123. Bhattacharya SK, Ramchandani S, Cervoni N, Szyf M. A mammalian protein with specific demethylase activity for mCpG DNA. Nature. 1999;397(6720):579–83.
124. Balada E, Ordi-Ros J, Serrano-Acedo S, Martinez-Lostao L, Vilardell-Tarres M. Transcript overexpression of the MBD2 and MBD4 genes in CD4+ T cells from systemic lupus erythematosus patients. J Leukoc Biol. 2007;81(6):1609–16.
125. Sedgwick B. Repairing DNA-methylation damage. Nat Rev Mol Cell Biol. 2004;5(2):148–57.
126. Jin SG, Guo C, Pfeifer GP. GADD45A does not promote DNA demethylation. PLoS Genet. 2008;4(3):e1000013.
127. Barreto G, Schafer A, Marhold J, et al. Gadd45a promotes epigenetic gene activation by repair-mediated DNA demethylation. Nature. 2007;445(7128):671–5.
128. Kangaspeska S, Stride B, Metivier R, et al. Transient cyclical methylation of promoter DNA. Nature. 2008;452(7183):112–5.
129. Hendrich B, Hardeland U, Ng HH, Jiricny J, Bird A. The thymine glycosylase MBD4 can bind to the product of deamination at methylated CpG sites. Nature. 1999;401(6750):301–4.
130. Bennett MT, Rodgers MT, Hebert AS, Ruslander LE, Eisele L, Drohat AC. Specificity of human thymine DNA glycosylase depends on N-glycosidic bond stability. J Am Chem Soc. 2006;128(38):12510–9.
131. Zhu B, Zheng Y, Angliker H, et al. 5-Methylcytosine DNA glycosylase activity is also present in the human MBD4 (G/T mismatch glycosylase) and in a related avian sequence. Nucleic Acids Res. 2000;28(21):4157–65.
132. Jost JP, Siegmann M, Sun L, Leung R. Mechanisms of DNA demethylation in chicken embryos. Purification and properties of a 5-methylcytosine-DNA glycosylase. J Biol Chem. 1995;270(17):9734–9.
133. Metivier R, Gallais R, Tiffoche C, et al. Cyclical DNA methylation of a transcriptionally active promoter. Nature. 2008;452(7183):45–50.
134. Rai K, Huggins IJ, James SR, Karpf AR, Jones DA, Cairns BR. DNA demethylation in zebrafish involves the coupling of a deaminase, a glycosylase, and gadd45. Cell. 2008;135(7):1201–12.

135. Bhutani N, Brady JJ, Damian M, Sacco A, Corbel SY, Blau HM. Reprogramming towards pluripotency requires AID-dependent DNA demethylation. Nature. 2010;463(7284):1042–7.
136. Popp C, Dean W, Feng S, et al. Genome-wide erasure of DNA methylation in mouse primordial germ cells is affected by AID deficiency. Nature. 2010;463(7284):1101–5.
137. Tutt Landolfi MM, Scollay R, Parnes JR. Specific demethylation of the CD4 gene during CD4 T lymphocyte differentiation. Mol Immunol. 1997;34(1): 53–61.
138. Kovtun IV, McMurray CT. Crosstalk of DNA glycosylases with pathways other than base excision repair. DNA Repair (Amst). 2007;6(4):517–29.
139. Li YQ, Zhou PZ, Zheng XD, Walsh CP, Xu GL. Association of Dnmt3a and thymine DNA glycosylase links DNA methylation with base-excision repair. Nucleic Acids Res. 2007;35(2): 390–400.
140. Boland MJ, Christman JK. Characterization of Dnmt3b:thymine-DNA glycosylase interaction and stimulation of thymine glycosylase-mediated repair by DNA methyltransferase(s) and RNA. J Mol Biol. 2008;379(3):492–504.
141. Yamazaki Y, Low EW, Marikawa Y, et al. Adult mice cloned from migrating primordial germ cells. Proc Natl Acad Sci USA. 2005;102(32): 11361–6.
142. Sato S, Yoshimizu T, Sato E, Matsui Y. Erasure of methylation imprinting of Igf2r during mouse primordial germ-cell development. Mol Reprod Dev. 2003;65(1):41–50.
143. Lees-Murdock DJ, Walsh CP. DNA methylation reprogramming in the germ line. Adv Exp Med Biol. 2008;626:1–15.
144. Tam PP, Zhou SX, Tan SS. X-chromosome activity of the mouse primordial germ cells revealed by the expression of an X-linked lacZ transgene. Development. 1994;120(10):2925–32.
145. Ginsburg M, Snow MH, McLaren A. Primordial germ cells in the mouse embryo during gastrulation. Development. 1990;110(2):521–8.
146. Kalra SK, Molinaro TA. The association of in vitro fertilization and perinatal morbidity. Semin Reprod Med. 2008;26(5):423–35.
147. Chen XK, Wen SW, Bottomley J, Smith GN, Leader A, Walker MC. In vitro fertilization is associated with an increased risk for preeclampsia. Hypertens Pregnancy. 2009;28(1):1–12.
148. Hansen M, Kurinczuk JJ, Bower C, Webb S. The risk of major birth defects after intracytoplasmic sperm injection and in vitro fertilization. N Engl J Med. 2002;346(10):725–30.

Part III

Assisted Reproduction Techniques

14 ART and Epigenetic Disorders: Should We Be Concerned?

Christopher N. Herndon and Paolo F. Rinaudo

Abstract

An ART treatment cycle – comprising a basic sequence of ovarian stimulation, oocyte retrieval, embryo culture, and transfer – is, by conventional measures, a routine and comparatively safe medical intervention. The greatest risks from ART derive from the complications associated with multiple pregnancies. Yet, studies indicate that even a singleton pregnancy from ART confers greater health risks than that of natural conceptions. In this section, we review the established associations of ART to rare epigenetic disorders of imprinting. The biologic mechanisms through which epigenetic programming might be altered within the process of ART are examined. The still unknown long-term health associations of ART past 30 years are considered in the framework of emerging and increasing compelling evidence that environmental conditions during the early development are an important determinant of health during later adult years.

Keywords

Epigenetics • ART • ICSI • Imprinting • Morbidity

14.1 Introduction

Since the first live birth from in vitro fertilization over 30 years ago, greater than three million children have been conceived through assisted reproductive technologies (ART) [1]. Over this interval, ART has emerged from a largely inefficient, experimental protocol to a highly efficacious therapeutic modality that is the standard of care treatment for many forms of infertility in developed countries. Conceptions from ART in this decade comprise an estimated 1-3% of live births in many developed countries [1]. Although established as an efficacious therapy, the safety and long-term health implications of in vitro fertilization and culture on children conceived by ART are not well known. Importantly, longitudinal follow-up outcomes for any offspring resulting from in vitro fertilization and culture do not

P.F. Rinaudo (✉)
Division of Reproductive Endocrinology and Infertility, Department of Obstetrics, Gynecology and Reproductive Sciences, University of California, San Francisco, CA, USA
e-mail: rinaudop@obgyn.ucsf.edu

C. Racowsky et al. (eds.), *Biennial Review of Infertility: Volume 2*,
DOI 10.1007/978-1-4419-8456-2_14, © Springer Science+Business Media, LLC 2011

extend past puberty, and the impact past adolescence remains entirely unknown [2–5]. In perspective of its wide and increasing utilization, the long-term health implications of ART are an issue of paramount relevance and concern to both the individual and society as a whole.

The emergence of ART as a therapeutic modality has been characterized by an extraordinary rapidity in its adoption, from proof of concept to clinical utilization in developed countries worldwide. Intracytoplasmic sperm injection (ICSI), the gamete micromanipulation technique that revolutionized the treatment of male factor infertility, was first reported in 1992 [6]. Within a few years, ICSI became widely adopted into clinical practice globally and currently it is utilized in >60% of cycles in the United States [7]. Similarly, preimplantation genetic diagnosis (PGD), the technique that allows genetic testing of an embryo following extraction of one or more cells, is now widely offered by clinical centers despite comparatively limited reporting of follow-up outcomes of live births [8]. Driving this progressive development and application of technology in the clinical are the hopes and desperation of infertile couples [9]. The social and biological drives to conceive are powerful and compelling and infertile couples are often willing to accept new therapies, however unproven, that may give them a chance to have a biological offspring.

In this section, we summarize the known risks and complications of ART, focusing on the reporting of increased risk of two rare epigenetic disorders of imprinting. We cite evidence using animal models to provide insights on the biologic mechanisms by which epigenetic programming might be altered through the process of ART. In this background, we introduce the concept that the environment of early development has the potential to profoundly affect the phenotype in later life. The still unknown long-term health associations of ART are considered within emerging and increasing unavoidable evidence that environmental conditions during the early development are a significant determinant of health in later adult life.

14.2 Complications of ART

An ART treatment cycle – comprising a basic sequence of ovarian stimulation, oocyte retrieval, embryo culture, and transfer – is, by conventional measures, a routine and safe medical intervention. Complications at that time of treatment cycle are infrequent and include ovarian hyper stimulation (OHSS), bleeding or infection from oocyte retrieval, and torsion of the stimulated ovaries. The majority of these complications, although serious, are rarely associated with significant long-term morbidity and mortality. Significant adverse reactions from medications are exceedingly rare.

The greatest health risks associated with ART are unquestionably attributable to multiple gestations that result from the transfer practice of more than one embryo to optimize per cycle pregnancy rates. In 2008, twinning and higher order multiple gestations accounted for approximately one third of live births from ART in the United States [7]. The cost of medical care associated with multiple pregnancies thus exceeds by far the cost of ART treatment itself [10, 11]. Beyond the significant maternal, fetal, and neonatal risks of multiple gestations, studies have convincingly demonstrated that perinatal risk of singleton pregnancies from ART is higher than natural conceptions [12–14]. ART singleton pregnancies have greater risks of preterm delivery and low birth weight, after adjustment to maternal age, parity, ethnicity, or other cofounding variables.

Significantly, there is a 30% increased risk of congenital anomalies among children conceived by ART (3–4%), in comparison to the background rate (2–3%) in pregnancies conceived in vivo [12, 13, 15]. Despite initial concern, the incidence of congenital anomalies does not appear to be higher among ART cycles in which ICSI is performed [16], although an slightly increased risk of hypospadias has been reported [17]. It remains unclear if the increased incidence of congenital anomalies following ART is attributable to the intervention itself or the intrinsic predisposition of the infertile state [18]. Indeed, subfertile couples who conceive without medical interventions are predisposed to increased incidence of a series of pregnancy complications, including preeclampsia, *abruptio placentae*, preterm birth, and perinatal mortality [19].

The first definite evidence that ART alters pregnancy outcomes came through the early reporting of an association of monozygotic twinning (MZT) with ART. Studies have reported the incidence of MZT following ART as 1.9–2.5% [20, 21], a rate consistently over a background incidence for spontaneous conceptions, generally reported to be around 0.4%. The mechanisms conferring this increased risk are not understood. Extension to blastocyst culture is the most consistent risk factor identified, although use of ICSI and micromanipulation has also been reported [22].

14.3 Epigenetic Regulation

While the role played by Darwinian selective pressure in determining trait inheritance is uncontested, modern biology suggests that the environment and life experience of an individual can modify future progeny, ironically somewhat rehabilitating the early and now widely debunked Lamarckan theory of inheritance. The field of epigenetics (epi- Greek: επί- over, above -genetics) studies the changes in gene expression, gene activity, and phenotype caused by mechanisms not involving base pair changes in the underlying DNA sequence [23–25]. Epigenetics can be viewed as the link between environment and genes. This seminal concept was proposed by Waddington in the 1950s, far in advance of the current interest in the field [26]. The concept of canalization was used to account for phenotypic changes that occur too rapidly to be explained by the natural progression of evolutionary changes in DNA sequence.

The mechanisms and control of the epigenetic alternations of DNA are still being unraveled. Three mechanisms are thought to be involved:

1. DNA methylation.
2. Posttranslational modification of histone proteins and remodeling of chromatin.
3. RNA-based mechanisms.

The first identified and by far the best studied of these three modifications is DNA methylation, in which a methyl group is added to a cytosine base located 5′ to a guanosine, commonly referred to as "CpG" (p indicates the phosphate group linking the two bases). Importantly, not all the CpG dinucleotides are methylated. An area of the genome (usually at least 200 bp long) with high incidence of CpGs (greater than 50%) is referred to as "CpG island." Approximately half of the CpG islands are located near the transcription start site of genes, particularly for housekeeping genes; these CpGs are generally not methylated or have low levels of methylation. The remaining 50% of CpG islands are intragenic or intergenic and are believed to represent the transcription start site of noncoding RNAs [27]; these CpG islands are usually methylated [25].

Generally speaking, methylation silences gene transcription through structural blocking of transcriptional factor binding to DNA by the presence of a methyl group [28]. DNA methylation is responsible for X chromosome inactivation, silencing of imprinted genes, and silencing of repetitive and transposable elements. A few genes, such as IGF2 and IGF2R, are activated by methylation [29]. Methylation is catalyzed by DNA methyltransferases (DNMT), acting in conjunction with interacting corepressors, transcription factors, and methyl-CpG-binding proteins. DNMT1 is a sequence independent methyltransferase and acts to conserve the patterns of methylation status in the process of DNA replication and cell division in somatic cells [30]. Two isoforms, DNMT3A and DNMT3B, are responsible for de novo methylation during the process of gametogenesis and early life. Recently, the existence of active DNA demethylation has been documented [31–33].

Methylation is only one epigenetic marker; epigenetic mechanisms include postranslational modifications of histone tails through addition of an acetyl, methyl, phosphate group, or more rarely, by ubiquitination, sumoylation, ADP-ribosylation, deimination, and noncovalent proline isomerization. Histone modifications work often in conjunction or, occasionally, independently of DNA methylation [25]. The histone tail modifications work through changing the affinity of the basic histone proteins to the acidic DNA. Acetylation, for example, neutralizes the positive charge of lysine, promoting disassociation of the histone protein from the negatively charged DNA, resulting in a more open chromatin conformation. Generally speaking, DNA is least transcriptionally active when it is methylated and bound with unacetylated histones.

The "histone code" is extremely complex and just being deciphered. The challenge of its study is exemplified by the complexity of multiple levels of modifications that can coexist. For example, arginine residues can be mono or demethylated while lysine residues can accept one, two, or three methyl residues [23, 34, 35]. An additional epigenetic control at the chromatin level is performed by two family of chromatin remodeling complexes. The Brahma/SWI/SNF complex alters the position of nucleosomes along the DNA, whereas the SNF2H/ISWI complex mobilizes nucleosomes.

A third model of epigenetic control involves noncoding RNAs (ncRNA, reviewed by Mattick et al. [36]). It has become apparent that the eukaryotic genome can be envisioned as an "RNA machine," in which the vast nonprotein-coding segments of DNA are important for generating abundant ncRNAs which play a central role in genetic and epigenetic processes. In fact, transcription factors and proteins involved in epigenetic modification (e.g., DNMTs and methyl DNA-binding domain proteins) can bind RNA. RNA can also contribute to chromatin structural organization [36].

A unique feature of the epigenome is its plasticity. While epigenetic marks are maintained through cellular mitosis and are considered stable, they can be reversibly modified by the environment. For example, it is clear that there are important epigenetic changes associated with aging. Overall, aging is associated with global DNA hypomethylation and isolated hypermethylation of specific loci [37]. In addition, epigenetic programming can change during specific windows of sensitivity.

In a seminal study, rat pups which received higher level of grooming (pup licking) and nursing behaviors (arched-back nursing) from their mothers were found to have diminished expression of corticotropin-releasing hormone and a blunted response to stress [38]. These differences in their adrenocortical axis emerged during the first week of life and persisted through the remainder of their adult lives. Offspring who received less grooming and reinforcement behaviors differed from the offspring who received more grooming in the methylation of just a single CpG dinucleotide in the promoter of the glucocorticoid receptor [38]. Remarkably, these differences were reversed through cross-fostering with rat mothers who exhibited high levels of grooming and nursing behaviors. Furthermore, the stress-response phenotype was also modified at the molecular level through central infusion of a histone deacetylase inhibitor.

14.4 Imprinting Disorders

The reporting of an association of ART to two rare disorders of imprinting opened a new perspective into the effect of ART on early development [39, 40]. Imprinting refers to the differential expression of genes dependent on parental inheritance. As a diploid species, humans contain two sets of autosomal genes, a copy inherited from each parental gamete. In classical Mendelian inheritance, the genes from each parent are expressed in the offspring in equal measure, independent of parental origin. In a small handful of known genetic disorders, the disease phenotype is dependent on uniparental expression. The concept of genomic imprinting was elegantly illustrated in experiments in which diploid uniparental murine embryos (either two male or two female pronuclei) failed to undergo normal embryogenesis in comparison to control embryos (with one male and one transplanted female pronucleus) [41].

The first link of ART to an imprinting disorder was a report in 2002 of two cases of Angelmann syndrome (AS, OMIM 105830), a rare disorder with an overall prevalence in the general population of approximately 1 in 15,000 [42]. The syndrome is characterized by severe developmental delays, learning disabilities, profound speech impairment, ataxia, microcephaly, and seizures. Affected individuals typically exhibit a pathogenomic demeanor that has been characterized as the "happy puppet syndrome," manifested by frequent laughter, excitable personality, and affectionate nature. AS results from loss of maternal expression of UBE3A gene within 15q11-q13 [43]. This loss of maternal expression most commonly results from a deletion within 15q11-q13 (~70%), but can also result in mutations in the UBE3A gene (~11%) or paternal disomy (7%). Epimutations, or abnormalities of epigenetic marking rather than directly in the sequence of genomic DNA, account for 3% of AS cases or an overall incidence of approximately 1/300,000 cases in the general population [44].

To date, seven cases of AS have been reported in children conceived by ICSI or IVF [39]. Importantly, five of these seven AS cases were secondary to epigenetic mutation suggesting a strong correlation between AS and ART. The likelihood of these epimutations occuring by chance is estimated to be less than 1 in 20 million [40]. It is unknown whether the increased risk is attributable to embryo culture, gamete micromanipulation, and/or ovarian stimulation. It is additionally plausible that subfertile couples may be predisposed to AS. Cases of AS have been observed among subfertile couples who conceived spontaneously or after ovarian stimulation alone [45–47].

The second imprinting disorder found to be associated with ART is Beckwith–Wiedemann syndrome (BWS, OMIM 130650), a rare condition with an incidence of 1 in 13,700 live births. BWS is a heterogeneous disorder of overgrowth and characterized by macroglossia, anterior abdominal wall defects, visceromegaly, omphalocele, microcephaly, and embryonal tumors (Wilms' tumor, rhabdomyosarcoma, hepatoblastoma). Afflicted individuals in utero may present with polyhydraminos, enlarged placenta, and macrosomia. In 2003, three series were published reporting an association between BWS and ART [48–50]. To date, over 60 cases of BWS conceived through ART have been reported [39, 40]. A high percentage (>90%) of these cases have been associated with hypomethylation of the maternal allele, while 60% of BWS cases in the general population derive as a result of epimutations [39]. The affected imprinted region is located on chromosome 11 (11p15) and includes several genes and two differentially methylated regions (DMR1, DMR2) that are either paternally expressed (IGF2, KCNQ10T1) or maternally expressed (H19, CDKN1C, KCNQ1). The overall prevalence of BWS following ART has been estimated to be approximately 1 in 4,000, a four to fivefold higher level than in the background population [51]; the relative risk is increased to 14-fold if only epimutation-associated cases are considered. While these numbers are worrisome, it should be noted that an association of BWS is not conclusive, as a few cohort studies have not found a correlation between BWS and ART [52, 53]. The rare incidence and sporadic occurrence of imprinting disorders make it challenging to establish a clear association. In addition, the closer scrutiny and surveillance of offspring from ART may lead to a greater detection of the disorders in comparison to natural conceptions.

Although not an imprinted disorder, the incidence of retinoblastoma (RB) in ART children is noteworthy. One study found a nearly fivefold increase in RB in ART children compared to the general population [54]. The occurrence of this tumor of the retina requires two separate mutations: the first mutation ("first hit") is inherited, and the second is acquired somatically [55]. It is possible that methylation changes following in vitro culture could alter the single functional copy of the RB gene. While the presence of epigenetic abnormalities was not evaluated in RB cases among ART offspring, hypermethylation of RB gene has been associated with the development of RB [56, 57]. Of note, a large Danish cohort study detected no cases of RB among 6,052 IVF singletons [52].

14.5 Are There Epigenetic Disturbances Following ART?

Compelling evidence indicates that stressful environmental conditions during sensitive periods of early development may predispose to chronic disease later in life [58]. The premise of this postulate, known as the developmental origin of health and disease (DOHAD) hypothesis, is that the plasticity of the conceptus to its environment is an adaptive response, conferring a survival advantage in low resource environments. In a different, high resource environment later in life, these adaptations may predispose to metabolic and cardiovascular dysfunction [59, 60]. In particular, the increased incidence of low birth weight among ART children is a reason of concern [61]. Low birth weight is an indicator of in utero stress. Barker's hypothesis was formulated from observations that regions of Britain with the greatest incidence of low birth weight correlated tightly to areas with the highest rates of cardiovascular disease [58, 62]. Subsequent epidemiologic studies in other countries have widely supported this association [63]. Fetuses exposed to famine in early gestation during wartime Holland had a threefold higher risk of heart disease in fetuses exposed (3.0 OR, 95% CI 1.2–8.8) [64].

Low birth weight has additionally been associated with other vascular morbidity including cerebrovascular disease and hypertension [65, 66]. In Scotland, incidence of stroke was found to be inversely proportional to birth weight [67]. An association of low birth weight and hypertension appears to be present, but the effect appears modest. In one study, a 1 kg decrease in birth weight was correlated with a 2–4 mmHg increase in systolic blood pressure [68].

Epidemiologic studies are compelling, but are limited by potential confounding variables. Controlled animal studies have confirmed the associations reported in epidemiological studies. Maternal undernourishment in rats and sheep during the period of conception and implantation, for example, leads to hypertension and cardiovascular dysfunction in offspring [69–71]. While the exact mechanisms responsible to alter the developmental pattern of the organism are unknown, epigenetic alterations are believed to play a fundamental role. This concept has particular relevance to ART, as gametes and preimplantation embryos are exquisitely sensitive to the environment and susceptible to epigenetic alterations.

The agouti viable (A^{vy}) mouse is an important animal model because it displays a labile and easily observable epigenetic state [72]. DNA methylation has been established to modulate in this mouse the transcriptional activity of agouti protein, which decreases melanin production by melanocytes. As such, the coat color of the agouti (=yellow) mouse is a highly useful tool for assessing whether phenotypic variability is attributable to epigenetic modifications. Mice without methylation at the intracisternal type-A particle element (IAP) of the agouti gene have increased agouti protein and therefore have a yellow coat color. In contrast, mice with increased IAP methylation do not have agouti protein production and have a brown coat color (a.k.a. pseudoagouti). The phenotype from epigenetic modifications is not restricted strictly to coat color. Pseudoagouti mice are lean and have normal glucose homeostasis, whereas yellow mice are obese, insulin-resistant, glucose-intolerant, and show a predisposition to diabetes [73]. Importantly, stresses of a different nature (presence of methyl supplement in the diet or in vitro preimplantation culture) result in change in DNA methylation [72, 74–77]. Specifically, in vitro culture of zygotes results in decrease in IAP methylation (and therefore in increase of yellow mice) compared to natural mating [72]. No difference in IAP methylation (and coat color) was observed in pups resulting from embryo transfer alone, indicating that the culture conditions caused hypomethylation of the agouti locus.

Epigenetic modifications are increasingly recognized to underlie a number of disease states beyond imprinting disorders. Human malignancies have been found to have global genomic hypomethylation (with activation of endogenous retroviral elements, oncogenes, and loss of imprinting) as well as hypermethylation of tumor suppressor genes [78]. Exposure to chemicals that function as reproductive endocrine disruptors (e.g., diethylstilbestrol, vinclozolin, and bisphenol A) is associated with specific epigenetic changes [79]. Even syndromes characterized by birth defects including ICF syndrome (immunodeficiency, centromere instability, and facial anomalies syndrome), ATRX syndrome (X-linked a-thalassemia – mental retardation syndrome [ATRX]), and Rubinstein–Taybi syndrome have characteristics of birth defect and have been attributed to epigenetic anomalies [80]. These associations raise the question is the increase in birth defects observed in offspring from ART have an underlying epigenetic contribution.

Limited studies of early adulthood are available in context of young age of the majority of ART children. Developmental outcomes and physical health in early childhood and during adolescent appear, however, to be comparable to naturally conceived children [81–83]. However, recent evidence suggests that pubertal children (mean age 12.6 years old) conceived by ART have increased blood pressure, are 2.5 times more likely to have fasting glucose levels in the highest quartile (≥5.2 mmol/L, 95% CI 1.2–5.2) [3], and have disturbed body fat composition [2, 4]. Although the alterations are mild, the findings are concerning because they may represent sentinel observations, hinting towards the possibility of clinically significant increased risks of metabolic abnormalities and chronic disease later in life.

Recent studies have begun to explore differences in epigenetic programming among human embryos conceived in vitro. Katari et al. examined global methylation patterns at CpG sites using a microarray approach on samples of placenta and cord blood from ten children conceived in vitro vs. 13 children in vivo [84]. Although significant variability and overlaps in methylation patterns were observed between groups, offspring from in vitro conceptions had globally lower mean levels of methylation at CpG sites in placental DNA and higher levels of methylation in DNA from cord blood samples in comparison to natural conceptions. Of note, several of the differentially methylated genes reported by Katari et al. have been implicated in chronic metabolic disorders, including Type II diabetes mellitus and obesity [84].

14.6 How ART Might Predispose to Epigenetic Problems

Our understanding of the time course of epigenetic regulation in humans is almost entirely extrapolated from analysis of imprinted loci in murine models. For a review, see ref. [30]. In summary, the epigenome is first reorganized after fertilization and again during gametogenesis to enable a sex-appropriate imprinted gene pattern. Following fertilization, embryos undergo a genome-wide demethylation; the male pronucleus is actively demethylated before zygotic genome activation, while the female pronucleus is passively demethylated in a process that requires DNA replication. At the blastocyst stage, there is a rapid remethylation process. Imprinted genes markings are normally unaffected by this process.

The second wave of epigenetic reorganization occurs only in the primordial germ cells (PGC), starting on day 13 of embryonic life in the mouse [30]. During this phase, the entire PGC genome, including imprinted genes, is demethylated and then remethylated in a sex-specific manner, so that eggs and sperm will have the appropriate respective imprinted marks. The time course for remethylation of gametes is different for the two sexes. Maternal imprints are established during the development of the oocyte, from primordial to maturation of antral follicles. While the imprinting process progresses over time with increasing oocyte diameter, different imprinted genes complete the process at different times and, for several imprinted genes, the process is not completed until ovulation [85, 86]. In contrast, the imprinted gene pattern of spermatozoa is completed much earlier, at the prospermatogonial stage [87].

Disruption at different points during this process results in varying degrees of epigenetic aberrations. Incomplete erasure of the imprints can result in epigenetic inheritance to the next generation. More specifically, an epigenetic modification could be transmitted to the offspring if one epigenetic mark is not erased in the parental germ cells. Alternatively, a novel epigenetic error could occur after fertilization and before specification of PGC [88]. Notably, ART interventions encompass both critical periods of epigenetic remodeling [80, 89]. Potential mechanisms by which ART could lead to epigenetic errors include (Table 14.1):

Hormonal superovulation. Differences in DNA methylation of imprinted genes have been identified among oocytes from stimulated ovaries, both in mice and humans [90]. Importantly, a dose–response effect was noted when mice oocytes were stimulated with different doses

Table 14.1 Potential mechanisms that can lead to increased incidence of epigenetic disorders following ART

Mechanism
Use of hormones to downregulate pituitary function and to stimulate ovary for supernumerary oocyte production
In vitro growth and/or in vitro maturation of oocytes
Use of immature sperm
Use of sperm from infertile man carrying a mutation
Asynchrony between uterus and embryo
Use of ICSI
In vitro culture
Cryopreservation of either gametes or embryos

of gonadotropins; higher gonadotropins were associated with increased alteration of imprinting gene methylation [85]. These experimental studies provide why patients undergoing ovarian stimulation alone have an higher incidence of AS [45]. Furthermore, the findings point to the benefit of the adoption of less aggressive ovarian stimulation protocols.

14.6.1 In Vitro Growth and In Vitro Maturation of Oocytes

The processes of in vitro growth (IVG) and in vitro maturation (IVM) are complex and with different efficiency in different species – see for review [91]. Live offspring have been obtained following IVG/IVM of mice primordial follicles [92]. On the contrary, only isolated preantral follicles have been grown in nonrodent species [91]. In humans, the process of IVM involves the maturation of germinal vesicle (GV) oocytes to metaphase II (MII), with primary clinical indications for women with PCOS or fertility preservation in patients preparing to undergo cytotoxic cancer therapy [93]. Although a small study detected no increase in congenital malformation in children conceived by IVM [94], a mouse study found significant histone acetylation changes in MII oocytes and early cleavage embryos, after IVM [95].

14.6.2 Sperm from Infertile Men

An increased prevalence of epigenetic defects could be present in the gametes of infertile couples, and thus predispose offspring of those individuals to epigenetic and imprinting errors [45, 80]. Sperm from oligospermic men has been demonstrated to contain a higher percentage of imprinting alterations [96].

14.6.3 Extraction and Injection of Immature Sperm

While common for severely oligospermic patients, extraction of sperm from the epididymis or testis is occasionally performed in patients with prior vasectomy or obstructive azoospermia. While it appears that imprinted gene marks have already been established at the spermatogonial stage [97], genes involved in spermatogenesis are methylated only at the level of the epididymis [87] and the spermatid is transcriptionally active [88]. In this way, the final epigenetic programming may not be present in nonejaculated spermatozoa. For these reasons, and because one study found an increased incidence of congenital malformation [98], injection of round spermatid injection (ROSI) is considered experimental.

14.6.4 Asynchrony Between Uterus and Embryo

Human blastocysts reach the uterus 5 days postfertilization. Blastocyst transfer was introduced to facilitate embryo selection and to better synchronize the embryo and the uterine receptivity. However, human embryos are routinely transferred into the uterus at the cleavage stage with good success. Importantly, asynchronous embryo transfer in sheep is associated with decreased implantation and altered growth trajectory of the implanted embryos [99]. In particular, transfer of embryos to an advanced uterine environment results in change in fetal muscle development [100], a phenomenon that may be epigenetically regulated [101].

14.6.5 Intracytoplasmic Sperm Injection

ICSI differs in multiple obvious aspects compared to in vivo fertilization. Beside the lack of the physiologic sperm egg interaction, ICSI entitles the introduction of the sperm tail into the ooplasm which may effect oocyte cellular pathways and result in suboptimal sperm nuclear decondensation [102]. In addition, ICSI zygotes exhibit shorter calcium oscillations with altered pattern [103]. The cleavage of the ICSI embryos occurs at a slower rate; the resulting blastocysts have reduced cell numbers and reduced hatching rate. While several reports suggested that fertilization by ICSI was associated with increase in imprinting errors [42, 104], a recent study did not find an increased incidence of chromatin or methylation errors in ICSI embryos compared to embryos fertilized through conventional IVF [105]. It is still possible that ICSI plays an indirect role, by allowing the creation of embryos with immature or suboptimal male gametes, a fact that could not occur in vivo.

14.6.6 In Vitro Culture of Preimplantation Embryos

Compelling evidence from animal models indicates that in vitro culture is in fact a stressful and unfavorable state for embryos. Rodent studies underline that the development rate and global patterns of gene expression are abnormal in mice embryos cultured in vitro [106, 107]. A lower number of trophectodermal cells are found in mouse blastocysts conceived in vitro in comparison to in vivo controls [107]. Suboptimal oxygen concentrations and culture medium increase aberrant gene expression [108]. Mouse fetuses generated by IVF display delayed fetal development in comparison to controls. In particular, culture in suboptimal conditions (using Whitten's medium, WM) resulted in a more severe phenotype as opposed to culture in optimized conditions (K simple optimized medium with amino acids, $KSOM_{AA}$) [109]. Intriguing are the behavioral abnormalities observed in mice offspring in vitro culture. Offspring of mice cultured for 2 days in vitro (from the two-cell stage to the blastocyst stage) in different media ($KSOM_{AA}$ or WM) showed decreased anxiety and decreased memorization of spatial information. These behavioral changes were not observed before 3 months of age (corresponding to the postpubertal age in humans) [110]. Similarly, one-cell mouse embryos cultured for 4 days in KSOM medium in the presence of 10% fetal calf serum or 1 g/L bovine serum albumin showed specific behavioral alterations in anxiety and deficiencies in implicit memories [111]. Disturbingly, fetal cord serum was used in several human IVF laboratories until recently [112].

Extension of embryo culture until the preimplantation stage is associated with epigenetic alterations. In the rodent model, Doherty et al. [113] showed that the H19 gene is imprinted and exclusively expressed from the maternal allele in vivo. However, mouse blastocysts that develop in vitro show biallelic expression. After culture of two-cell embryos to the blastocyst stage in WM, the normally silent paternal H19 allele is aberrantly expressed; in contrast, as in the in vivo situation, little paternal expression is observed after culture in $KSOM_{AA}$ medium. IVF and embryo culture can generate abnormal epigenetic marks at levels of histones as well as modify global DNA methylation patterns [114]. In mice, changes in global DNA methylation from embryo culture are evident as early as the two-cell stage [115].

Studies in sheep and cattle conceived through ART show an increased incidence of elevated birth weight and increased perinatal morbidity, a condition known as the "large offspring syndrome" (LOS), reviewed by Sinclair et al. [116]. Although the differences in size levels off at 1 year of age, examination of in vitro conceived animals revealed abnormal organ and skeletal development [117]. LOS is associated with epigenetic changes including alterations of global methylation levels [118, 119] and specifically a lack of methylation at IGF2 receptor, an imprinted gene in mice [120]. Hiendleder et al. analyzed the effects of two in vitro fertilization protocols (IVF1 and IVF2) on the phenotype and tissue methylation levels in bovine fetuses [119]. The two protocols differed only in the amount of follicle-stimulating hormone, luteinizing hormone, and cow serum in the culture medium. IVF1 fetuses were similar to controls fertilized in vivo, but IVF2 fetuses were significantly heavier and longer, with increased heart and liver weights, displaying an overgrowth phenotype. Quantification of genomic 5-methylcytosine by capillary electrophoresis indicated that both IVF1 and IVF2 fetuses differed from in vivo controls [118, 119]. Lastly, there were significant differences in DNA hypomethylation in liver and muscle of IVF1 fetuses and significant hypermethylation in liver of IVF2 fetuses.

14.6.7 Cryopreservation of Gametes/Embryos

Mouse oocytes subjected to vitrification show an increase in H3K9 methylation and H4K5 acetylation [121]. This epigenetic alteration could be secondary to the freezing and thawing process or to the use of cryoprotectants. One study found that the methyltransfer activity of DNMT3a is stimulated by the addition of dimethyl sulfoxide (DMSO), a cryprotectant commonly used in vitrification or cryopreservation process [122]. It should, however, be noted that epidemiological evidence suggests reduced perinatal morbidity in children born after cryopreservation of embryos or oocytes [123]. Reasons to explain the better outcome include the lack of adverse effect of hormone stimulation and the fact that embryos surviving freezing and thawing might be of better quality than fresh embryos.

14.7 Conclusions

At our current state of knowledge, the vast majority of children conceived by ART are healthy and the established epigenetic risks from IVF are confined to two rare and sporadic disorders. Although both conditions are associated with profound disability, the absolute risks of AS and BWS are remote. In this context, these disorders are unlikely to defer prospective infertile couples from pursuing treatment. For many patients, ART represent the only therapeutic option to have a genetically linked child. The detection of an association to these imprinting disorders may, however, have a broader value as the proverbial canary in the coal mine, heralding the presence of other epigenetic alterations that may not be manifested until later in life.

Are there reasons to be concerned? Animal studies strongly suggest that stress in specific windows of development can be associated with long-term health complications. The low birth weight outcomes associated with ART live births may predispose to a greater extent of vascular and metabolic disorders. The late stages of gametogenesis and early embryo development are a highly sensitive window for potential epigenetic programming influenced by environmental states. Studies in animal models and initial studies in humans suggest that multiple aspects of the process of ART can result in epigenetic dysregulation. The current evidence endorses the important need for longitudinal studies for surveillance of the health outcome of ART conceptions as well as basic research geared to understanding the mechanisms that can lead to epigenetic errors. Unfortunately, despite million of people suffering from fertility-related problems, the NIH in 2009 spent only 75 million dollars out of a 31.2 billion budget (0.002%) to fund research related to infertility [124]. In addition, given the profound effects of culture media on embryo gene expression, it is worrisome that the composition of commercial proprietary media used for human IVF is not disclosed. Until the risks and safety of ART are better defined, its use should be reserved, as with any medical treatment, to patients with clear indication after exhausting other more conservative therapeutic interventions. Research and interventions to optimize in vitro culture and other aspects of ART may have potential to translate to lower risk of disease of later life with attendant lower morbidity, mortality, and economic cost.

Acknowledgment This work is supported by NICHD grant R01 HD 062803 - 01 A1 to PFR.

References

1. de Mouzon J, Lancaster P, Nygren KG, et al. World collaborative report on Assisted Reproductive Technology, 2002. Hum Reprod. 2009;24(9):2310–20.
2. Ceelen M, van Weissenbruch MM, Roos JC, Vermeiden JP, van Leeuwen FE, Delemarre-van de Waal HA. Body composition in children and adolescents

born after in vitro fertilization or spontaneous conception. J Clin Endocrinol Metab. 2007;92(9): 3417–23.
3. Ceelen M, van Weissenbruch MM, Vermeiden JP, van Leeuwen FE, Delemarre-van de Waal HA. Pubertal development in children and adolescents born after IVF and spontaneous conception. Hum Reprod. 2008;23(12):2791–8.
4. Ceelen M, van Weissenbruch MM, Vermeiden JP, van Leeuwen FE, Delemarre-van de Waal HA, Ceelen M. Cardiometabolic differences in children born after in vitro fertilization: follow-up study. J Clin Endocrinol Metab. 2008;93(5):1682–8.
5. Ceelen M, van Weissenbruch MM, Vermeiden JP, van Leeuwen FE, Delemarre-van de Waal HA. Growth and development of children born after in vitro fertilization. Fertil Steril. 2008;90(5):1662–73.
6. Palermo G, Joris H, Devroey P, Van Steirteghem AC. Pregnancies after intracytoplasmic injection of single spermatozoon into an oocyte. Lancet. 1992; 340(8810):17–8.
7. SART Member Clinics. Clinic summary report for 2008. 2010. Accessed 7 Oct 2010.
8. Handyside AH, Kontogianni EH, Hardy K, Winston RM. Pregnancies from biopsied human preimplantation embryos sexed by Y-specific DNA amplification. Nature. 1990;344(6268):768–70.
9. Atwood J, Dobins S. Storm clouds are coming: ways to help couples reconstruct the crisis of infertility. Contemp Fam Ther. 1992;14(5):385–403.
10. Collins J, Graves G. The economic consequences of multiple gestation pregnancy in assisted conception cycles. Hum Fertil (Camb). 2000;3(4):275–83.
11. Chambers GM, Chapman MG, Grayson N, Shanahan M, Sullivan EA. Babies born after ART treatment cost more than non-ART babies: a cost analysis of inpatient birth-admission costs of singleton and multiple gestation pregnancies. Hum Reprod. 2007;22(12): 3108–15.
12. Jackson RA, Gibson KA, Wu YW, Croughan MS. Perinatal outcomes in singletons following in vitro fertilization: a meta-analysis. Obstet Gynecol. 2004;103(3):551–63.
13. Helmerhorst FM, Perquin DA, Donker D, Keirse MJ. Perinatal outcome of singletons and twins after assisted conception: a systematic review of controlled studies. BMJ. 2004;328(7434):261.
14. McGovern PG, Llorens AJ, Skurnick JH, Weiss G, Goldsmith LT. Increased risk of preterm birth in singleton pregnancies resulting from in vitro fertilization-embryo transfer or gamete intrafallopian transfer: a meta-analysis. Fertil Steril. 2004;82(6): 1514–20.
15. Hansen M, Bower C, Milne E, de Klerk N, Kurinczuk JJ. Assisted reproductive technologies and the risk of birth defects – a systematic review. Hum Reprod. 2005;20(2):328–38.
16. Lie R, Lyngstadass A, Orstavik K. Birth defects in children conceived by ICSI compared with children conceived by other IVF-methods; a meta-analysis. Int J Epidemiol. 2005;34:696–701.
17. Wennerholm UB, Bergh C, Hamberger L, et al. Incidence of congenital malformations in children born after ICSI. Hum Reprod. 2000;15(4):944–8.
18. Brinton LA, Westhoff CL, Scoccia B, et al. Causes of infertility as predictors of subsequent cancer risk. Epidemiology. 2005;16(4):500–7.
19. Horsthemke B, Ludwig M. Assisted reproduction: the epigenetic perspective. Hum Reprod Update. 2005;11(5):473–82.
20. Sills ES, Moomjy M, Zaninovic N, et al. Human zona pellucida micromanipulation and monozygotic twinning frequency after IVF. Hum Reprod. 2000;15(4): 890–5.
21. Blickstein I, Jones C, Keith LG. Zygotic-splitting rates after single-embryo transfers in in vitro fertilization. N Engl J Med. 2003;348(23):2366–7.
22. Skiadas CC, Missmer SA, Benson CB, Gee RE, Racowsky C. Risk factors associated with pregnancies containing a monochorionic pair following assisted reproductive technologies. Hum Reprod. 2008;23(6):1366–71.
23. Delcuve GP, Rastegar M, Davie JR. Epigenetic control. J Cell Physiol. 2009;219(2):243–50.
24. Robertson KD. DNA methylation and human disease. Nat Rev Genet. 2005;6(8):597–610.
25. Gibney ER, Nolan CM. Epigenetics and gene expression. Heredity. 2010;105(1):4–13.
26. Waddington C. The strategy of genes. London: George Allen & Unwin; 1957.
27. Illingworth R, Kerr A, Desousa D, et al. A novel CpG island set identifies tissue-specific methylation at developmental gene loci. PLoS Biol. 2008;6(1):e22.
28. Bird A, Wolffe A. Methylation-induced repression-belts, braces, and chromatin. Cell. 1999;99:451–4.
29. Li E, Beard C, Jaenisch R. Role for DNA methylation in genomic imprinting. Nature. 1993;366:362–5.
30. Reik W, Dean W, Walter J. Epigenetic reprogramming in mammalian development. Science. 2001; 293(5532):1089–93.
31. Bhutani N, Brady JJ, Damian M, Sacco A, Corbel SY, Blau HM. Reprogramming towards pluripotency requires AID-dependent DNA demethylation. Nature. 2010;463(7284):1042–7.
32. Szyf M. The early life environment and the epigenome. Biochim Biophys Acta. 2009;1790(9): 878–85.
33. Okada Y, Yamagata K, Hong K, Wakayama T, Zhang Y. A role for the elongator complex in zygotic paternal genome demethylation. Nature. 2010;463(7280): 554–8.
34. Jenuwein T, Allis CD. Translating the histone code. Science. 2001;293(5532):1074–80.
35. Peterson CL, Laniel MA. Histones and histone modifications. Curr Biol. 2004;14(14):R546–51.
36. Mattick JS, Amaral PP, Dinger ME, Mercer TR, Mehler MF. RNA regulation of epigenetic processes. Bioessays. 2009;31(1):51–9.
37. Calvanese V, Lara E, Kahn A, Fraga MF. The role of epigenetics in aging and age-related diseases. Ageing Res Rev. 2009;8(4):268–76.

38. Weaver I, Cervoni N, Champagne F, et al. Epigenetic programming by maternal behavior. Nat Neurosci. 2004;7(8):847–54.
39. Manipalviratn S, DeCherney A, Segars J. Imprinting disorders and assisted reproductive technology. Fertil Steril. 2009;91(2):305–15.
40. Amor DJ, Halliday J. A review of known imprinting syndromes and their association with assisted reproduction technologies. Hum Reprod. 2008;23(12):2826–34.
41. McGrath J, Solter D. Completion of mouse embryogenesis requires both the maternal and paternal genomes. Cell. 1984;37(1):179–83.
42. Cox G, Burger J, Lip V, et al. The risk of major birth defects after intracytoplasmic sperm injection may increase the risk of imprinting defects. Am J Hum Genet. 2002;71:162–4.
43. Kishino T, Lalande M, Wagstaff J. UBE3A/E6-AP mutations cause Angelman syndrome. Nat Genet. 1997;15:70–3.
44. Buiting K, Gross S, Lich C, Gillessen-Kaesbach G, el-Maari O, Horsthemke B. Epimutations in Prader-Willi and Angelman syndromes: a molecular study of 136 patients with an imprinting defect. Am J Hum Genet. 2003;72:571–7.
45. Ludwig M, Katalinic A, Gross S, Sutcliffe A, Varon R, Horsthemke B. Increased prevalence of imprinting defects in patients with Angelman syndrome born to subfertile couples. J Med Genet. 2005;42(4):289–91.
46. Sutcliffe AG, Peters CJ, Bowdin S, et al. Assisted reproductive therapies and imprinting disorders – a preliminary British survey. Hum Reprod. 2006;21(4):1009–11.
47. Doornbos ME, Maas SM, McDonnell J, Vermeiden JP, Hennekam RC. Infertility, assisted reproduction technologies and imprinting disturbances: a Dutch study. Hum Reprod. 2007;22(9):2476–80.
48. DeBaun MR, Niemitz EL, Feinberg AP. Association of in vitro fertilization with Beckwith–Wiedemann syndrome and epigenetic alterations of LIT1 and H19. Am J Hum Genet. 2003;72(1):156–60.
49. Gicquel C, Gaston V, Mandelbaum J, Siffroi JP, Flahault A, Le Bouc Y. In vitro fertilization may increase the risk of Beckwith–Wiedemann syndrome related to the abnormal imprinting of the KCN1OT gene. Am J Hum Genet. 2003;72(5):1338–41.
50. Maher ER, Brueton LA, Bowdin SC, et al. Beckwith–Wiedemann syndrome and assisted reproduction technology (ART). J Med Genet. 2003;40(1):62–4.
51. Halliday J, Oke K, Breheny S, Algar E, Amor D. Beckwith–Wiedemann syndrome and IVF: a case-control study. Am J Hum Genet. 2004;75:526–8.
52. Lidegaard O, Pinborg A, Andersen AN. Imprinting diseases and IVF: Danish National IVF cohort study. Hum Reprod. 2005;20(4):950–4.
53. Kallen B, Finnstrom O, Nygren KG, Olausson PO. In vitro fertilization (IVF) in Sweden: risk for congenital malformations after different IVF methods. Birth Defects Res A Clin Mol Teratol. 2005;73(3):162–9.
54. Moll AC, Imhof SM, Cruysberg JR, Schouten-van Meeteren AY, Boers M, van Leeuwen FE. Incidence of retinoblastoma in children born after in-vitro fertilization. Lancet. 2003;361:309–10.
55. Knudson Jr AG. Mutation and cancer: statistical study of retinoblastoma. Proc Natl Acad Sci USA. 1971; 68(4):820–3.
56. Greger V, Passarge E, Hopping W, Messmer E, Horsthemke B. Epigenetic changes may contribute to the formation and spontaneous regression of retinoblastoma. Hum Genet. 1989;83(2):155–8.
57. Greger V, Debus N, Lohmann D, Hopping W, Passarge E, Horsthemke B. Frequency and parental origin of hypermethylated RB1 alleles in retinoblastoma. Hum Genet. 1994;94(5):491–6.
58. Barker D. Mothers, babies and health in later life. 2nd ed. Glasgow: Churchill Livingstone; 1998.
59. Gluckman PD, Lillycrop KA, Vickers MH, et al. Metabolic plasticity during mammalian development is directionally dependent on early nutritional status. Proc Natl Acad Sci USA. 2007;104(31):12796–800.
60. Rinaudo PF, Lamb J. Fetal origins of perinatal morbidity and/or adult disease. Semin Reprod Med. 2008;26(5):436–45.
61. Schieve LA, Meikle SF, Ferre C, Peterson HB, Jeng G, Wilcox LS. Low and very low birth weight in infants conceived with use of assisted reproductive technology. N Engl J Med. 2002;346(10):731–7.
62. Barker D, Winter P, Osmond C, Margetts B, Simmonds S. Weight in infancy and death from ischaemic heart disease. Lancet. 1989;2:577–80.
63. Barker DJ. Coronary heart disease: a disorder of growth. Horm Res. 2003;59 Suppl 1:35–41.
64. Roseboom TJ, van der Meulen JH, Osmond C, et al. Coronary heart disease after prenatal exposure to the Dutch famine, 1944–45. Heart. 000;84(6):595–8.
65. Morley R. Fetal origins of adult disease. Semin Fetal Neonatal Med. 2006;11:73–8.
66. Rich-Edwards JW, Kleinman K, Michels KB, Stampfer MJ, Manson JE, Rexrode KM, et al. Longitudinal study of birth weight and adult body mass index in predicting risk of coronary heart disease stroke in women. BMJ. 2005;330:1115–8.
67. Lawlor D, Ronalds G, Clark H, Smith G, Leon D. Birth weight is inversely associated with incident coronary heart disease and stroke among individuals born in the 1950s: findings from the Aberdeen children of the 1950s prospective cohort study. Circulation. 2005;112:1414–8.
68. Law C, Shiell A. Is blood pressure inversely related to birth weight? The strength of evidence from a systematic review of the literature. J Hypertens. 1996;14:935–41.
69. Edwards LJ, McMillen IC. Periconceptional nutrition programs development of the cardiovascular system in the fetal sheep. Am J Physiol. 2002; 283(3):R669–79.
70. Gardner DS, Pearce S, Dandrea J, et al. Peri-implantation undernutrition programs blunted angiotensin II evoked baroreflex responses in young adult sheep. Hypertension. 2004;43(6):1290–6.
71. Kwong WY, Wild AE, Roberts P, Willis AC, Fleming TP. Maternal undernutrition during the preimplantation period of rat development causes blastocyst

abnormalities and programming of postnatal hypertension. Development. 2000;127(19):4195–202.
72. Morgan HD, Jin XL, Li A, Whitelaw E, O'Neill C. The culture of zygotes to the blastocyst stage changes the postnatal expression of an epigentically labile allele, agouti viable yellow, in mice. Biol Reprod. 2008;79(4):618–23.
73. Duhl DM, Vrieling H, Miller KA, Wolff GL, Barsh GS. Neomorphic agouti mutations in obese yellow mice. Nat Genet. 1994;8(1):59–65.
74. Cooney CA, Dave AA, Wolff GL. Maternal methyl supplements in mice affect epigenetic variation and DNA methylation of offspring. J Nutr. 2002;132 (8 Suppl):2393S–400.
75. Wolff GL, Kodell RL, Moore SR, Cooney CA. Maternal epigenetics and methyl supplements affect agouti gene expression in Avy/a mice. FASEB J. 1998;12(11):949–57.
76. Dolinoy DC, Huang D, Jirtle RL. Maternal nutrient supplementation counteracts bisphenol A-induced DNA hypomethylation in early development. Proc Natl Acad Sci USA. 2007;104(32):13056–61.
77. Dolinoy DC, Weidman JR, Waterland RA, Jirtle RL. Maternal genistein alters coat color and protects Avy mouse offspring from obesity by modifying the fetal epigenome. Environ Health Perspect. 2006;114(4): 567–72.
78. Gopalakrishnan S, Van Emburgh BO, Robertson KD. DNA methylation in development and human disease. Mutat Res. 2008;647(1–2):30–8.
79. Ho SM, Tang WY. Techniques used in studies of epigenome dysregulation due to aberrant DNA methylation: an emphasis on fetal-based adult diseases. Reprod Toxicol. 2007;23(3):267–82.
80. Niemitz EL, Feinberg AP. Epigenetics and assisted reproductive technology: a call for investigation. Am J Hum Genet. 2004;74(4):599–609.
81. Wagenaar K, Ceelen M, van Weissenbruch MM, Knol DL, Delemarre-van de Waal HA, Huisman J. School functioning in 8- to 18-year-old children born after in vitro fertilization. Eur J Pediatr. 2008;167(11): 1289–95.
82. Ludwig A, Katalinic A, Thyen U, Sutcliffe AG, Diedrich K, Ludwig M. Neuromotor development and mental health at 5.5 years of age of singletons born at term after intracytoplasmatic sperm injection ICSI: results of a prospective controlled single-blinded study in Germany. Fertil Steril. 2009;91(1): 125–32.
83. Ludwig AK, Katalinic A, Thyen U, Sutcliffe AG, Diedrich K, Ludwig M. Physical health at 5.5 years of age of term-born singletons after intracytoplasmic sperm injection: results of a prospective, controlled, single-blinded study. Fertil Steril. 2009;91(1):115–24.
84. Katari S, Turan N, Bibikova M, et al. DNA methylation and gene expression differences in children conceived *in vitro* or *in vivo*. Hum Mol Genet. 2009;18(20):3769–78.
85. Market-Velker BA, Zhang L, Magri LS, Bonvissuto AC, Mann MR. Dual effects of superovulation: loss of maternal and paternal imprinted methylation in a dose-dependent manner. Hum Mol Genet. 2009;19(1):36–51.
86. Lucifero D, Mann MR, Bartolomei MS, Trasler JM. Gene-specific timing and epigenetic memory in oocyte imprinting. Hum Mol Genet. 2004;13(8): 839–49.
87. Ariel M, Cedar H, McCarrey J. Developmental changes in methylation of spermatogenesis-specific genes include reprogramming in the epididymis. Nat Genet. 1994;7(1):59–63.
88. De Rycke M, Liebaers I, Van Steirteghem A. Epigenetic risks related to assisted reproductive technologies: risk analysis and epigenetic inheritance. Hum Reprod. 2002;17(10):2487–94.
89. Grace KS, Sinclair KD. Assisted reproductive technology, epigenetics, and long-term health: a developmental time bomb still ticking. Semin Reprod Med. 2009;27(5):409–16.
90. Sato A, Otsu E, Negishi H, Utsunomiya T, Arime T. Aberrant DNA methylation of imprinted loci in superovulated oocytes. Hum Reprod. 2007;22:26–35.
91. Picton HM, Harris SE, Muruvi W, Chambers EL. The in vitro growth and maturation of follicles. Reproduction. 2008;136(6):703–15.
92. Eppig JJ, O'Brien MJ. Development in vitro of mouse oocytes from primordial follicles. Biol Reprod. 1996;54(1):197–207.
93. Siristatidis CS, Maheshwari A, Bhattacharya S. In vitro maturation in sub fertile women with polycystic ovarian syndrome undergoing assisted reproduction. Cochrane Database Syst Rev. 2009(1):CD006606.
94. Buckett WM, Chian RC, Holzer H, Dean N, Usher R, Tan SL. Obstetric outcomes and congenital abnormalities after in vitro maturation, in vitro fertilization, and intracytoplasmic sperm injection. Obstet Gynecol. 2007;110(4):885–91.
95. Wang N, Le F, Zhan QT, et al. Effects of in vitro maturation on histone acetylation in metaphase II oocytes and early cleavage embryos. Obstet Gynecol Int. 2010;2010:989278.
96. Kobayashi H, Sato A, Otsu E, et al. Aberrant DNA methylation of imprinted loci in sperm from oligospermic patients. Hum Mol Genet. 2007;16(21): 2542–51.
97. Reik W, Walter J. Genomic imprinting: parental influence on the genome. Nat Rev Genet. 2001;2:21–32.
98. Zech H, Vanderzwalmen P, Prapas Y, Lejeune B, Duba E, Schoysman R. Congenital malformations after intracytoplasmic injection of spermatids. Hum Reprod. 2000;15(4):969–71.
99. Wilmut I, Sales DI. Effect of an asynchronous environment on embryonic development in sheep. J Reprod Fertil. 1981;61(1):179–84.
100. Maxfield EK, Sinclair KD, Dunne LD, et al. Temporary exposure of ovine embryos to an advanced uterine environment does not affect fetal weight but alters fetal muscle development. Biol Reprod. 1998;59(2):321–5.
101. Rupp RA, Singhal N, Veenstra GJ. When the embryonic genome flexes its muscles. Eur J Biochem. 2002;269(9):2294–9.

102. Markoulaki S, Kurokawa M, Yoon SY, Matson S, Ducibella T, Fissore R. Comparison of Ca^{2+} and CaMKII responses in IVF and ICSI in the mouse. Mol Hum Reprod. 2007;13(4):265–72.
103. Kurokawa M, Fissore RA. ICSI-generated mouse zygotes exhibit altered calcium oscillations, inositol 1, 4, 5-trisphosphate receptor-1 down-regulation, and embryo development. Mol Hum Reprod. 2003;9(9):523–33.
104. Orstavik KH, Eiklid K, van der Hagen CB, et al. Another case of imprinting defect in a girl with Angelman syndrome who was conceived by intracytoplasmic semen injection. Am J Hum Genet. 2003;72(1):218–9.
105. Santos F, Hyslop L, Stojkovic P, et al. Evaluation of epigenetic marks in human embryos derived from IVF and ICSI. Hum Reprod. 2010;25(9):2387–95.
106. Rinaudo P, Schultz R. Effects of embryo culture on global pattern of gene expression in preimplantation mouse embryos. Reproduction. 2004;128:301–11.
107. Giritharan G, Talbi S, Donjacour A, Di Sebastiano F, Dobson AT, Rinaudo PF. Effect of in vitro fertilization on gene expression and development of mouse preimplantation embryos. Reproduction. 2007;134(1):63–72.
108. Rinaudo P, Giritharan G, Talbi S, Dobson A, Schultz R. Effects of oxygen tension on gene expression in preimplantation mouse embryos. Fertil Steril. 2006;86 Suppl 4:1252–65.
109. Delle Piane L, Lin W, Liu X, et al. Effect of the method of conception and embryo transfer procedure on mid-gestation placenta and fetal development in an IVF mouse model. Hum Reprod. 2010;25(8):2039–46.
110. Ecker DJ, Stein P, Xu Z, et al. Long-term effects of culture of preimplantation mouse embryos on behavior. Proc Natl Acad Sci USA. 2004;101(6):1595–600.
111. Fernandez-Gonzalez R, Moreira P, Bilbao A, et al. Long-term effect of in vitro culture of mouse embryos with serum on mRNA expression of imprinting genes, development, and behavior. Proc Natl Acad Sci USA. 2004;101(16):5880–5.
112. Dugan KJ, Shalika S, Smith RD, Padilla SL. Comparison of synthetic serum substitute and fetal cord serum as media supplements for in vitro fertilization: a prospective, randomized study. Fertil Steril. 1997;67(1):166–8.
113. Doherty AS, Mann MR, Tremblay KD, Bartolomei MS, Schultz RM. Differential effects of culture on imprinted H19 expression in the preimplantation mouse embryo. Biol Reprod. 2000;62(6):1526–35.
114. Li T, Vu TH, Ulaner GA, et al. IVF results in de novo DNA methylation and histone methylation at an Igf2-H19 imprinting epigenetic switch. Mol Hum Reprod. 2005;11(9):631–40.
115. Shi W, Haaf T. Aberrant methylation patterns at the two-cell stage as an indicator of early developmental failure. Mol Reprod Dev. 2002;63(3):329–34.
116. Sinclair KD, Young LE, Wilmut I, McEvoy TG. In-utero overgrowth in ruminants following embryo culture: lessons from mice and a warning to men. Hum Reprod. 2000;15 Suppl 5:68–86.
117. Walker SK, Hartwich KM, Robinson JS. Long-term effects on offspring of exposure of oocytes and embryos to chemical and physical agents. Hum Reprod Update. 2000;6(6):564–77.
118. Hiendleder S, Mund C, Reichenbach HD, et al. Tissue-specific elevated genomic cytosine methylation levels are associated with an overgrowth phenotype of bovine fetuses derived by in vitro techniques. Biol Reprod. 2004;71(1):217–23.
119. Hiendleder S, Wirtz M, Mund C, et al. Tissue-specific effects of in vitro fertilization procedures on genomic cytosine methylation levels in overgrown and normal sized bovine fetuses. Biol Reprod. 2006;75(1): 17–23.
120. Young L, Fernandes K, McEvoy T, et al. Epigenetic change in IGF2R is associated with fetal overgrowth after sheep embryo culture. Nat Genet. 2001;27: 153–4.
121. Yan LY, Yan J, Qiao J, Zhao PL, Liu P. Effects of oocyte vitrification on histone modifications. Reprod Fertil Dev. 2010;22(6):920–5.
122. Yokochi T, Robertson KD. Dimethyl sulfoxide stimulates the catalytic activity of de novo DNA methyltransferase 3a (Dnmt3a) in vitro. Bioorg Chem. 2004;32(4):234–43.
123. Wennerholm UB, Soderstrom-Anttila V, Bergh C, et al. Children born after cryopreservation of embryos or oocytes: a systematic review of outcome data. Hum Reprod. 2009;24(9):2158–72.
124. NIH. 2009. http://report.nih.gov/rcdc/categories/Default.aspx.

15 Novel Approaches of Sperm Selection for ART: The Role of Objective Biochemical Markers of Nuclear and Cytoplasmic Integrity and Sperm Function

Gabor Huszar and Denny Sakkas

Abstract

With the technological advancements in assisted reproduction treatment, it is now feasible to cause fertilization and pregnancy by injection of a single spermatozoon into the oocyte via the ICSI method. The ultimate goal in this respect is the selection of a spermatozoon that has genetic and cellular attributes comparable to those sperm that interact with the zona pellucida under physiological or conventional IVF fertilization conditions. In light of this aim, this review focuses largely on objective biochemical markers within the nuclear and cytoplasmic compartment of spermatozoa, which define and reflect sperm developmental and genetic characteristics that are optimal for fertilization as well as for paternal contribution to the developing embryo. The ICSI sperm selection methods, including those based on hyaluronic acid binding and high-magnification visualization, are discussed along with the research evidence that supports the interrelated developmental and genetic integrity of the selected sperm.

Furthermore, the review examines the use of other sperm diagnostics which may guide us in the treatment of male factor infertility patients. The diagnostic techniques examined include those focusing on the sperm nuclear integrity, in particular the Sperm Chromatin Structure Assay (SCSA).

The fundamental information being generated from more molecular and biochemical-based analysis of sperm will create a basis for identifying key deficiencies in spermatozoa that might be implicated in the defective sperm function observed in a significant proportion of infertile males and may aid in both diagnosis and treatment.

D. Sakkas (✉)
IVF Laboratories, Department of Obstetrics, Gynecology and Reproductive Sciences, Yale University School of Medicine, New Haven, CT, USA
e-mail: denny.sakkas@yale.edu

C. Racowsky et al. (eds.), *Biennial Review of Infertility: Volume 2*,
DOI 10.1007/978-1-4419-8456-2_15, © Springer Science+Business Media, LLC 2011

Keywords
Sperm nucleus • Spermatogenesis • Spermiogenesis • Intracytoplasmic sperm injection • Male infertility • Protamine • Hyaluronic acid • Apoptosis

15.1 Introduction

Infertility has been commonly defined as failure to conceive after 12 months of regular intercourse. Based on this definition, the prevalence of infertility has been calculated to be 10–15% [1]. A multicenter study conducted by the World Health Organization (WHO) concluded that in 20% of infertile couples, the predominant cause of infertility is the male factor, while in a further 27% of couples both partners contribute [1]. In the 2008 national US statistics, 35% of the IVF-ET cycles reported in the United States were diagnosed with male factor infertility either as a single (17%) or combined (18%) diagnosis [2]. While these statistics underlie the importance of male factor in reproduction, the clinical and analytical methodologies used to diagnose male infertility are still evolving [3].

Semen analysis is routinely used to evaluate the male partner of the infertile couple. Although widely used parameters for normal semen measurements have been published by the WHO, the current normal values for sperm concentration, motility, and morphology fail to meet rigorous clinical, technical, and statistical standards. With the advent of ICSI [4], the onus to understand the biology of which sperm fertilized the egg and the ongoing research focusing on biochemical markers of sperm function [5] have taken higher prominence, as the pathology in male factor infertility patients, who require ICSI treatment, is likely to be of higher complexity.

There are, however, valid concerns about the use of ICSI in these low fertility patients [6], even though large follow-up studies do not show any major differences between ICSI, IVF, and normal conceptions [7]. In this chapter, we examine the current and new methods available to identify and select the optimal sperm to be selected to fertilize the oocyte.

15.2 Beyond Routine Sperm Analysis

15.2.1 Sperm Biochemical Markers

A major approach in the discovery of sperm biochemical markers, independently from sperm concentration and motility in the semen, is based on the recognition that there are objective markers of sperm function that focus on elements of spermatogenesis and spermiogenesis that are abnormal in the process of sperm development from spermatogonium to spermatozoa. One of the first recognized morphological markers was cytoplasmic retention, which was measured by the excess cytoplasm in sperm; biochemically, this observation translated to an increased sperm creatine phosphokinase (CK) activity [8]. The variation in CK activity in the various semen samples has been well documented, as well as the fact that sperm recovered from pellets of density gradient centrifugation had substantially lower CK content [9]. A logistic regression analysis of 180 couples with oligozoospermic husbands when treated with intrauterine insemination indicated that the increased levels of CK activity in these oligospermic men predicted a lower likelihood for pregnancy [8].

The connection between arrested cytoplasmic extrusion and diminished sperm fertilizing function was also established by experiments using CK-immunocytochemistry of sperm-hemizona complexes; only the sperm with clear heads without cytoplasmic retention were bound to the hemizona [10]. This important finding led to a concept, described in the latter part of this chapter, relating to one of the new methods available for sperm selection.

Other aspects of the spermatogenetic and spermiogenetic processes, including (a) specific protein expression in human sperm (for example the HspA2 chaperone); (b) persistent histones which indicate abnormal histone-transition protein-protamine replacement process; (c) apoptotic processes; (d) and reactive oxygen species (ROS) production within the sperm or in the surrounding seminal fluid [5, 11–13] will all be assessed in relation to novel methods of sperm selection.

15.2.2 Sperm Nuclear DNA Integrity

Over the past two decades, a number of tests have been introduced for the analysis of sperm nuclear DNA fragmentation [14, 15]. These tests include TdT-mediated-dUTP Nick-End Labeling (TUNEL) [16], COMET [17], chromomycin A3 (CMA3) [18], in situ nick translation [19, 20], DBD-FISH (DNA breakage detection fluorescence in situ hybridization) [21], the sperm chromatin dispersion test (SCD) [22], and the Sperm Chromatin Structure Assay (SCSA) [23].

One of the important questions related to sperm DNA fragmentation analysis is the type of breaks occurring in the DNA strands. First, whether the breaks are single or double-stranded and what is needed to detect them. The different tests therefore sometimes require an initial step of denaturation in order to detect DNA breaks: such as the SCSA [24, 25], SCD [22], or COMET at acid or alkaline pH. Other tests such as TUNEL [16] (in situ nick translation [19]) and COMET at neutral pH [26] do not require an initial denaturation step and, therefore, measure single-stranded or double-stranded DNA breaks directly. In general, single-stranded DNA damage provides a better prognosis and is easier to repair than double-stranded DNA damage. Single-stranded DNA fragmentation may be caused by unrepaired DNA nicks generated during the process of meiosis chromatin remodeling. It might be also caused by oxygen radical-induced damage. Double-stranded DNA damage is more likely to lead to failure of an individual sperm to pass on its paternal DNA [27].

Regarding tests that measure DNA damage directly, some controversy still exists regarding which test is best [28]. A recent study reported by Borini et al. [29] showed that sperm DNA fragmentation values in aliquots of the same sperm fraction used for IVF, measured by TUNEL, were significantly correlated with pregnancy outcome. This is in sharp contrast to the results reported by Bungum et al. [15] who found no correlation between sperm DNA fragmentation values in the samples used for IVF, as measured by the SCSA test, and pregnancy outcome. Another misconception is that TUNEL is unique to apoptosis, which is studied in many sperm DNA assessment papers; this correlation to apoptosis in sperm is an overestimation of this test's capability [30].

15.2.3 SCSA Issues and Usefulness

In 1980, Evenson et al. [31] published a pioneering paper in Science entitled "Relation of mammalian sperm chromatin heterogeneity to fertility" in which they used flow cytometry measurements of heated sperm nuclei to reveal a significant decrease in resistance to in situ denaturation of spermatozoal DNA in samples from bulls, mice, and humans of low or questionable fertility when compared with others of high fertility. They then went on to suggest that flow cytometry of heated sperm nuclei and testing of DNA chain integrity could provide a new and independent determinant of male fertilizing potential and the ability of sperm to provide paternal contribution.

The SCSA test has been extensively studied to date from the clinical point of view [31–36]. The SCSA test measures sperm susceptibility to DNA denaturation after exposure to a mild acid. DNA of sperm with normal chromatin structure do not denature, while if the DNA is somewhat damaged and contains breaks, DNA strands can reach different degrees of denaturation, which is detected after mild acid treatment and with acridine orange staining [35]. The degree of DNA damage is measured by flow cytometry and is expressed as a DNA Fragmentation Index or DFI. Previous studies indicate that a DFI value >27% is associated with pregnancy failure in ART [37, 38]. However, recent reports challenge the predictive value of the SCSA test [15, 39, 40].

One possible reason for the discrepancy between studies is the variability of sperm concentrations within the samples studied. In other words, for fertilization to occur, there is a minimal threshold number of normal fertile sperm that are necessary. If this amount of fertile sperm is present (the threshold level depends on the conception model), the additional presence of nonfertile sperm, as assessed by SCSA or any other equivalent test, whether 20, 40, or 70% of the total sperm content of the semen, is irrelevant. The importance of examining nuclear DNA integrity is clearly highlighted as numerous studies have emphasized its relationship to human fertility success [28, 41, 42].

In animal studies, an inverse correlation was shown between increasing levels of DNA damage inducers, such as heat and radiation, and good reproductive outcome. For example, the studies by Ahmadi and Ng [43, 44] showed that fertilization rates, blastocyst development, and the rates of live births are very much related to the degree of DNA damage secondary to controlled amounts of radiation.

In relation to natural conception and intrauterine insemination rather than fertility treatments by conventional IVF or IVF-ICSI, if an advanced sperm selection method is used, the ICSI results are not related to the results of DNA integrity within the whole sperm sample. The single final determinant of pregnancy success is the quality of sperm DNA in the actual fertilizing spermatozoa.

15.2.4 Sperm Preparation by Gradient Centrifugation

The two-phase gradient centrifugation and fractionations of sperm is based on the specific gravity differences between normally developed spermatozoa (ie. sperm with completed cytoplasmic retention and a head containing only DNA plus plasma membrane), as opposed to sperm affected by dysmaturation (excess cytoplasm in the sperm head). Normal sperm will sediment in the pellet, whereas the lighter, dysmature sperm with cytoplasmic retention will remain at the interface or in the top portion of the gradient media.

In 1988, a paper by Aitken and Clarkson [45] demonstrated that centrifugal pelleting of unselected sperm fractions from human ejaculates caused the production of ROS (superoxide and hydroxyl radicals) within the pellet. ROS production has induced irreversible damage to the spermatozoa and impairment of their fertilizing ability. Superoxide radicals cause peroxidation of sperm plasma membrane phospholipids [46] and elevated superoxide production, through a membrane-bound NADPH oxidase system, which has been implicated in defective sperm function at the cellular level [47].

As an alternative concept, addressing the question whether all sperm are equally affected by ROS propagation, using the sperm biochemical markers, three related points were addressed in the Huszar laboratory [9]. First, a relationship was found between cytoplasmic retention as measured by CK activity and ROS production. Thus, retention of the excess cytoplasm was proportional with the ROS production. The second point with respect to the CK and ROS production was the fact that sperm fractions purified by Percoll gradient centrifugation showed lower ROS production and CK content. Third, in order to study whether the iatrogenic cause of increased ROS production indeed propagates from spermatozoa to spermatozoa, the following experiments were performed. Semen pairs [A and B] were studied by first assessing the sperm destruction by ROS following measurement of malonyldialdehyde (MDA), an end product of sperm lipid peroxidation. The two semen samples were assayed independently, and the mixture of the two samples was also subjected to MDA assessment. All three semen fractions (A, B, and A+B) were then centrifuged for 10 min, and the sperm pellets were incubated at 37°C for 30 min. Further, the MDA has been remeasured in all three samples. The data indicated that the aggregate MDA levels were the same as in the original A and B semen samples before the mixing, centrifugation, and incubation of the two semen samples, whether the initial MDA measurements were high (ROS present) or low [9].

Thus, we could deduce that in the case of iatrogenic generation, the propagation of the ROS production does not apparently apply to the normally developed sperm without cytoplasmic retention. Further, based on the data, Huszar and colleagues concluded that the increased sperm MDA levels and ROS production are apparently not "acquired," but arise from an "inborn" error of spermatogenesis and spermiogenesis [9]. This experiment was carried out in 1993–1994, yet the data, with respect to "inborn errors" and the role of objective biochemical markers in the detection of sperm function and fertility, have remained valid and confirmed in the ensuing years with more studies [5, 31, 48].

Using the various sperm biochemical attributes, it has been confirmed that sperm quality is improved by density gradient centrifugation techniques. In addition to the decline of ROS and CK levels in sperm following gradient centrifugation [5, 45, 49], Gandini and coworkers measured DFI and HDS on both the raw and gradient semen purified aliquots [39, 50]. They found that enriched cell suspensions contained sperm with better motility, morphology, SCSA, and DFI. The Sakkas laboratory had also shown that when sperm samples from different men were prepared using density gradient techniques and stained using the CMA3 fluorochrome, which indirectly demonstrates a decreased presence of protamine, or with in situ DNA nick translation which examines for the presence of endogenous DNA nicks, a significant ($P<0.001$) decrease in both CMA3 positivity and DNA strand breakage was observed [9, 20, 48, 51, 52].

Another technology that could aid in the preparation of sperm populations is microfluidics [53]. It has been reported that the use of a microfluidic device, designed with two parallel laminar flow channels that could preferentially separate motile spermatozoa into a separate outlet, increased sperm motility in a sample from 44 to 98% and morphology from 10 to 22% following processing [54]. This microfluidic device provided a novel method for isolating motile, morphologically normal spermatozoa from semen samples without centrifugation. This may limit some of the iatrogenic preparation problems described earlier. This technology may also prove useful in isolating motile spermatozoa from oligozoospermic samples, even with high amounts of nonmotile gamete and/or nongamete cell contamination.

15.2.5 Considerations Related to Men with Excessive Semen ROS Production

Sperm preparation for assisted reproduction in men with high seminal ROS may improve sperm quality if media containing antioxidants such as reduced glutathione and catalase/EDTA is used [55–57]. Such an approach may improve the quality of gametes used by protecting the spermatozoa from high oxidative stress.

In case of oxidative stress-related infertility, the appropriate treatment strategy is the elimination of the underlying cause, whether lifestyle and environmental factors that enhance oxidative stress, infections and antibiotic treatment, or use of sperm for IVF-ICSI arising from the testicular sperm extraction (TESE sperm). It is also advisable to avoid using cryopreserved spermatozoa which are sensitive to DNA damage [58].

Regarding the utilization of TESE sperm, it is established that sperm originating in the adluminal area are protected from oxidative attack, whereas most ROS-initiated DNA fragmentation occurs during epididymal storage [59]. In studies of sperm DNA integrity within the same individuals in ejaculated sperm or epididymal sperm, there were significant improvements in sperm DNA quality in TESE samples [60, 61]. Thus, the use of testicular sperm in men with poor DNA quality is recommended if more conservative treatments such as antioxidant administration had failed.

Another approach is offered by the hyaluronic acid-mediated sperm selection, as it will be described later, at selection for single sperm for IVF/ICSI. The rationale for this approach is as follows: (a) A close correlation has been shown between ROS production and cytoplasmic retention which represent gamete dysmaturity [9]. Thus, it is expected that dysmature sperm, which produces and/or have been affected by ROS, would have a high amount of DNA degradation, and due to the arrested spermiogenesis, would not bind to hyaluronic acid, and (b) Sperm selection by HA-binding is also helpful as hyaluronic acid-bound sperm is also devoid of excess persistent histones, DNA fragmentation, and the apoptotic process. Thus, sperm selection by deselection of dysmature spermatozoa and positive selection of normally developed spermatozoa with low or no ROS production is an appropriate and practical solution [5, 10, 83].

15.2.6 Impact of Sperm Chromatin Maturation on Sperm Function

Protamine replacement of histones and transition proteins may also facilitate the modulation of the expression pattern of the genome, as well as the imprinting pattern of the gamete [62, 63]. This methylation lends variability to the paternal genome during zygotic gene expression events with individual consequences in developmental effects. There are several studies on the impact of sperm chromatin methylation levels in IVF success regarding both fertilization and pregnancy rates. Some support the idea that children conceived by ART do not show a higher degree of imprinting variability. The present understanding with respect to chromatin methylation during the remodeling process is not complete, but it is known that the DNA methylation and chromatin recycling, during the histone-to-protamine exchange, are important [63].

15.3 Source of Sperm for Assisted Reproduction

It could be argued that whatever sperm preparation technique is used, the protection of ejaculated spermatozoa may be late due to the testicular and epididymal exposure to ROS. Posttesticular sperm DNA damage induced by hydroxyl radicals or after exposure to ionizing radiation is associated with nucleotide damage. In the first stage, the damage produced is of the 8-OHdG type, followed by double-stranded DNA fragmentation that may be mediated by caspases and endonucleases. The implications of combined nucleotide damage and DNA strand fragmentation, in addition to its diagnostic value (oxygen radical-induced damage may be treated with antioxidants), are the fact that this type of DNA fragmentation causes a diminished sperm functional integrity because the great majority of the sperm cells will be affected [27].

In line with the above discussion regarding ROS-damaged sperm, most negative effects may be avoided by using testicular sperm. A number of reports indicate that sperm DNA damage is significantly lower in the seminiferous tubules compared to the cauda epididymis or ejaculated sperm [59, 60]. The use of testicular sperm in couples with repeated pregnancy failure in ART, and high sperm DNA fragmentation in semen, resulted in a significant increase in pregnancy rates [61, 64]. Moreover, pregnancy rates in first cycles of TESA-ICSI are relatively high [27]. These results are consistent with the notion that in couples with long-standing infertility, or repeated pregnancy failure in ART without an apparent cause, sperm DNA fragmentation could be an underlying factor. Thus, use of testicular sperm with very low levels of sperm DNA fragmentation reduces the burden of sperm DNA repair by the oocyte. In the majority of cases, sperm DNA damage occurs or is increased in the epididymis and, therefore, DNA fragmentation levels in testicular sperm originating in the seminiferrous tubuli could be relatively lower [61]. With respect to sperm in the seminiferous tubuli and in the epididymis, it is relevant to consider that both in horses and in humans, sperm development with respect to cytoplasmic extrusion and HspA2 expression occurs within the adluminal area [63]. Thus, regarding TESE spermatozoa, the usefulness of this approach is limited to the location of the testicular origin, i.e., whether sperm extracted from the testes would originate in the seminiferous tubuli, in which the spermatozoa was already released from the adluminal compartment after all aspects of the sperm cellular development have been completed [63].

15.4 Deselection of Spermatozoa with Apoptotic Marker Proteins

The presence of apoptotic sperm in the ejaculate was shown by the Sakkas laboratory and has since been verified by a number of other studies, for example, Fas, phosphatidylserine, Bcl-XL, p53, etc. [51, 65–67]. The expression of these apoptotic marker proteins on the surface membrane of ejaculated spermatozoa indicates that this phenomenon could be utilized to select non-apoptotic spermatozoa from semen samples [68]. A novel and promising technique of annexin V-conjugated microbeads (ANMB) – magnetic-activated cell sorting (MACS) – has been shown to remove spermatozoa with phosphatidylserine externalization (marker of apoptosis) and produce a higher quality nonapoptotic sperm fraction [68]. Furthermore, these nonapoptotic cells display higher fertilization rates when used in animal models for IVF and ICSI.

15.5 Sperm Chromatin Maturation and its Importance

The formation of mature spermatozoa is a unique process involving a series of developmental steps in both the nuclear and cytoplasmic compartments including histone-transition protein-protamine replacement. In this process, first somatic histones are replaced by testis-specific histone variants, which are then replaced by transition proteins (TP1 and TP2) in a process that involves extensive DNA rearrangement and remodeling [69]. A greater than tenfold compaction of sperm chromatin is achieved during the final phases of spermatogenesis when the histone that is bound to DNA is almost completely replaced by protamine 1 and protamine [70].

Earlier studies showed an association between diminished histone-transition protein-protamine exchanges that may be detected by aniline blue staining of the excess persistent lysine-rich histones [71–75]. Accordingly, based on the variations in sperm maturity, staining intensity was light, intermediate, and dark tone and represent sperm with mature, moderately immature, and severely immature developmental status, respectively [30].

It is clear that sperm chromatin is essential for sperm function and subsequent embryonic development because defects in sperm chromatin are linked to natural reproductive malfunctions like spontaneous abortion as well as assisted reproductive failure [15, 73]. DNA damage is the main cause of implantation failure in embryos derived from healthy eggs fertilized by protamine compromised sperm [74, 76].This requirement for histone-to-protamine exchange in order to maintain chromatin integrity facilitates the correct folding of DNA and preserves DNA chain integrity. The relationship between persistent histones and DNA degradation was highlighted in a recent report from the Huszar laboratory. In sperm with dark aniline blue staining, representing extensive levels of persistent histones, there was a lack of fluorescence in situ hybridization (FISH) chromosome probe binding [77]. Thus, deficiency in sperm chromatin development, improper DNA folding, and consequentially diminished DNA chain integrity caused diminished FISH probe binding, as there were limited number of long DNA sequences that would facilitate the binding of FISH probes. In addition, environmental stress also can disturb chromatin maturation and ultimately lead to an abnormal chromatin structure that is incompatible with fertility [12, 75].

15.6 Sperm Binding to Hyaluronic Acid

Various biochemical sperm markers indicate that human sperm bound to HA exhibit attributes similar to that of zona pellucida-bound sperm, including minimal DNA fragmentation, normal shape, no persistent histones, and low frequency of chromosomal aneuploidies [5]. Jakab et al. [78] reported that the frequency of chromosomal aneuploidies in HA-bound spermatozoa was significantly decreased after the HA-mediated sperm selection, regardless of the frequency of chromosomal aberrations in the initial semen. It was suggested that clinical use of HA-mediated sperm selection could ultimately solve the pertinent problem of ICSI with increased frequency of aneuploidies in the offspring when the ICSI is performed with embryologist-selected sperm from samples with high proportion of dysmature spermatozoa.

Subsequently, a number of studies have now indicated that HA-bound sperm used in the ICSI procedure may lead to increased implantation rates. In one such study, Parmegiani et al. [79] showed that in 293 couples treated with HA-ICSI vs. 86 couples treated with conventional ICSI (historical control group), all outcome measures of fertilization, embryo quality, implantation, and pregnancy were the same or improved in the HA-bound sperm group. The implantation rate was increased from 10.3% in conventional ICSI to 17.1% in the HA group. The authors concluded that if multicenter randomized studies confirm the beneficial effects on ICSI outcome, HA could be considered as a routine choice for "physiologic" sperm selection prior to ICSI. A smaller clinical trial assessing the same technology by Worrilow et al. [80] has also shown that clinical pregnancy rates are improved when using HA-selected sperm compared to conventional ICSI. Furthermore, the sperm HA-binding score (the proportion of sperm that underwent plasma membrane remodeling in spermatogenesis and binds to hyaluronic acid) is an important diagnostic indicator. Men with <55% binding score would particularly benefit, as their ICSI success rates were improved by (20–30% higher pregnancy rates) by using the HA-mediated sperm selection [80]. Thus, it is important that in IVF programs, the Andrology Laboratory performs the sperm-HA-binding test for the husbands of IVF-ICSI couples and that the IVF team triages the couples according to their HA-binding score. This score provides the information on the proportion of sperm with attributes of dysmaturity, such as DNA fragmentation, chromosomal aneuploidies, persistent histones, cytoplasmic retention, and lack of HA-binding ability, consequential to dysmaturity.

Another aspect of the markers of sperm development is the enhancement of sperm with normal morphology in the HA-bound sperm fraction. Studies in the Huszar laboratory indicated that there was a 2–3-fold enrichment of Tygerberg normal sperm compared to the respective semen sperm fraction, which, interestingly, agreed with the finding of the Tygerberg group with respect to the enrichment of normal morphology sperm in the zona pellucida-bound vs. semen sperm fraction [81].

15.6.1 Selection of Single Sperm for ICSI by Hyaluronic Acid (HA) Binding: Normally Developed Spermatozoa Selectively Bind to Solid State HA

The data on biochemical markers have also revealed that the sperm membrane remodeling process is inherently related to upstream spermatogenetic and spermiogenetic events. First, the Huszar group looked at the sperm markers of LDH-C, cytoplasmic retention, DNA integrity, sperm shape, chromatin abnormalities, apoptotic markers, and enzymes [5]. Sperm with cytoplasmic retention (arrested cellular maturation) showed a positive signal with these probes; however, sperm aliquots that were bound to a hyaluronic acid-coated slide contained no sperm with the positive signals for any of the dysmaturity and DNA degradation markers.

Furthermore, in a more refined experiment, semen aliquots were smeared on glass slides and the sperm were fixed for the various markers. Another aliquot of the same semen was incubated on hyaluronic acid-coated slides. After the 15 min binding process, the unbound sperm were gently rinsed off, and the HA-bound fraction was fixed. Finally, both the whole semen fraction on glass slides and the HA-bound sperm fraction on the HA-coated slides were stained for the biochemical markers and were evaluated. In the semen sperm fraction, there were sperm with cytoplasmic retention, DNA degradation (detected in individual spermatozoa with DNA-nick translation), aberrant shape, and persistent histones with aniline blue staining, whereas in the HA-bound sperm fraction, there was no presence of sperm with any of the cytoplasmic or nuclear defects [5, 9].

15.6.2 Sperm Dysmaturity and Persistent Histones

Regarding the interrelationship between persistent histones and arrested sperm development, a recent report by the Huszar laboratory indicates that diminished sperm fertility and reduced paternal contribution of sperm to the embryo may not originate only in the arrested histone – protamine remodeling, but along with the persistent histones, there are other associated factors of dysmaturity in the same spermatozoa [30]. In these double staining studies, a method was developed: First, sperm are stained with aniline blue for probing persistent histones. Second, after recording the aniline blue-stained sperm fields, and a subsequent destaining step, the same sperm are probed for sperm shape, for cytoplasmic retention with creatine kinase immuno-staining, for the apoptotic process with caspase 3 immunostaining, and for DNA chain fragmentation with in situ DNA-nick translation.

The evaluation of the same sperm after the first and second probes convincingly showed an approximately 75% agreement between the aniline blue staining patterns whether light (no probe presence), intermediate (some probe detection), and dark staining (heavy probe presence) and of the various other biochemical probes and sperm morphology. This indicated that indeed there is a relationship between the attributes of arrested development or dysmaturity within the same sperm. Also, the experiment demonstrated that the nuclear and cytoplasmic as well as the early and late events of sperm development are related. It also suggests that persistent histones and arrested chromatin modulation fail to initiate protamine transport and proper DNA folding in the nucleus and are associated with the events contributing to diminished sperm function. Thus, the data support the idea that the later manifestations of arrested sperm development may originate in common upstream events of early spermatogenesis [30].

15.6.3 Does Sperm HA-Binding Test Predict High DNA Integrity in the HA-Bound Sperm?

A recent example of DNA integrity in the HA-selected sperm was developed by acridine orange [AO] staining of HA-bound spermatozoa, a reagent which provides green fluorescence for DNA with high chain integrity and orange fluorescence for damaged DNA. Baker et al. reported previously that the zone pellucida-bound sperm has mostly green fluorescence [82]. In the Huszar laboratory, the AO assay was performed with sperm bound to the HA-spot of the PICSI dish, which is used for ICSI sperm selection in IVF laboratories. The data indicated, using the very fine Polyscience Inc. acridine orange, that literally 100% of the hundreds of HA-bound sperm were of green fluorescence. Thus, whether we probe DNA integrity with nick translation or acridine orange reagent, the DNA of HA-bound sperm had high integrity and no cellular dysmaturity defects [5, 83]. Thus, one more experiment supports the concept that HA-mediated sperm selection by the PICSI dish is an optimal tool for ICSI sperm selection.

Regarding the HA-mediated ICSI sperm selection, in addition to the DNA integrity, there is now focus on the increase in chromosomal aneuploidies with the embryologist-selected sperm, as the aneuploidy frequencies are 3–4 times higher in the ICSI offspring. Pointing out the relationship between meiotic and late spermiogenetic events, it was shown that sperm with cytoplasmic retention defects and sperm dysmaturity also have increased frequencies of chromosomal aneuploidies with a significant correlation at the level of $r>0.75$, $P<0.001$ [84]. Thus, these data, along with the experiments by Jakab et al. with FISH studies of >20,000 spermatozoa [78], suggest that the filtering effect of the zona pellucida has been reconstructed and tested by hyaluronic acid binding. No matter how high the aneuploidy frequency was in the initial semen sperm fraction, in the sperm bound, and removed from HA, there was a 4–6x decline in disomy and diploidy frequencies within the 0.1–0.2% normal range, which is customary in babies conceived with natural conception or with conventional IVF [5, 78].

15.6.4 Relationship Between the Various Biochemical Sperm Markers of Dysmaturity and Diminished Sperm Function

Along with sperm dysmaturity, that is detectable by defects of the histone-transition protein-protamine replacement, and by the consequential strong aniline blue staining due to excess histone retention (which also has consequences in DNA folding and DNA chain vulnerability/integrity), there were several other sperm attributes that are associated with arrested cellular development contributing to diminished sperm fertilizing potential.

The key elements, confirmed with objective biochemical markers, include (a) Cytoplasmic retention. Indeed, high sperm creatine kinase activity of oligozoospermic men treated with intrauterine insemination has predicted the lack of pregnancies, independently from sperm concentration and motility [85]; (b) The diminished expression of the HspA2 chaperone protein. Men with low sperm HspA2 levels failed to achieve pregnancy in couples treated with conventional IVF in two independent studies, one in a Yale-Norfolk collaboration and one of a Yale IVF study [86, 87]; (c) Men with sperm cytoplasmic retention and low HspA2 expression had a higher incidence of sperm with aniline blue staining, indicating elevated content of histones; (d) In semen samples with increased frequency of spermatozoa with cytoplasmic retention, there were increased levels of sperm creatine kinase, and aniline blue staining; (e) Sperm with cytoplasmic retention have a higher rate of aneuploidy with a statistically significant relationship (i.e., sperm with cytoplasmic retention vs. Y disomy: $R=0.78$, $P=<0.001$) [84]; (f) Further, with the establishment that sperm, after the decondensation step necessary for FISH or DNA integrity studies, maintain their initial shape as it was in semen [88], an association was demonstrated between sperm shape and aneuploidies within the same spermatozoa.

Conversely, study of hyaluronic acid (HA)-bound spermatozoa that underwent spermiogenetic plasma membrane remodeling has indicated that the HA-bound sperm lacked any of the attributes of arrested sperm development, including cytoplasmic retention, no persistent histones, and no DNA fragmentation (detected by two methods: in situ DNA-nick translation, and acridine orange fluorescence), and had improved Tygerberg strict morphology (approximately 3× enrichment of normal sperm vs. the semen sperm population), as well as normal frequency of chromosomal aneuploidies, regardless how elevated the aneuploidy and diploidy levels were in the semen sperm fraction [5, 9, 77, 78, 89].

Finally, regarding the validation of the sperm characteristics discussed above, there are two points of interest. First, in a study of comparing sperm binding to hemizonae and HA, there was a high correlation and a significant relationship ($r=0.76$, $P<0.001$), which validates the HA-binding assay and reinforces the idea that the formation of the zona pellucida and HA receptors are related during the spermiogenetic plasma membrane remodeling [5]. The location of these receptors is also common in the acrosomal region, as sperm binding to the zona pellucida and HA follows identical patterns [5, 9]. Second, it was recently published that sperm with dark aniline blue staining show no DNA staining with probes for in situ fluorescence hybridization, or with a DNA probe [77]. The data suggest that sperm with high levels of persistent histones and diminished protamine content suffer major DNA chain fragmentations, thus the FISH probes are unable to bind and the fragmented DNA dissipates from sperm during the multiple steps of the FISH process.

15.7 Other Sperm Selection Techniques

15.7.1 Sperm Selection by Sperm Charge Properties

The Aitken group recently reported a novel electrophoretic sperm isolation device utilizing a separation strategy based on sperm size and electronegative charge. The suspensions generated by the electrophoretic separation technique contained motile, viable, and morphologically normal spermatozoa, while exhibiting low levels of DNA damage. Reportedly, the electrophoretic sperm isolation procedure is both time- and cost-effective [90] and the first pregnancy using this method for a couple suffering from extensive sperm DNA damage was reported [91].

15.7.2 Intracytoplasmic Morphologically Selected Sperm Injection (IMSI)

In 2001, Bartoov et al. [92] reported the selection of spermatozoa with normal nuclei to improve the pregnancy rate with intracytoplasmic sperm injection. They went on to verify this technique by performing ICSI using morphologically normal sperm, strictly defined by high-power light microscopy ($x > 6{,}000$). Sixty-two couples, with at least two previous consequent pregnancy failures after ICSI, underwent a single ICSI trial preceded by morphological selection of spermatozoa with normal nuclei. Fifty of these couples were matched with couples who underwent a routine ICSI procedure at the same IVF center and exhibited the same number of previous ICSI failures. The matching study revealed that the pregnancy rate after modified ICSI was significantly higher than that of the routine ICSI procedure (66.0 vs. 30.0%).

More recently, Antinori et al. [93] conducted a prospective randomized study to assess the advantages of intracytoplasmic morphologically selected sperm injection (IMSI) over the conventional ICSI procedure. A total of 446 couples with 3 years of primary infertility, the woman aged 35 years or younger, without workup for female factor and husbands of severe oligoasthenoteratozoospermia were randomized to eye selected ICSI ($n=219$; group 1) and IMSI ($n=227$; group 2) treatment groups. The data showed that IMSI resulted in a higher clinical pregnancy rate (39.2 vs. 26.5%; $P=0.004$) than ICSI. In spite of their initial poor reproductive prognosis, patients with two or more previous failed attempts benefited from IMSI in terms of pregnancy (29.8 vs. 12.9%; $P=0.017$) and miscarriage rates (17.4 vs. 37.5%).

Hazout et al. [94] also reported a positive association between high-magnification selection of sperm cells with normal nuclear shape and pregnancy outcome in patients with repeated conventional ICSI failures. In a subgroup of patients ($n=72$) involved in the study, a noticeable improvement in clinical outcomes (implantation and birth rates) was observed both in patients with an elevated (>40%) and moderate (30–40%) degree of sperm DNA fragmentation and in those with normal sperm DNA status (<30%) using the TUNEL assay.

The use of IMSI appears promising [95]. Some drawbacks are, however, present; in particular, the belief that it is a complicated technique that cannot be routinely performed [96]. Future simplification of the selection procedure by automated ICSI may, however, be possible. As the high-magnification approach is increasingly used, more studies examining high magnification selected sperm and their respective levels of cytoplasmic retention, persistent histones, DNA chain integrity, aneuploidy rates, tyrosine phosphorylation, or apoptotic markers should be performed.

Another microscopic technology that may show promise is the birefringence analysis of the sperm head. Gianaroli et al. [97] previously postulated that this could represent both a diagnostic tool and a novel method for sperm selection. Recently, they performed a prospective randomization including 71 couples with severe male factor infertility and performed ICSI using polarized light for sperm selection which permitted analysis of the birefringence sperm head [98]. Twenty-three patients had their oocytes injected with acrosome-reacted spermatozoa, 26 patient's oocytes were injected with nonacrosome-reacted spermatozoa, and in 22 patients with both reacted and nonreacted spermatozoa. They found no effect on the fertilizing capacity and embryo development of either type of sperm, whereas the implantation rate was higher in oocytes injected with reacted spermatozoa (39.0%) vs. those injected with nonreacted spermatozoa (8.6%). The implantation rate was 24.4% in the group injected with both reacted and nonreacted spermatozoa.

15.8 Future Technologies

A number of novel new technologies are being developed in sperm selection for classical IVF or IVF-ICSI. An example is Raman Spectroscopy which noninvasively distinguish the DNA packaging and protamine content between normal and abnormal cells [99]. Differences identified include the vibrational marker modes that Raman spectra of individual sperm cells can distinguish and this may be used to assess the efficiency of DNA packaging for each cell. The attributes followed are the relative protein content per sperm cell and DNA packaging efficiencies throughout wide ranges for sperm cells with both normal and abnormal shapes. Data indicate that single-cell Raman spectroscopy could be a valuable tool in assessing the quality of sperm cells.

Other molecular techniques may allow the future analysis of sperm populations. For example, DNA methylation patterns of key developmental genes have been shown to differ in spermatozoa and this may impact embryo development. In addition, the fundamental information being generated from Proteomic [100] and RNA [101] analysis of sperm will also create a basis for identifying key points in spermatozoa that might be implicated in the defective sperm function observed in a significant proportion of infertile males and aid in both diagnosis and treatment.

References

1. World health organization laboratory manual for examination of human semen. Cambridge: Cambridge University Press; 1992.
2. Society of Assisted Reproduction Technologies (SART). Clinic summary report. 2008. http://www.sartcorsonline.com.
3. Jequier AM. Clinical andrology – still a major problem in the treatment of infertility. Hum Reprod. 2004;19(6):1245–9.
4. Palermo G, Joris H, Devroey P, Van Steirteghem AC. Pregnancies after intracytoplasmic injection of single spermatozoon into an oocyte. Lancet. 1992;340(8810):17–8.
5. Huszar G, Jakab A, Sakkas D, et al. Fertility testing and ICSI sperm selection by hyaluronic acid binding: clinical and genetic aspects. Reprod Biomed Online. 2007;14(5):650–63.
6. Devroey P, Van Steirteghem A. A review of ten years experience of ICSI. Hum Reprod Update. 2004;10(1):19–28.
7. Ponjaert-Kristoffersen I, Bonduelle M, Barnes J, et al. International collaborative study of intracytoplasmic sperm injection-conceived, in vitro fertilization-conceived, and naturally conceived 5-year-old child outcomes: cognitive and motor assessments. Pediatrics. 2005;115(3):e283–9.
8. Huszar G, Vigue L. Spermatogenesis-related change in the synthesis of the creatine kinase B-type and M-type isoforms in human spermatozoa. Mol Reprod Dev. 1990;25(3):258–62.
9. Huszar G, Vigue L. Correlation between the rate of lipid peroxidation and cellular maturity as measured by creatine kinase activity in human spermatozoa. J Androl. 1994;15(1):71–7.
10. Huszar G, Vigue L, Oehninger S. Creatine kinase immunocytochemistry of human sperm-hemizona complexes: selective binding of sperm with mature creatine kinase-staining pattern. Fertil Steril. 1994;61(1):136–42.
11. Huszar G, Stone K, Dix D, Vigue L. Putative creatine kinase M-isoform in human sperm is identified as the 70-kilodalton heat shock protein HspA2. Biol Reprod. 2000;63(3):925–32.
12. Aoki VW, Emery BR, Liu L, Carrell DT. Protamine levels vary between individual sperm cells of infertile human males and correlate with viability and DNA integrity. J Androl. 2006;27(6):890–8.
13. Seli E, Sakkas D. Spermatozoal nuclear determinants of reproductive outcome: implications for ART. Hum Reprod Update. 2005;11(4):337–49.
14. Perreault SD, Aitken RJ, Baker HW, et al. Integrating new tests of sperm genetic integrity into semen analysis: breakout group discussion. Adv Exp Med Biol. 2003;518:253–68.
15. Bungum M, Humaidan P, Axmon A, et al. Sperm DNA integrity assessment in prediction of assisted reproduction technology outcome. Hum Reprod. 2007;22(1):174–9.
16. Gorczyca W, Traganos F, Jesionowska H, Darzynkiewicz Z. Presence of DNA strand breaks and increased sensitivity of DNA in situ to denaturation in abnormal human sperm cells: analogy to apoptosis of somatic cells. Exp Cell Res. 1993;207(1):202–5.
17. Hughes CM, Lewis SE, McKelvey-Martin VJ, Thompson W. A comparison of baseline and induced DNA damage in human spermatozoa from fertile and infertile men, using a modified comet assay. Mol Hum Reprod. 1996;2(8):613–9.
18. Manicardi GC, Bianchi PG, Pantano S, et al. Presence of endogenous nicks in DNA of ejaculated human spermatozoa and its relationship to chromomycin A3 accessibility. Biol Reprod. 1995;52(4):864–7.
19. Bianchi PG, Manicardi GC, Bizzaro D, Bianchi U, Sakkas D. Effect of deoxyribonucleic acid protamination on fluorochrome staining and in situ nick-translation of murine and human mature spermatozoa. Biol Reprod. 1993;49(5):1083–8.

20. Tomlinson MJ, Moffatt O, Manicardi GC, Bizzaro D, Afnan M, Sakkas D. Interrelationships between seminal parameters and sperm nuclear DNA damage before and after density gradient centrifugation: implications for assisted conception. Hum Reprod. 2001;16(10):2160–5.
21. Fernandez JL, Vazquez-Gundin F, Delgado A, et al. DNA breakage detection-FISH (DBD-FISH) in human spermatozoa: technical variants evidence different structural features. Mutat Res. 2000;453(1):77–82.
22. Fernandez JL, Muriel L, Rivero MT, Goyanes V, Vazquez R, Alvarez JG. The sperm chromatin dispersion test: a simple method for the determination of sperm DNA fragmentation. J Androl. 2003;24(1): 59–66.
23. Virro MR, Larson-Cook KL, Evenson DP. Sperm chromatin structure assay (SCSA) parameters are related to fertilization, blastocyst development, and ongoing pregnancy in in vitro fertilization and intracytoplasmic sperm injection cycles. Fertil Steril. 2004;81(5):1289–95.
24. Evenson D, Wixon R. Meta-analysis of sperm DNA fragmentation using the sperm chromatin structure assay. Reprod Biomed Online. 2006;12(4):466–72.
25. Evenson DP, Wixon R. Data analysis of two in vivo fertility studies using sperm chromatin structure assay-derived DNA fragmentation index vs. pregnancy outcome. Fertil Steril. 2008;90(4):1229–31.
26. Singh NP, Danner DB, Tice RR, McCoy MT, Collins GD, Schneider EL. Abundant alkali-sensitive sites in DNA of human and mouse sperm. Exp Cell Res. 1989;184(2):461–70.
27. Sakkas D, Alvarez JG. Sperm DNA fragmentation: mechanisms of origin, impact on reproductive outcome, and analysis. Fertil Steril. 2010;93(4):1027–36.
28. Barratt CL, Aitken RJ, Bjorndahl L, et al. Sperm DNA: organization, protection and vulnerability: from basic science to clinical applications – a position report. Hum Reprod. 2010;25(4):824–38.
29. Borini A, Tarozzi N, Bizzaro D, et al. Sperm DNA fragmentation: paternal effect on early post-implantation embryo development in ART. Hum Reprod. 2006;21(11):2876–81.
30. Sati L, Ovari L, Bennett D, Simon SD, Demir R, Huszar G. Double probing of human spermatozoa for persistent histones, surplus cytoplasm, apoptosis and DNA fragmentation. Reprod Biomed Online. 2008;16(4):570–9.
31. Evenson DP, Darzynkiewicz Z, Melamed MR. Relation of mammalian sperm chromatin heterogeneity to fertility. Science. 1980;210(4474):1131–3.
32. Evenson D, Jost L. Sperm chromatin structure assay: DNA denaturability. Meth Cell Biol. 1994;42(Pt B): 159–76.
33. Evenson D, Jost L, Gandour D, et al. Comparative sperm chromatin structure assay measurements on epiillumination and orthogonal axes flow cytometers. Cytometry. 1995;19(4):295–303.
34. Evenson DP. Flow cytometry of acridine orange stained sperm is a rapid and practical method for monitoring occupational exposure to genotoxicants. Prog Clin Biol Res. 1986;207:121–32.
35. Evenson DP. Flow cytometric analysis of male germ cell quality. Meth Cell Biol. 1990;33:401–10.
36. Evenson DP, Larson KL, Jost LK. Sperm chromatin structure assay: its clinical use for detecting sperm DNA fragmentation in male infertility and comparisons with other techniques. J Androl. 2002;23(1):25–43.
37. Larson KL, DeJonge CJ, Barnes AM, Jost LK, Evenson DP. Sperm chromatin structure assay parameters as predictors of failed pregnancy following assisted reproductive techniques. Hum Reprod. 2000;15(8):1717–22.
38. Larson-Cook KL, Brannian JD, Hansen KA, Kasperson KM, Aamold ET, Evenson DP. Relationship between the outcomes of assisted reproductive techniques and sperm DNA fragmentation as measured by the sperm chromatin structure assay. Fertil Steril. 2003;80(4):895–902.
39. Gandini L, Lombardo F, Paoli D, et al. Full-term pregnancies achieved with ICSI despite high levels of sperm chromatin damage. Hum Reprod. 2004;19(6): 1409–17.
40. Bungum M, Humaidan P, Spano M, Jepson K, Bungum L, Giwercman A. The predictive value of sperm chromatin structure assay (SCSA) parameters for the outcome of intrauterine insemination, IVF and ICSI. Hum Reprod. 2004;19(6):1401–8.
41. Zini A, Libman J. Sperm DNA damage: clinical significance in the era of assisted reproduction. CMAJ. 2006;175(5):495–500.
42. Spano M, Seli E, Bizzaro D, Manicardi GC, Sakkas D. The significance of sperm nuclear DNA strand breaks on reproductive outcome. Curr Opin Obstet Gynecol. 2005;17(3):255–60.
43. Ahmadi A, Ng SC. Fertilizing ability of DNA-damaged spermatozoa. J Exp Zool. 1999;284(6): 696–704.
44. Ahmadi A, Ng SC. Fertilization and development of mouse oocytes injected with membrane-damaged spermatozoa. Hum Reprod. 1997;12(12):2797–801.
45. Aitken RJ, Clarkson JS. Significance of reactive oxygen species and antioxidants in defining the efficacy of sperm preparation techniques. J Androl. 1988;9(6): 367–76.
46. Aitken RJ, Clarkson JS. Cellular basis of defective sperm function and its association with the genesis of reactive oxygen species by human spermatozoa. J Reprod Fertil. 1987;81(2):459–69.
47. Alvarez JG, Touchstone JC, Blasco L, Storey BT. Spontaneous lipid peroxidation and production of hydrogen peroxide and superoxide in human spermatozoa. Superoxide dismutase as major enzyme protectant against oxygen toxicity. J Androl. 1987;8(5): 338–48.
48. Sakkas D, Manicardi GC, Tomlinson M, et al. The use of two density gradient centrifugation techniques and the swim-up method to separate spermatozoa with chromatin and nuclear DNA anomalies. Hum Reprod. 2000;15(5):1112–6.

49. Mortimer D. Sperm preparation techniques and iatrogenic failures of in-vitro fertilization. Hum Reprod. 1991;6(2):173–6.
50. Spano M, Cordelli E, Leter G, Lombardo F, Lenzi A, Gandini L. Nuclear chromatin variations in human spermatozoa undergoing swim-up and cryopreservation evaluated by the flow cytometric sperm chromatin structure assay. Mol Hum Reprod. 1999; 5(1):29–37.
51. Oehninger S, Morshedi M, Weng SL, Taylor S, Duran H, Beebe S. Presence and significance of somatic cell apoptosis markers in human ejaculated spermatozoa. Reprod Biomed Online. 2003;7(4):469–76.
52. Morrell JM, Moffatt O, Sakkas D, et al. Reduced senescence and retained nuclear DNA integrity in human spermatozoa prepared by density gradient centrifugation. J Assist Reprod Genet. 2004;21(6): 217–22.
53. Beebe D, Wheeler M, Zeringue H, Walters E, Raty S. Microfluidic technology for assisted reproduction. Theriogenology. 2002;57(1):125–35.
54. Schuster TG, Cho B, Keller LM, Takayama S, Smith GD. Isolation of motile spermatozoa from semen samples using microfluidics. Reprod Biomed Online. 2003;7(1):75–81.
55. Donnelly ET, McClure N, Lewis SE. Glutathione and hypotaurine in vitro: effects on human sperm motility, DNA integrity and production of reactive oxygen species. Mutagenesis. 2000;15(1):61–8.
56. Griveau JF, Le Lannou D. Effects of antioxidants on human sperm preparation techniques. Int J Androl. 1994;17(5):225–31.
57. Chi HJ, Kim JH, Ryu CS, et al. Protective effect of antioxidant supplementation in sperm-preparation medium against oxidative stress in human spermatozoa. Hum Reprod. 2008;23(5):1023–8.
58. Donnelly ET, Steele EK, McClure N, Lewis SE. Assessment of DNA integrity and morphology of ejaculated spermatozoa from fertile and infertile men before and after cryopreservation. Hum Reprod. 2001;16(6):1191–9.
59. Steele EK, McClure N, Maxwell RJ, Lewis SE. A comparison of DNA damage in testicular and proximal epididymal spermatozoa in obstructive azoospermia. Mol Hum Reprod. 1999;5(9):831–5.
60. Suganuma R, Yanagimachi R, Meistrich ML. Decline in fertility of mouse sperm with abnormal chromatin during epididymal passage as revealed by ICSI. Hum Reprod. 2005;20(11):3101–8.
61. Greco E, Scarselli F, Iacobelli M, et al. Efficient treatment of infertility due to sperm DNA damage by ICSI with testicular spermatozoa. Hum Reprod. 2005;20(1):226–30.
62. Aoki VW, Carrell DT. Human protamines and the developing spermatid: their structure, function, expression and relationship with male infertility. Asian J Androl. 2003;5(4):315–24.
63. Miller D, Brinkworth M, Iles D. Paternal DNA packaging in spermatozoa: more than the sum of its parts? DNA, histones, protamines and epigenetics. Reproduction. 2010;139(2):287–301.
64. Alvarez J. Aplicaciones clinicas del estudio de fragmentacion del DNA espermatico. Revista Argentina de Andrologia. 2008;5:354–363.
65. Sakkas D, Moffatt O, Manicardi GC, Mariethoz E, Tarozzi N, Bizzaro D. Nature of DNA damage in ejaculated human spermatozoa and the possible involvement of apoptosis. Biol Reprod. 2002;66(4): 1061–7.
66. Cayli S, Sakkas D, Vigue L, Demir R, Huszar G. Cellular maturity and apoptosis in human sperm: creatine kinase, caspase-3 and Bcl-XL levels in mature and diminished maturity sperm. Mol Hum Reprod. 2004;10(5):365–72.
67. Mahfouz RZ, Sharma RK, Said TM, Erenpreiss J, Agarwal A. Association of sperm apoptosis and DNA ploidy with sperm chromatin quality in human spermatozoa. Fertil Steril. 2009;91(4):1110–8.
68. Said TM, Grunewald S, Paasch U, et al. Advantage of combining magnetic cell separation with sperm preparation techniques. Reprod Biomed Online. 2005; 10(6):740–6.
69. Ward WS, Coffey DS. DNA packaging and organization in mammalian spermatozoa: comparison with somatic cells. Biol Reprod. 1991;44(4):569–74.
70. Braun RE. Packaging paternal chromosomes with protamine. Nat Genet. 2001;28(1):10–2.
71. Dadoune JP. The nuclear status of human sperm cells. Micron. 1995;26(4):323–45.
72. Steger K, Failing K, Klonisch T, et al. Round spermatids from infertile men exhibit decreased protamine-1 and -2 mRNA. Hum Reprod. 2001;16(4):709–16.
73. Filatov MV, Semenova EV, Vorob'eva OA, Leont'eva OA, Drobchenko EA. Relationship between abnormal sperm chromatin packing and IVF results. Mol Hum Reprod. 1999;5(9):825–30.
74. Aoki VW, Moskovtsev SI, Willis J, Liu L, Mullen JB, Carrell DT. DNA integrity is compromised in protamine-deficient human sperm. J Androl. 2005; 26(6):741–8.
75. Carrell DT, Emery BR, Hammoud S. Altered protamine expression and diminished spermatogenesis: what is the link? Hum Reprod Update. 2007;13(3): 313–27.
76. Ramos L, van der Heijden GW, Derijck A, et al. Incomplete nuclear transformation of human spermatozoa in oligo-astheno-teratospermia: characterization by indirect immunofluorescence of chromatin and thiol status. Hum Reprod. 2008;23(2):259–70.
77. Ovari L, Sati L, Stronk J, Borsos A, Ward DC, Huszar G. Double probing individual human spermatozoa: aniline blue staining for persistent histones and fluorescence in situ hybridization for aneuploidies. Fertil Steril. 2010;93(7):2255–61.
78. Jakab A, Sakkas D, Delpiano E, et al. Intracytoplasmic sperm injection: a novel selection method for sperm with normal frequency of chromosomal aneuploidies. Fertil Steril. 2005;84(6):1665–73.
79. Parmegiani L, Cognigni GE, Bernardi S, Troilo E, Ciampaglia W, Filicori M. "Physiologic ICSI": hyaluronic acid (HA) favors selection of spermatozoa without DNA fragmentation and with normal nucleus, resulting in improvement of embryo quality. Fertil Steril. 2010;93(2):598–604.

80. Worrilow K, Huynh H, Bower J, Peters A, Johnston JB. The clinical impact associated with the use of PICSI TM-derived embryos. Fertil Steril. 2006; 86(3):S62.
81. Menkveld R, Franken DR, Kruger TF, Oehninger S, Hodgen GD. Sperm selection capacity of the human zona pellucida. Mol Reprod Dev. 1991; 30(4):346–52.
82. Liu DY, Baker HW. Human sperm bound to the zona pellucida have normal nuclear chromatin as assessed by acridine orange fluorescence. Hum Reprod. 2007;22(6):1597–602.
83. Yagci A, Murk W, Stronk J, Huszar G. Spermatozoa bound to solid state hyaluronic acid show chromatin structure with high DNA chain integrity: an Acridine Orange Fluorescence Study. J Androl. 2010;31: 566–72.
84. Kovanci E, Kovacs T, Moretti E, et al. FISH assessment of aneuploidy frequencies in mature and immature human spermatozoa classified by the absence or presence of cytoplasmic retention. Hum Reprod. 2001;16(6):1209–17.
85. Huszar G, Vigue L, Corrales M. Sperm creatine kinase activity in fertile and infertile oligospermic men. J Androl. 1990;11(1):40–6.
86. Huszar G, Vigue L, Morshedi M. Sperm creatine phosphokinase M-isoform ratios and fertilizing potential of men: a blinded study of 84 couples treated with in vitro fertilization. Fertil Steril. 1992;57(4):882–8.
87. Ergur AR, Dokras A, Giraldo JL, Habana A, Kovanci E, Huszar G. Sperm maturity and treatment choice of in vitro fertilization (IVF) or intracytoplasmic sperm injection: diminished sperm HspA2 chaperone levels predict IVF failure. Fertil Steril. 2002; 77(5):910–8.
88. Celik-Ozenci C, Catalanotti J, Jakab A, et al. Human sperm maintain their shape following decondensation and denaturation for fluorescent in situ hybridization: shape analysis and objective morphometry. Biol Reprod. 2003;69(4):1347–55.
89. Huszar G, Sbracia M, Vigue L, Miller DJ, Shur BD. Sperm plasma membrane remodeling during spermiogenetic maturation in men: relationship among plasma membrane beta 1, 4-galactosyltransferase, cytoplasmic creatine phosphokinase, and creatine phosphokinase isoform ratios. Biol Reprod. 1997; 56(4):1020–4.
90. Ainsworth C, Nixon B, Aitken RJ. Development of a novel electrophoretic system for the isolation of human spermatozoa. Hum Reprod. 2005;20(8):2261–70.
91. Ainsworth C, Nixon B, Jansen RP, Aitken RJ. First recorded pregnancy and normal birth after ICSI using electrophoretically isolated spermatozoa. Hum Reprod. 2007;22(1):197–200.
92. Bartoov B, Berkovitz A, Eltes F. Selection of spermatozoa with normal nuclei to improve the pregnancy rate with intracytoplasmic sperm injection. N Engl J Med. 2001;345(14):1067–8.
93. Antinori M, Licata E, Dani G, et al. Intracytoplasmic morphologically selected sperm injection: a prospective randomized trial. Reprod Biomed Online. 2008;16(6):835–41.
94. Hazout A, Dumont-Hassan M, Junca AM, Cohen Bacrie P, Tesarik J. High-magnification ICSI overcomes paternal effect resistant to conventional ICSI. Reprod Biomed Online. 2006;12(1):19–25.
95. Nadalini M, Tarozzi N, Distratis V, Scaravelli G, Borini A. Impact of intracytoplasmic morphologically selected sperm injection on assisted reproduction outcome: a review. Reprod Biomed Online. 2009;19 Suppl 3:45–55.
96. Cohen-Bacrie P, Dumont M, Junca AM, Belloc S, Hazout A. Indications for IMSI. J Gynécol Obstét Biol Reprod. 2007;36 Suppl 3:S105–8.
97. Gianaroli L, Magli MC, Collodel G, Moretti E, Ferraretti AP, Baccetti B. Sperm head's birefringence: a new criterion for sperm selection. Fertil Steril. 2008;90(1):104–12.
98. Gianaroli L, Magli MC, Ferraretti AP, et al. Birefringence characteristics in sperm heads allow for the selection of reacted spermatozoa for intracytoplasmic sperm injection. Fertil Steril. 2010;93(3):807–13.
99. Huser T, Orme CA, Hollars CW, Corzett MH, Balhorn R. Raman spectroscopy of DNA packaging in individual human sperm cells distinguishes normal from abnormal cells. J Biophotonics. 2009; 2(5):322–32.
100. Aitken RJ, Baker MA. The role of proteomics in understanding sperm cell biology. Int J Androl. 2008;31(3):295 302.
101. Ostermeier GC, Goodrich RJ, Diamond MP, Dix DJ, Krawetz SA. Toward using stable spermatozoal RNAs for prognostic assessment of male factor fertility. Fertil Steril. 2005;83(6):1687–94.

16 The Role of the Oocyte in Remodeling of Male Chromatin and DNA Repair: Are Events During the Zygotic Cell Cycle of Relevance to ART?

Liliana Ramos and Peter de Boer

Abstract

Transmission of male genetic material through highly differentiated and specialized sperm cells is a highly dynamic process, in which the zygote plays a major role. Chromatin remodeling and DNA repair are involved, both during spermatid nuclear elongation and after gamete fusion at chromatin remodeling from a protamine dominated towards a nucleosomal chromatin state. Roles for DNA repair are further envisaged for zygotic G1 and S-phases, with an active role of the maternal complement toward the male PN. In this chapter, findings from mainly the mouse, extending into paternal DNA demethylation in the zygote, have been integrated. Although biological insight into the roles of the oocyte toward chromatin of the sperm cell is developing, there is a gap between the current knowledge for mouse and the observations made on human sperm DNA and chromatin, fertilization efficiency (after IVF and ICSI), and the subsequent zygote and cleavage stage development of human embryos. In part, this is due to the use of normal mouse sperm for research, whereas in male factor infertility, the fraction of normal gametes can be sharply reduced. On the other hand, human oocytes will not be homogeneous in chromatin remodeling and DNA repair capacity. Nevertheless, there are enough experimental data in transmission biology to make a plea for more careful monitoring of DNA and chromatin in ART children and adults.

L. Ramos (✉)
Department of Obstetrics and Gynecology, Radboud University Nijmegen Medical Center, Nijmegen, The Netherlands
e-mail: l.ramos@obgyn.umcn.nl

C. Racowsky et al. (eds.), *Biennial Review of Infertility: Volume 2*,
DOI 10.1007/978-1-4419-8456-2_16, © Springer Science+Business Media, LLC 2011

Keywords
ART • Base excision repair • Chromosomes • Nucleus decondensation • DNA demethylation • DNA damage • DNA repair • Double-strand breaks • Embryo, epigenetics • Gametes • GammaH2AX • Fertilization • Histones • Homologous recombination repair • ICSI • Immunofluorescence • Imprinting • Matrix-associated regions • DNA methylation • Mutagenesis • Nonhomologous end joining • Nucleosomes • Nucleotide excision repair • Oocytes • Oxydative stress • Pronucleus • Protamines • Polycomb proteins • Spermatozoa • Spermiogenesis • S-phase • Synchrony • Zygote

16.1 Introduction

In recent years, exciting new insights have been made regarding mouse/human gametes: (a) nonrandom distribution of nucleosomes in sperm, (b) different DNA repair requirements between the parental chromosome sets, (c) DNA demethylation involves DNA repair, and (d) the presence of small RNA molecules in sperm.

Seemingly unrelated, these findings all touch upon one underlying aspect: the transmission of genetic and nongenetic (epigenetic) information to the next generation. Although already a topic fascinating for biologists, it gains in medical relevance due to the widespread and increasing use of artificial reproductive techniques (ART). As a consequence, ART babies are often conceived from gametes that in normal reproduction would never have functioned. What are the de novo genetic and epigenetic effects of this type of reproduction? The answer to this question is currently largely unknown, but the new studies yield strong handholds that can guide and focus future research.

Although in ART, the term fertilization is used synonymous to pronucleus formation (2PN), it is actually a more lengthy process that encompasses both cytoplasmic and nuclear fusion, hence includes first cleavage. Fusion between male and female pronuclei is never obtained, only apposition, in the human earlier after gamete fusion than in the mouse. The two chromosome sets do not intermingle at the spindle and only gradually mix in next rounds of cell division [1].

The premise of this chapter is that, in ART, the borders of the normal interaction between gametes are stretched due to the use of gametes that in vivo would never play a role. The biological insight that is required is not readily available as experimental mouse models use normal sperm cells [2–4]. When in the mouse an experimental condition such as unprotected sperm freezing is applied, detrimental phenotypic effects arise [5]. The problem in ART is exacerbated because of the fundamental differences between human spermatogenesis and that of experimental animals (rodents and farm animals) that usually have very homogeneous sperm populations. On the contrary, human sperm, especially in cases of male factor sub- and infertility, is among the most variable cell populations to be found in the body [6].

This chapter will focus mainly on mouse data concerning the remodeling of sperm chromatin by the zygote, particularly during sperm pronucleus formation. Thereafter, repair of DNA damage and removal of DNA methylation will be covered, ending with differences in DNA replication between male and female pronuclei as associated with DNA repair. At the end, we will introduce information from human sperm and embryo culture that can be interpreted against the presented background of mouse data. Although much uncertainty remains, the conclusion is probably justified that the first 26 h of our existence will hallmark our life more than at any other short period of time.

16.2 Male Chromatin Remodeling, Preparation in the Male Germline

Chromatin remodeling during the nuclear elongation phase of spermiogenesis and chromatin remodeling after sperm entry in a number of aspects are mirror images. Loss of nucleosomes, hence histones, and acquiring protamines to stabilize the DNA lead to chromatin condensation needed for sperm formation. Male chromatin decondensation in the zygote involves the reverse order, though at a much higher rate. No protamines, as observed at the level of immune fluorescence (IF), are retained in zygotic male chromatin [7]. Nucleosomes consist of an octamer of four histone molecules, of which each is present twice (two times a H2A-H2B dimer and twice a H3-H4 dimer) and around which 146 bp of DNA is wrapped [8].

Both stages involve Topoisomerase II (TopoII) inflicted DNA-double-strand (dsDNA) breakage and ligation (zygote: [9–11]; elongating spermatids: [12, 13]). During spermiogenesis, a nucleosomal chromatin state is only selectively lost [14–17]. Where protamines dominate, high DNA content doughnut-like toroids are formed [18]. These are believed to encompass only one loop domain of about 50 kb that is attached to a nuclear matrix [19]. The current insight is that as TopoII religates its break [20], most TopoII-induced cuts, needed to alleviate supercoiling of nucleosomal DNA, will not require backing up by other DNA repair systems. The extent of non-ligated TopoII-induced breaks present in elongating spermatids is currently hardly known [21]. PARP-1 and PARG are involved in the regulation of polyribosylation of chromatin proteins in mouse elongating spermatids [22]. This is an argument for active DNA break repair at this stage. In man, PARP activity was established by situ histochemistry on testis sections [23, 24]; the presence of PARP-1, PARP-2, and PARP-9 was determined on sperm by western blotting [25]. Also, transition proteins (that form an intermediary chromatin state after histone shedding [26]) and protamines are supposed to act as DNA-stabilizing factors. Experimental proof for this has been obtained for transition protein 1 [27]. In a classical mouse mutagenesis study, Marchetti and Wyrobek analyzed the effect of diepoxybutane (DEB), a bifuctional alkylating agent that induces inter- and intrastrand DNA crosslinks as the basis of its mutagenicity. DEB is the metabolite of 1,3 butadiene, a tobacco smoke mutagen [28]. Postmeiotic male germ cell stages were exposed and chromosome abnormalities were observed in the zygote at the first cleavage division. In agreement with the standing concept, DNA repair decreases from the onset of chromatin remodeling in elongating spermatid nuclei on until completion of spermiogenesis. Our understanding of DNA metabolism in this important phase of male reproduction is rudimentary. This is illustrated by the reported decline in dsDNA breaks upon inhibition of TopoII beta by etoposide [29]. The anticancer cell drug etoposide inhibits the ligation of the TopoII-induced dsDNA break. In the zygote, and in agreement with expectation, etoposide treatment induced persistent dsDNA breaks [10].

There is no proof for stabilization of free dsDNA ends during the later stages of spermiogenesis, the current opinion being that religation is complete [29]. Techniques to make this an absolute statement are currently lacking. As already mentioned in this section, from human and mouse sperm mutagenesis studies [30–33], it has been deduced that DNA breaks induced at these later remodeling stages and in sperm are not repaired in situ upon induction, but are processed by the oocyte after sperm penetration [34]. The statement that dsDNA break repair is principally impossible in sperm chromatin can, however, not be made, although it is unlikely yet alone for the adaptation of chromatin structure that accompanies DNA repair [35, but see 25]. Methods to measure DNA breaks directly (by neutral and alkaline comet assay, TUNEL assay) and indirectly (by Sperm Chromatin Structure Assay [SCSA] and sperm chromatin dispersion [SCD] tests) are by far not accurate enough to test human sperm for active DNA repair [36, 37].

We do know for a long time that during spermatid nucleus elongation, replacement of nucleosomes by protamines is not complete, less so for the human than for mouse. Before the advent of chromatin immunoprecipitation followed by DNA identification, histones have been determined by gel electrophoresis [14, 38], by IF on artificially expanded sperm nuclei [39, 40], and by IF on the expanding mouse sperm nucleus before and after gamete fusion [41]. The most plausible explanations for their presence are the restoration of the embryonic somatic chromosome architecture [41] and determining gene function towards embryo pattern formation [16, 17].

16.3 Male Chromatin Remodeling, Paternal vs. Maternal Histones

Expansion of sperm chromatin in the oocyte initially involves reduction of the protamine cysteine S-S bridges and acceptance of the shed protamines by an unknown maternal mechanism [42]. For mammalian oocytes, reduced glutathion (GSH) acts as the reductor of protamines, and without this step, no shedding of protamines is possible [43, 44]. In the toad *Xenopus*, the chromatin chaperone nucleoplasmin 2 (NPM2) is implicated in the removal of protamines [45, 46]. When testing this gene by maternal depletion in the mouse [47], no effect on sperm decondensation was shown. Instead, heterochromatin organization around the primary oocyte nucleolus and zygote nucleolus precursor bodies and fusion product (that was absent) failed. In the mouse, no maternal mutation for sperm nuclear decondensation has yet been picked up. As a parallel to the in vitro situation, where heparan and heparan sulfate can decondense the sperm nucleus, Romanato et al. showed the presence of heparan sulfate in the mouse oocyte, suggesting a role in nuclear expansion, as it does in vitro on sperm [48, 49].

When nucleosomes are built on free DNA, histone dimer assembly complexes (also called chaperones) are involved. Some are specific for one of the two major histone 3 (H3) variants contained in the H3–H4 dimer that, as a tetramer, forms the core of the nucleosome [50]. Dimers between H3.1/3.2 and H4 are used during DNA replication; dimers between H3.3 and H4 are used in all other circumstances involving de novo nucleosome assembly such as transcription. HIRA, a replication-independent H3.3–H4 specific chaperone, was found in the mouse remodeling sperm nucleus after gamete fusion (using IF [7]). In line with the absence of DNA replication at this early stage, the male PN did not stain with an antibody specific for H3.1/3.2, which, as expected, was detected at the onset of paternal DNA synthesis [7]. Proof for the exclusive use of H3.3 in male chromatin remodeling was obtained when the corresponding mRNA probe with HA tag was injected in the zygote, and specific staining of the male PN was obtained [51]; for a review on the role of H3.3 in reproduction and development see [52].

As histones are among the most conserved proteins in biology, the mouse-derived H3.1 antibody used above also detects the human protein. The fact that histones are more abundant in human sperm compared to mouse sperm was used to probe for this protein by IF after heterologous ICSI between human sperm and mouse oocytes [15]. H3.1 could be followed in male chromatin up to the start of DNA replication. Thereafter, massive de novo nucleosome formation, using H3.1/H3.2-H4 dimers, obscures the sperm-specific nucleosome signal. These experiments were repeated in human tripronuclear (3PN) zygotes, collected in the early PN stage which is before S-phase. Male and female PNs could easily be recognized on the basis of the density of H3.1 signal, heavier staining being observed in the female PN. Hence, transfer of sperm histones to the male PN was shown again [15, 41]. The meaning of paternal histones for embryo development has received support from the analysis of the epigenome of the human sperm nucleus [16, 17].

From earlier sperm chromatin research, it was already known that nucleosome density could vary within one gene [53]. The advent of chromatin immuno precipitation (CHIP) on chip technology, connecting histone modification with DNA sequence technology, was thereafter used to decipher the whole sperm epigenome, i.e., histone occupancy/density in combination with histone modification [16, 17]. One conclusion is shared: genes that play a role in embryonic cell differentiation and pattern formation and are non-transcribed during the cleavage divisions are under suppression of the Polycomb complex, as deduced by promoters that are more heavily occupied with nucleosomes. The Polycomb signature is picked up because of their H3 N-tail posttranslational modification (PTM). The H3 N-tail mark trimethylation of lysine 27 (H3K27me3) stands for methyltransferase activity of Polycomb repressive complex 2 (PRC2), hence gene suppression by Polycomb repressive complex 1 (PRC1). Contrary to Hammoud and coworkers, Bryszinska and colleges found that nucleosomes were present everywhere in the genome, though at a low density. A regular distribution of histones (i.e., nucleosomes) over the genome would be compatible with the 50 kb spaced sensitivity for endogenous endonucleases in mouse sperm nuclei [19]. Digestion of more open chromatin at matrix-associated regions (MARs), which leads to the indicated regular loop domain representing DNA fragments, is then made possible because of the association between matrix association and nucleosome occupancy. Taking the evidence together, is it highly likely that histones do play a role in the transmission of nuclear information via the male germline, other than by DNA code. The histone landscape of the sperm nucleus also gives testimony to past functioning by showing increased density of nucleosomes at promoter sites of genes involved in spermatogenesis. These nucleosomes were picked up because of the di and trimethylated states of H3 lysine 4 (H3K4me2 and 3), a mark of gene activity [16, 17].

As introduced by the above examples, PTMs, both by general nuclear characterization as obtained by IF and by analysis at the level of the gene, can be used to read the functional status of both the gene and chromatin domains [54–56]. So, different chromatin states, constitutively inactive (heterochromatic) vs. facultatively inactive or active, can be illustrated by PTMs at lysine (K) residues of particularly the N-tails of H3 and 4. When staining by IF for these N-tail modifications, a superficial picture of the overall state of chromatin is obtained, annexed to the development of constitutive heterochromatin that usually is found around the centromeres.

When these methods were applied to mouse zygotes, it was soon apparent that male and female pronuclei greatly differ for H3, H4 lysine methyl PTMs: these are strikingly underrepresented in the male PN [7, 57–59]. This observation is known as the epigenetic asymmetry of the zygote. What happens during the first cleavage divisions, as nicely illustrated by Puschendorf et al., is that the overall histone PTM pattern is equalized between male- and female-derived chromosomes [60]. Theoretically, this agrees with the notion, like for DNA methylation [61, 62], that under the influence of oocyte cytoplasm, male and female chromatin becomes more equal to each other at the onset of cell differentiation from the blastocyst inner cell mass. Epigenetic asymmetry has also been described in human 3 PN zygotes [63].

16.4 Male Chromatin Remodeling, DNA Repair is Involved

The evidence for DNA breaks during paternal chromatin remodeling in the mouse oocyte is based on inhibition of TopoII [9–11]. TopoII beta has been found in the late stage of sperm nucleus remodeling and early female PN. TopoII alpha was not found there, but was abundant on the secondary oocyte metaphase II chromosomes, where TopoII beta was absent [64]. Nucleosome deposition and protamine shedding most likely occur simultaneously and commence within 30 min after gamete fusion [7]. Remodeling starts at the posterior (caudal) side of the sperm nucleus, which first unfolds after fusion with IVF [7] and after ICSI in the Rhesus monkey [65]. As soon as nucleosomes appear, the H2A variant H2AX apparently is incorporated (next to H2A), as gammaH2AX focal staining (the common expression for phosphorylation of H2AX at serine 139) is routinely observed at this stage in the mouse [10]. After an initial stage of chromatin expansion, condensation takes place, a process that can be followed by the H3S10Ph marker [10, 41]. The most likely explanation for this phenomenon is that as male chromatin remodeling occurs, female chromosomes are in anaphase/telophase of the second meiotic division [42]. Male chromatin apparently does not entirely escape the influence of a lowering level of MPF (maturation promoting factor, alias for CDC2/cyclin B). If oocyte activation is incomplete and a metaphase II spindle is maintained, this process ends with premature chromosome condensation (PCC) [66]. The male chromatin contraction phase that normally occurs [42] allows a sharp delineation of large gammaH2AX foci, which are induced by sperm irradiation in a dose-dependent manner [10]. These large foci are taken to represent dsDNA breaks for which gammaH2AX is a chromatin indicator [67, 68]. Large foci are also induced by the inhibition of TopoII religation by etoposide [10]. Also, many small gammaH2A foci can be seen; these are not induced by ionizing irradiation of sperm before entry [10]. The meaning of small gammaHAX foci is uncertain, maybe indicating other DNA irregularities such as bulky DNA lesions that challenge nucleotide excision repair (NER) [69]. An indication for DNA repair of this male stage was found long before, using UV-irradiated mouse sperm, by spotting the uptake of radioactive (3H) Thymidine in the male PN 3–4 h after setting up in vitro fertilization [70]. DNA synthesis is typical for NER that repairs UV-induced DNA helix distortions. Also, very much unlike the situation in somatic nuclei, UV irradiation of sperm before fertilization results into structural chromosome-type abnormalities (the abnormality occurs before S-phase, is doubled during S-phase, and is scored by morphology at first mitosis) [71].

The use of oocyte genotypes that are deficient for specific DNA repair routes can yield unexpected information into the matter of DNA repair in male chromatin remodeling after gamete fusion. Classical DNA.PKcs-dependent nonhomologous end joining (NHEJ), one of the major routes to repair dsDNA breaks [72, 73], usually is tested in hypomorphs of the DNA.PKcs holoenzyme, such as spontaneously found in the BALB/c and C.B17 mouse genetic backgrounds (with 10% activity) [74]. In the C.B17 scid mouse, only residual NHEJ activity remains [75]. These oocyte genotypes show more male gammaH2AX large foci when using the same source of mouse sperm [76]. This effect is exacerbated when sperm is irradiated before IVF. Hence, NHEJ is involved in sperm chromatin remodeling in the mouse. This defect also leads to high levels of chromosome abnormalities at the first cleavage division [76, 77]. The high levels of gammaH2AX foci (around one per nucleus for both control mouse and human sperm [10, 78]), compared to the very low levels in somatic cell nuclei [79], are testimony to the fact that dsDNA repair is a normal event during male chromatin remodeling after gamete fusion.

This high level of foci is an underestimate of the real number of dsDNA breaks dependant on active DNA repair (as contrasted to just TopoII religation). Using the heterologous ICSI model to count gammaH2AX foci of human sperm in mouse oocytes [78], sperm selected by ICSI criteria from normospermic and oligospermic donors was compared. Average levels of foci were about the same. Only the fraction of sperm without foci was smaller in the oligospermic donors. Strikingly abnormal male patterns of gammaH2AX were found when nonmotile sperm was selected. Also, an intense H2AX phosphorylation was often imposed upon female chromatin. This result is one of the warnings against the use of ejaculated nonmotile sperm in human ICSI.

Using heterologous in vitro fertilization and cytogenetic techniques at first cleavage, Tateno et al. [80] showed hamster oocytes to faithfully repair (and misrepair) radiation-induced DNA damage to human sperm, enabling dose–response curves to be made for misrepaired dsDNA breaks that lead to structural chromosomes abnormalities. Human sperm was more irradiation sensitive than were hamster and mouse sperm [30]. More experiments are necessary to monitor chromosomal stability in human fertilization [81]. Unfortunately, the only human zygotes ethically suitable for experimental use, such as monopronuclear and tripronuclear ones, occur at a reduced rate. Most instructive would be studies on zygotes evolving from severe male factor infertility.

It seems that oocyte activation can relate to the fidelity of break repair management during male chromatin remodeling. Using an oligo-astheno-teratozoospermia (OAT) mouse model, Baart et al. [66] observed that after ICSI with cauda epididymal sperm, absence of activation with resulting PCC was relatively common. Often, abnormal male chromosomes were produced with many acentric (without centromere) fragments and composite multicentrics in the same male complement. Both lack of dsDNA break repair and illegitimate religation of breaks had occurred, a cytogenetic picture typical for NHEJ malfunctioning. This result could suggest that oocyte activation by the sperm affects male chromatin remodeling, maybe with implications for DNA repair.

16.5 Paternal DNA Demethylation and DNA Repair at Zygotic G1, Is There a Link?

From mouse mutagenesis studies, we know for long that zygotes at the early PN stage are extremely sensitive to DNA insult [82]. Sensitivity for irradiation increases when the pronuclei have been formed [83] and decreases towards S-phase [84]. Recent research into active paternal demethylation of DNA is shedding some light on this matter, although as expected major uncertainties remain.

By using an antibody against 5 methyl cytosine, in the mouse, the phenomenon of active paternal DNA demethylation after gamate fusion has been discovered [85, 86]. This observation was subsequently proven by bisulfite sequencing [87] and shown to be sequence-specific such that already differences were noted between two types of retrotransposons [88]. Active demethylation also occurs in the human PN [89] and is not genome wide. In mouse and man, methylation of paternal (and also maternal) imprinting control regions (ICRs) is preserved. The demethylation reaction extends over most of the first cell cycle, as shown by an in situ reporter construct [90]. For a period of time now, demethylation has been linked to DNA repair activity [91]. At zygotic Gap1 (G1, pre S-phase) in the mouse, spontaneous gammaH2AX foci only occur in the male PN and never in the female one [10, 76, 88]. At this stage, these foci were found to sharply increase in the male PN in the presence of aphidicolin, an inhibitor of many DNA polymerases [88]. As S-phase has not yet commenced and DNA repair often involves DNA synthesis, this may suggest a DNA repair event associated with the removal of the so-called fifth base (5 methyl cytosine) in order to demethylate CpG dimers in paternal chromatin. In the absence of aphidicolin, DNA synthesis was shown (by an in situ nick translation assay) both at the sperm chromatin remodeling stage (in keeping with the earlier statement that DNA repair is involved with sperm chromatin remodeling) and in the G1 PN [88].

Another interesting observation by Wossidlo and coworkers is colocalization at G1 of the universal DNA repair enzyme PARP-1 with gammaH2AX, in a focal pattern indicative for dsDNA repair. It was subsequently found that a chromatin bound form of the repair enzyme XRCC1, which as PARP-1 can both function in base excision repair (BER) and in DNA.PKcs-independent NHEJ (hence dsDNA repair [92]), is present in the male PN before S-phase, at the time of active demethylation of 5 methyl cytosine [93]. The puzzle of male DNA metabolism at zygote G1 is further enhanced by the BER-inducing mutagen methyl methane sulfonate (MMS), which is capable of strongly enhancing the number of PARP-1 gammaH2AX colocalizations [88]. The mutagenic effect of MMS on mouse sperm is long known [71], leading to chromosome-type abnormalities in the mouse zygote, a result that cannot be explained on the basis of classical somatic cell cytogenetics. Similar to the experiments involving UV-irradiated mouse sperm, in the zygote, repair upon mutagenic treatments that lead to transitory single-strand breaks (which is the case with BER and NER) leads to chromosome-type abnormalities that in somatic nuclei are mainly caused by dsDNA breaks. A further riddle is that after a low dose of 0.5 Gy X-rays, the female G1 PN is more sensitive to the induction of chromosome abnormalities than the male one, a result not expected as spontaneous gammaH2AX foci are absent [10, 83, 88]. Apparently, repair is more directed towards the male PN. Final proof for the involvement of DNA repair with paternal CpG demethylation will await the use of gene knockout mouse models.

Recently, an alternative approach, based on siRNA gene knockout technology for candidate proteins and a reporter construct to stain for unmethylated CpG residues, was developed [90]. By this procedure, proteins involved with RNA polymerase II elongation (i.e., transcription), such as

Elp1, 3 and 4, were found to affect active paternal demethylation.

16.6 A Role for the Zygote in Maintenance of Imprinting

After many years of molecular research into the control mechanisms that ensure monoallelic inheritance from both the mother and the father, the CpG methylation status of the differentially methylated region (DMR) of the imprint control regions (ICRs) has proven to be a reliable indicator of the epigenetic status of the germline. By axioma, the methylation status of the ICR must be resistant to the paternally active and maternally passive demethylation that results into largely demethylated genomes at the blastocyst stage [62]. Hirasawa et al. confirmed this expectation at the blastocyst stage, combining methylation sensitive (bisulfite) sequencing with allele differentiation enabled by an intraspecies mouse cross, using two paternally imprinted ICRs (of the *H19* and *Rasgrf1* gene clusters) and two maternally imprinted ones [94]. When the maintenance DNA methylase DNMT1 was not present in both the oocyte and in the embryo (using a null-allele from the father), the CpG methylation imprint was eradicated [94]. Apart from mechanistic copying of the methylation status during DNA replication, there is active though selective protection of the methylated status at the zygote stage. This has been illustrated in zygotes from oocytes that lack the germ cell-specific protein Stella [95]. Maternal absence of Stella, as observed in late zygotes, affected both maternal and paternal imprints though not systematically. Such embryos develop poorly beyond the maternal to zygote transition (the activation of the embryonic genome) that in the mouse is at the late 2-cell stage and between the 4 and 8-cell stage in the human [96, 97]. Another DNA-interacting protein has recently been discovered (Zfp57, member of a family of transcription factors) that clearly shows a maternal effect as to maintenance of the mCpG mark at the DMR [98]. Both paternally and maternally imprinted ICRs were affected, but as for Stella, not systematically. Zpf57 already affects the methylation status of a maternally imprinted ICR in the oocyte (such as the *Snrpn* gene, linked to the human Prader-Willi and Angelman imprinting syndromes). The gene-specific aspect in protection for demethylation is also illustrated by the fact that for the *H19* DMR, the 5 methyl cytosine-binding protein MBD3 is needed to maintain imprinting during preimplantation development [99].

As expected, matters are more complicated, as has nicely been demonstrated by Terranova and coworkers. Another reflection of the imprinting status is chromatin organization. Around the Beckwith Wiedemann syndrome (*Kcnq1*)-imprinted gene cluster, paternal silencing is already found at the late zygote stage, due to the involvement of Polycomb proteins and histone-repressive PTMs colocalizing with the inactivating RNA transcript [100]. These authors did not determine the CpG methylation status of the ICR (the promoter region of the functional-inactivating Kcnq1ot1 RNA). Summarizing, the message must be that the oocyte is mandatory for fine regulation of imprinting maintenance. In the mouse, the stability of both male and female imprinting maintenance was in a gonadotrophin dose-dependent mode affected by the induction of superovulation [101]. In this light, the increase in imprinting disorders associated with ART is of significance [102].

16.7 Is Zygotic S-Phase a Backup System to Further Repair Male DNA?

The classical cytogenetic outcomes of dsDNA breaks during S-phase and the G2 phase of the cell cycle are chromatid-type chromosome abnormalities in which the chromatid is the unit of breakage. When the break occurs before S-phase, the replication machinery simply copies the abnormality leading to a chromosome-type exchange. When misrepair involves the union of two ends of different chromatids, a so-called chromatid exchange occurs by which four chromatids now adhere (sister segment by sister segment) in a so-called quadriradial. These changes always lead to mosaicsm in the preimplantation embryo. The chromosomal make up of the two daughter blastomeres now depends on the orientation of centromeres in the cleavage spindle, always leading to blastomere inequality for the genetic content of the two involved chromosomes. Derijck et al. [76] observed that extremely low doses of the free radicals generating mutagen 4-nitroquinoline 1-oxide (4NQO) in an oocyte impaired for homologous recombination dsDNA break repair (HRR, by ablation of *Rad54/Rad54B*) resulted into a high incidence of quadriradials, especially in the male PN. This is another indication for the genetic vulnerability of male DNA. This finding nicely combines with the long-standing fact that de novo human reciprocal translocations in great majority are from the male germline [103]. At this moment and incorporating the available information from spermatogenesis, the zygote is the most likely stage at which these occur. Compared with other mammals, the human has a high frequency of de novo occurrence of reciprocal translocations (1:2,000 by classical cytogenetics analysis on amniocentesis cases) [104].

Because the presence of gammaH2AX symbolizes ongoing repair activity, foci on zygote metaphase chromosomes (involving one or two chromatids) means transportation of the repair event to the next cell generation. Using two mutagens on S-phase zygotes, 4NQO and X-rays and maternally defective DNA repair genotypes, it was found that especially targeting HRR yields transmission a majority of male chromatin repair foci to the two-cell stage [76]. Ablation of *Rad54/Rad54b* in combination with these mutagenic treatments leads to a sharp increase of stalled replication forks in especially the male PN, as if the zygote expects problems in male DNA replication mainly [76]. A likewise indication for the sensitivity of male S-phase for obstruction in DNA metabolism was reported by Wossidlo and coworkers in the mouse. At this stage (as in G1), the gammaH2AX focal response to the DNA polymerase inhibitor aphidicolin, indicating stalled replication forks, is much stronger in the male PN than in the female one [88].

Paternal replication problems likely underlie impaired first cleavage in two OAT mouse models that were used for ICSI to study testicular vs. cauda epididymal sperm cells. In the T(1;13)70H/T(1;13)1Wa double translocation heterozygous mouse, a full autosomal meiotic synapsis often is not achieved. The unsynapsed autosomal chromatin then joins the sex body. When using cauda epididymal sperm, the majority (around 70%) of ICSI zygotes blocks in S-phase, the female PN adjusting to the male one that seems more severely affected. This problem is alleviated when testicular sperm is used [66]. The epididymal environment, by for instance ROS (reactive oxygen species), likely causes damage to the sperm nucleus that is fatal at DNA replication. This finding was subsequently confirmed in a mouse model, deficient for transition protein 1 and haploinsufficient for transition protein 2 (Tnp1,Tnp2; –/–, +/–) in which the error occurs during chromatin remodeling at spermatid nuclear elongation [105]. In the reduced amount of metaphase zygotes from cauda epididymal sperm, an elevated rate of chromosome abnormalities was found.

An element that is much overlooked and is predicted to relate to the difference in S-phase behavior between male and female PN is explained in a recent review on male transgenerational epimutation and genetic mutation [106]. Attention is given to the loop domain structure of sperm nuclei that can be interpreted as a prerequisite for zygotic DNA replication as is explained by Lemaitre et al. for *Xenopus* zygotes [107]. A dogma in cell biology is that per loop domain, one origin of replication is active. Hence, the process of DNA replication takes longer when loop domains are big, and shorter when loop domains are small. When the cell experiences difficulty in finishing S-phase, at metaphase an adjustment of loop domains towards shorter ones is made by imposing activity on existing MARs that then also become attached to the scaffold/nuclear matrix [107, 108]. These attachments now are in the memory system of the cell and the corresponding origins of replication will be used in forthcoming S-phases. In this way, differentiation problems of the male gamete could lead to S-phase obstacles in the zygote [106].

16.8 Indications from Human ART for Early Roles of Oocyte and Sperm in Determining Ongoing Embryonic Development

Direct observations on human chromatin remodeling and DNA damage responses in elongating spermatids, remodeling sperm nuclei after gamete fusion, and in pronuclei before, during, and after zygotic S-phase are largely lacking. For zygotes, ethical and legal implications prevent these experiments. However, data on fertilization, embryo development, and pregnancy from ART practice can sometimes be interpreted in the light of mouse experimental data on DNA repair and OAT sperm as presented here. However, seemingly contradictory results and alternative interpretations will remain in this complicated field.

16.8.1 Maternal vs. Paternal Factors

Sperm in situations of male factor infertility is more often not fully protaminated [39, 40, 109]. Earlier, it had been found that in a RNA FISH for protamines 1 and 2, the frequency of "positive" round spermatids was lower for infertile patients [110]. More recently, protamine 1 and 2 RNA levels in mature sperm were found to correlate positively with fertilization success in conventional IVF [111]. The etiology of these observations will have aspects in common with the earlier finding that the two human protamine species P1 and P2 that normally are present in a ratio of between 0.8 and 1.3 (P1/P2, [112–114]) in infertile patients often show deviations in both directions.

Larger ratios outnumber smaller ones [113]. A shortage of P2 relative to P1 has been reported in 40% and a shortage of P1 in 13.6% of infertile patients [114]. Generally, the standard spermiogram values, concentration, motility, and morphology are affected when P1/P2 ratios are deviant [115, 116]. A low level of P1 has more obvious clinical consequences [113, 116], affecting fertilization rates and implantation rates [112, 117]. Also, the presence of preP2 in spermatozoa seems to influence the chance of pregnancy, higher ratios of preP2 to P2 being favorable [112] despite the earlier finding that the level of preP2 positively correlates with the level of sperm DNA damage [118]. Principally, these observations show that the chromatin composition of sperm influences fertilization and implantation (causally or not). DNA damage, found in sperm with deviant P1/P2 ratios, could be one detrimental factor [115, 119]. Of notice, the P1/P2 ratio of prepared sperm of human donors with known fertility (90% PureSperm layer, PS) tends to be lower than 1.0 [120]. This tendency was confirmed by de Mateo et al. [109]. Interestingly, sperm from the 90% PS layer of OAT samples presented with a higher P1/P2 ratio than in fertile controls (1.02 and 0.93, respectively).

In ART literature, early paternal effects are separated from later paternal effects, the later ones suggested to be linked to DNA damage [121]. Mouse data on mutagenized normal sperm cells do agree with this subdivision. In an overview of several mutagens applied to sperm, Marchetti and coworkers calculate that when misrepair in the zygote yields more than four chromosome abnormalities at first cleavage, the result is preimplantation loss, which in the mouse will be apparent as delayed development from the morula stage on [122, 123]. Zygotes with fewer chromosome abnormalities are able to implant and lead to later embryonic death [123]. Irradiation of bull sperm that was subsequently researched in an IVF setup yielded a comparable result. The lowest dose of 1.25 Gy already resulted into embryonic death showing apoptotic blastomeres and leading to a shortage of day 7 blastocysts [124]. In the mouse, the kinetics of the first cleavage division have been reported not to be altered by radiation-induced sperm and early zygote DNA breakage (5 Gy [83, 125]). However, using a dose of 6 Gy and 3H Thymidine uptake to monitor S-phase progression, an effect on DNA replication hence the length of the first cleavage division was found in another mouse strain and shown to be under control of p53 [122, 126]. Mouse data on irradiated sperm can be of relevance for human ART because of the implicated oxidative stress.

Oxydative stress is a prime suspect for causing DNA damage in human sperm [127, 128]. Zini et al. have, in a review and meta analysis, evaluated the existing literature on a possible relation between the level of (directly and indirectly) measured DNA damage in spermatozoa and reproductive outcome in ART. They found the patient sperm DNA damage level to be associated with an increased risk for pregnancy loss [129]. As an argument for a negative role for the epididymal environment including length of storage, testicular sperm has been shown to improve fertility when DNA damage was dominant in ejaculated sperm [130].

Eight-oxoguanine (8-oxoG) is the accepted genotoxic indicator for oxidative DNA stress. In an oocyte donation program to which younger women contributed, the effect of the level of 8-oxoG in the sperm nucleus on embryo development in ART could be determined, not being hindered by variation in oocyte quality. Marked levels of oxidative stress in sperm were found to affect zygotes using PN grading by nucleolus precursor body numbers and positions and were visible in day 3 blastomere symmetry [131]. However, stalled pronuclear development as was found when cauda epididymal sperm from OAT mouse models was used for ICSI [66, 105] is rarely encountered in human ART practice.

Conclusively, sperm nuclear effects, both on the level of DNA and of chromatin protein distribution, can lead to early and late embryonic effects. Early paternal effects of course are also related to centrosome and tubuline aster behavior, which together with oocyte activation could be summed up as the non-nuclear paternal contribution [121, 132], which is of a lesser concern in the context of this review.

In an IVF setting, early zygote/embryo events can be recorded by time lapse microscopy. This technology has been stimulated by the search for early predictors of normal development. The value of zygote PN observation has been touched upon above, but also synchrony of the division from 2 to 4 blastomeres has been used to assess embryo development [133].

One rationale is that when S-phase encounters difficulties in the sphere of DNA management, sperm nuclear structure, this may well lead to delayed first cleavage as in human ART pronuclear blocks are rare. In many laboratories, indications for the value of early first cleavage for predicting pregnancy have been obtained [134–140]. Direct demonstration of a longer duration of DNA replication would involve a difference in the frequency of stalled replication forks between early and late cleavage human embryos. Of note here is that corrected for the lag phase of sperm entry in IVF, the first cell cycle in IVF is 1 h longer than an ICSI cycle (27 vs. 26 h) [141]. Also, differences between IVF and ICSI have been observed around the second cleavage division that is less synchronous after ICSI [141]. Nevertheless, and despite the value of synchrony of cleavage for reproductive success [132, 133] and the expected larger load of detrimental paternal factors with ICSI, no differences in efficiency between IVF vs. ICSI have been found.

This leads to the paradox in ART. On a casuistic basis, there is almost no limit to the source of the sperm cell (testis, epididymis, ejaculate), and within certain margins with respect to head morphology and motility, to achieve reproductive success [140, 142–145]. On the other hand, male inheritance assumes a more differentiated landscape, with the likely involvement of histone occupancy, the presence of microRNA species [146], and DNA damage to affect heredity. These aspects, for instance DNA damage, may well be more serious at older age [23, 147] as is also indicated by an oocyte donation program that avoids bias for the maternal factor [148, 149].

16.9 Conclusion

This review serves to show to what extent DNA and chromatin remodeling is occurring in late spermiogenesis and in the zygote. Roles for male and female gametes are strikingly divided. There are many indications that more male information is transferred than purely genetically defined. No formal proof for a role of nucleosomes with histone code in male transmission is yet available, although the circumstantial evidence for such a function is apparent. Further research must show the significance of other information carriers such as small RNA species and nucleus loop domain organization.

From the active role of the oocyte in the remodeling of sperm chromatin annex DNA repair, it follows that male–female interaction is important for the correct transmission of genetic material [76, 77]. Next to a role shortly after gamete fusion, DNA repair is likely involved with the active demethylation of paternal mCpG sequences. Also, the paternal chromatin structure must allow faithful replication of male DNA. The male nucleus changes that are involved, for instance, the adaptation of loop domains for DNA replication, are presently beyond our insight. On the female part, DNA repair functions are important for allowing normal embryonic development and for limiting the mutational load. A female role for epigenetic processing of male chromatin has always been expected and now has been proven in the mouse [60]. The understanding of gamete interaction as to chromatin processing to enable embryonic development is only just emerging. It would be wise when more attention is given to the genetic [150] and epigenetic [151, 152] variability by performing whole genome scans in both terrains in children born after ART.

Acknowledgments Godfried van der Heijden is thanked for comments on the setup of this chapter and Marieke de Vries for final comments and checking the text.

References

1. Mayer W, Smith A, Fundele R, Haaf T. Spatial separation of parental genomes in preimplantation mouse embryos. J Cell Biol. 2000;148(4):629–34.
2. Li MW, Willis BJ, Griffey SM, Spearow JL, Lloyd KC. Assessment of three generations of mice derived by ICSI using freeze-dried sperm. Zygote (Cambridge, England). 2009;17(3):239–51.
3. Caperton L, Murphey P, Yamazaki Y, et al. Assisted reproductive technologies do not alter mutation frequency or spectrum. Proc Natl Acad Sci USA. 2007; 104(12):5085–90.
4. Kimura Y, Yanagimachi R. Intracytoplasmic sperm injection in the mouse. Biol Reprod. 1995;52(4): 709–20.
5. Fernandez-Gonzalez R, Moreira PN, Perez-Crespo M, et al. Long-term effects of mouse intracytoplasmic sperm injection with DNA-fragmented sperm on health and behavior of adult offspring. Biol Reprod. 2008;78(4):761–72.
6. Lewis SE. Is sperm evaluation useful in predicting human fertility? Reproduction (Cambridge, England). 2007;134(1):31–40.
7. van der Heijden GW, Dieker JW, Derijck AA, et al. Asymmetry in histone H3 variants and lysine methylation between paternal and maternal chromatin of the early mouse zygote. Mech Dev. 2005;122(9):1008–22.
8. Bernstein E, Hake SB. The nucleosome: a little variation goes a long way. Biochem Cell Biol. 2006;84(4): 505–17.
9. Bizzaro D, Manicardi G, Bianchi PG, Sakkas D. Sperm decondensation during fertilisation in the mouse: presence of DNase I hypersensitive sites in situ and a putative role for topoisomerase II. Zygote (Cambridge, England). 2000;8(3):197–202.
10. Derijck AA, van der Heijden GW, Giele M, Philippens ME, VanBavel CC, de Boer P. gammaH2AX signalling during sperm chromatin remodelling in the mouse zygote. DNA Repair. 2006;5(8):959–71.
11. Tateno H, Kamiguchi Y. Chromosome analysis of mouse one-cell androgenones derived from a sperm nucleus exposed to topoisomerase II inhibitors at pre- and post-fertilization stages. Mutat Res. 2004; 556(1–2):117–26.
12. Laberge RM, Boissonneault G. On the nature and origin of DNA strand breaks in elongating spermatids. Biol Reprod. 2005;73(2):289–96.
13. McPherson SM, Longo FJ. Nicking of rat spermatid and spermatozoa DNA: possible involvement of DNA topoisomerase II. Dev Biol. 1993;158(1):122–30.
14. Gatewood JM, Cook GR, Balhorn R, Schmid CW, Bradbury EM. Isolation of four core histones from human sperm chromatin representing a minor subset of somatic histones. J Biol Chem. 1990;265(33):20662–6.
15. van der Heijden GW, Ramos L, Baart EB, et al. Sperm-derived histones contribute to zygotic chromatin in humans. BMC Dev Biol. 2008;8:34.
16. Hammoud SS, Nix DA, Zhang H, Purwar J, Carrell DT, Cairns BR. Distinctive chromatin in human sperm packages genes for embryo development. Nature. 2009;460(7254):473–8.
17. Brykczynska U, Hisano M, Erkek S, et al. Repressive and active histone methylation mark distinct promoters in human and mouse spermatozoa. Nat Struct Mol Biol. 2010;17(6):679–87.
18. Vilfan ID, Conwell CC, Hud NV. Formation of native-like mammalian sperm cell chromatin with folded bull protamine. J Biol Chem. 2004;279(19):20088–95.

19. Ward WS. Function of sperm chromatin structural elements in fertilization and development. Mol Hum Reprod. 2010;16(1):30–6.
20. Pommier Y, Leo E, Zhang H, Marchand C. DNA topoisomerases and their poisoning by anticancer and antibacterial drugs. Chem Biol. 2010;17(5):421–33.
21. Leduc F, Maquennehan V, Nkoma GB, Boissonneault G. DNA damage response during chromatin remodeling in elongating spermatids of mice. Biol Reprod. 2008;78(2):324–32.
22. Meyer-Ficca ML, Lonchar J, Credidio C, et al. Disruption of poly(ADP-ribose) homeostasis affects spermiogenesis and sperm chromatin integrity in mice. Biol Reprod. 2009;81(1):46–55.
23. El-Domyati MM, Al-Din AB, Barakat MT, El-Fakahany HM, Xu J, Sakkas D. Deoxyribonucleic acid repair and apoptosis in testicular germ cells of aging fertile men: the role of the poly(adenosine diphosphate-ribosyl)ation pathway. Fertil Steril. 2009;91(5 Suppl):2221–9.
24. Maymon BB, Cohen-Armon M, Yavetz H, et al. Role of poly(ADP-ribosyl)ation during human spermatogenesis. Fertil Steril. 2006;86(5):1402–7.
25. Jha R, Agarwal A, Mahfouz R, et al. Determination of Poly (ADP-ribose) polymerase (PARP) homologues in human ejaculated sperm and its correlation with sperm maturation. Fertil Steril. 2009;91(3):782–90.
26. Eirin-Lopez JM, Ausio J. Origin and evolution of chromosomal sperm proteins. Bioessays. 2009; 31(10):1062–70.
27. Levesque D, Veilleux S, Caron N, Boissonneault G. Architectural DNA-binding properties of the spermatidal transition proteins 1 and 2. Biochem Biophys Res Commun. 1998;252(3):602–9.
28. Marchetti F, Wyrobek AJ. DNA repair decline during mouse spermiogenesis results in the accumulation of heritable DNA damage. DNA Repair. 2008;7(4): 572–81.
29. Leduc F, Nkoma GB, Boissonneault G. Spermiogenesis and DNA repair: a possible etiology of human infertility and genetic disorders. Syst Biol Reprod Med. 2008;54(1):3–10.
30. Kamiguchi Y, Tateno H. Radiation- and chemical-induced structural chromosome aberrations in human spermatozoa. Mutat Res. 2002;504(1–2):183–91.
31. Matsuda Y, Yamada T, Tobari I. Studies on chromosome aberrations in the eggs of mice fertilized in vitro after irradiation. I. Chromosome aberrations induced in sperm after X-irradiation. Mutat Res. 1985; 148(1–2):113–7.
32. Matsuda Y, Tobari I. Repair capacity of fertilized mouse eggs for X-ray damage induced in sperm and mature oocytes. Mutat Res. 1989;210(1):35–47.
33. van Loon AA, Sonneveld E, Hoogerbrugge J, et al. Induction and repair of DNA single-strand breaks and DNA base damage at different cellular stages of spermatogenesis of the hamster upon in vitro exposure to ionizing radiation. Mutat Res. 1993;294(2):139–48.
34. Marchetti F, Wyrobek AJ. Mechanisms and consequences of paternally-transmitted chromosomal abnormalities. Birth Defects Res C Embryo Today. 2005;75(2):112–29.
35. Svetlova MP, Solovjeva LV, Tomilin NV. Mechanism of elimination of phosphorylated histone H2AX from chromatin after repair of DNA double-strand breaks. Mutat Res. 2010;685(1–2):54–60.
36. Barratt CL, Aitken RJ, Bjorndahl L, et al. Sperm DNA: organization, protection and vulnerability: from basic science to clinical applications – a position report. Hum Reprod (Oxford, England). 2010;25(4):824–38.
37. Santiso R, Muriel L, Goyanes V, Segrelles E, Gosalvez J, Fernandez JL. Evidence of modified nuclear protein matrix in human spermatozoa with fragmented deoxyribonucleic acid. Fertil Steril. 2007;87(1):191–4.
38. Gatewood JM, Cook GR, Balhorn R, Bradbury EM, Schmid CW. Sequence-specific packaging of DNA in human sperm chromatin. Science (New York, NY). 1987;236(4804):962–4.
39. Ramos L, van der Heijden GW, Derijck A, et al. Incomplete nuclear transformation of human spermatozoa in oligo-astheno-teratospermia: characterization by indirect immunofluorescence of chromatin and thiol status. Hum Reprod (Oxford, England). 2008; 23(2):259–70.
40. Zhang X, San Gabriel M, Zini A. Sperm nuclear histone to protamine ratio in fertile and infertile men: evidence of heterogeneous subpopulations of spermatozoa in the ejaculate. J Androl. 2006;27(3):414–20.
41. van der Heijden GW, Derijck AA, Ramos L, Giele M, van der Vlag J, de Boer P. Transmission of modified nucleosomes from the mouse male germline to the zygote and subsequent remodeling of paternal chromatin. Dev Biol. 2006;298(2):458–69.
42. McLay DW, Clarke HJ. Remodelling the paternal chromatin at fertilization in mammals. Reproduction (Cambridge, England). 2003;125(5):625–33.
43. Perreault SD, Barbee RR, Slott VL. Importance of glutathione in the acquisition and maintenance of sperm nuclear decondensing activity in maturing hamster oocytes. Dev Biol. 1988;125(1):181–6.
44. Perreault SD, Wolff RA, Zirkin BR. The role of disulfide bond reduction during mammalian sperm nuclear decondensation in vivo. Dev Biol. 1984;101(1):160–7.
45. Philpott A, Leno GH, Laskey RA. Sperm decondensation in Xenopus egg cytoplasm is mediated by nucleoplasmin. Cell. 1991;65(4):569–78.
46. Ohsumi K, Katagiri C. Characterization of the ooplasmic factor inducing decondensation of and protamine removal from toad sperm nuclei: involvement of nucleoplasmin. Dev Biol. 1991;148(1):295–305.
47. Burns KH, Viveiros MM, Ren Y, et al. Roles of NPM2 in chromatin and nucleolar organization in oocytes and embryos. Science (New York, NY). 2003;300(5619):633–6.
48. Romanato M, Cameo MS, Bertolesi G, Baldini C, Calvo JC, Calvo L. Heparan sulphate: a putative decondensing agent for human spermatozoa in vivo. Hum Reprod (Oxford, England). 2003;18(9):1868–73.
49. Romanato M, Julianelli V, Zappi M, Calvo L, Calvo JC. The presence of heparan sulfate in the mammalian

oocyte provides a clue to human sperm nuclear decondensation in vivo. Hum Reprod (Oxford, England). 2008;23(5):1145–50.
50. Margueron R, Reinberg D. Chromatin structure and the inheritance of epigenetic information. Nat Rev. 2010;11(4):285–96.
51. Torres-Padilla ME, Bannister AJ, Hurd PJ, Kouzarides T, Zernicka-Goetz M. Dynamic distribution of the replacement histone variant H3.3 in the mouse oocyte and preimplantation embryos. Int J Dev Biol. 2006;50(5):455–61.
52. Orsi GA, Couble P, Loppin B. Epigenetic and replacement roles of histone variant H3.3 in reproduction and development. Int J Dev Biol. 2009;53(2–3):231–43.
53. Gardiner-Garden M, Ballesteros M, Gordon M, Tam PP. Histone- and protamine-DNA association: conservation of different patterns within the beta-globin domain in human sperm. Mol Cell Biol. 1998;18(6): 3350–6.
54. Peters AH, Schubeler D. Methylation of histones: playing memory with DNA. Curr Opin Cell Biol. 2005;17(2):230–8.
55. Berger SL. The complex language of chromatin regulation during transcription. Nature. 2007;447(7143): 407–12.
56. Cheng X, Blumenthal RM. Coordinated chromatin control: structural and functional linkage of DNA and histone methylation. Biochemistry. 2010;49(14): 2999–3008.
57. Lepikhov K, Walter J. Differential dynamics of histone H3 methylation at positions K4 and K9 in the mouse zygote. BMC Dev Biol. 2004;4:12.
58. Liu H, Kim JM, Aoki F. Regulation of histone H3 lysine 9 methylation in oocytes and early pre-implantation embryos. Development (Cambridge, England). 2004;131(10):2269–80.
59. Ooi SL, Henikoff S. Germline histone dynamics and epigenetics. Curr Opin Cell Biol. 2007;19(3):257–65.
60. Puschendorf M, Terranova R, Boutsma E, et al. PRC1 and Suv39h specify parental asymmetry at constitutive heterochromatin in early mouse embryos. Nat Genet. 2008;40(4):411–20.
61. Corry GN, Tanasijevic B, Barry ER, Krueger W, Rasmussen TP. Epigenetic regulatory mechanisms during preimplantation development. Birth Defects Res C Embryo Today. 2009;87(4):297–313.
62. Weaver JR, Susiarjo M, Bartolomei MS. Imprinting and epigenetic changes in the early embryo. Mamm Genome. 2009;20(9–10):532–43.
63. van der Heijden GW, van den Berg IM, Baart EB, Derijck AA, Martini E, de Boer P. Parental origin of chromatin in human monopronuclear zygotes revealed by asymmetric histone methylation patterns, differs between IVF and ICSI. Mol Reprod Dev. 2009;76(1): 101–8.
64. St Pierre J, Wright DJ, Rowe TC, Wright SJ. DNA topoisomerase II distribution in mouse preimplantation embryos. Mol Reprod Dev. 2002;61(3):335–46.
65. Ramalho Santos J, Sutovsky P, Simerly C, et al. ICSI choreography: fate of sperm structures after monospermic rhesus ICSI and first cell cycle implications. Hum Reprod (Oxford, England). 2000;15(12): 2610–20.
66. Baart EB, van der Heijden GW, van der Hoeven FA, Bakker R, Cooper TG, de Boer P. Reduced oocyte activation and first cleavage rate after ICSI with spermatozoa from a sterile mouse chromosome mutant. Hum Reprod (Oxford, England). 2004;19(5):1140–7.
67. Rogakou EP, Pilch DR, Orr AH, Ivanova VS, Bonner WM. DNA double-stranded breaks induce histone H2AX phosphorylation on serine 139. J Biol Chem. 1998;273(10):5858–68.
68. Rogakou EP, Boon C, Redon C, Bonner WM. Megabase chromatin domains involved in DNA double-strand breaks in vivo. J Cell Biol. 1999;146(5):905–16.
69. Ray A, Mir SN, Wani G, et al. Human SNF5/INI1, a component of the human SWI/SNF chromatin remodeling complex, promotes nucleotide excision repair by influencing ATM recruitment and downstream H2AX phosphorylation. Mol Cell Biol. 2009;29(23): 6206–19.
70. Brandriff B, Pedersen RA. Repair of the ultraviolet-irradiated male genome in fertilized mouse eggs. Science (New York, NY). 1981;211(4489):1431–3.
71. Matsuda Y, Tobari I. Chromosomal analysis in mouse eggs fertilized in vitro with sperm exposed to ultraviolet light (UV) and methyl and ethyl methanesulfonate (MMS and EMS). Mutat Res. 1988;198(1): 131–44.
72. Hartlerode AJ, Scully R. Mechanisms of double-strand break repair in somatic mammalian cells. Biochem J. 2009;423(2):157–68.
73. Iliakis G. Backup pathways of NHEJ in cells of higher eukaryotes: cell cycle dependence. Radiother Oncol. 2009;92(3):310–5.
74. Okayasu R, Suetomi K, Yu Y, et al. A deficiency in DNA repair and DNA-PKcs expression in the radiosensitive BALB/c mouse. Cancer Res. 2000;60(16): 4342–5.
75. Biedermann KA, Sun JR, Giaccia AJ, Tosto LM, Brown JM. scid mutation in mice confers hypersensitivity to ionizing radiation and a deficiency in DNA double-strand break repair. Proc Natl Acad Sci USA. 1991;88(4):1394–7.
76. Derijck A, van der Heijden G, Giele M, Philippens M, de Boer P. DNA double-strand break repair in parental chromatin of mouse zygotes, the first cell cycle as an origin of de novo mutation. Hum Mol Genet. 2008;17(13):1922–37.
77. Marchetti F, Essers J, Kanaar R, Wyrobek AJ. Disruption of maternal DNA repair increases sperm-derived chromosomal aberrations. Proc Natl Acad Sci USA. 2007;104(45):17725–9.
78. Derijck AA, van der Heijden GW, Ramos L, Giele M, Kremer JA, de Boer P. Motile human normozoospermic and oligozoospermic semen samples show a difference in double-strand DNA break incidence. Hum Reprod (Oxford, England). 2007;22(9):2368–76.
79. Rothkamm K, Lobrich M. Evidence for a lack of DNA double-strand break repair in human cells

exposed to very low x-ray doses. Proc Natl Acad Sci USA. 2003;100(9):5057–62.
80. Tateno H, Kamiguchi Y, Watanabe S, Mikamo K, Sawada S. Relative biological effectiveness (RBE) of 252Cf fission neutrons for the induction of chromosome damage in human spermatozoa. Int J Radiat Biol. 1996;70(2):229–35.
81. Vanneste E, Voet T, Le Caignec C, et al. Chromosome instability is common in human cleavage-stage embryos. Nat Med. 2009;15(5):577–83.
82. Russel L, Saylors C. The relative sensitivity of various germcell stages of the mouse to radiation induced non-disjunction, chromosome losses and deficiencies. In: Sobels F, editor. Repair from genetic radiation damage and differential radiosensibility in germ cells. Oxford: Pergamon Press; 1963. p. 313–40.
83. Matsuda Y, Seki N, Utsugi-Takeuchi T, Tobari I. Changes in X-ray sensitivity of mouse eggs from fertilization to the early pronuclear stage, and their repair capacity. Int J Radiat Biol. 1989;55(2):233–56.
84. Grinfeld S, Jacquet P. An unusual radiation-induced G2 arrest in the zygote of the BALB/c mouse strain. Int J Radiat Biol Relat Stud Phys Chem Med. 1987;51(2):353–63.
85. Mayer W, Niveleau A, Walter J, Fundele R, Haaf T. Demethylation of the zygotic paternal genome. Nature. 2000;403(6769):501–2.
86. Santos F, Hendrich B, Reik W, Dean W. Dynamic reprogramming of DNA methylation in the early mouse embryo. Dev Biol. 2002;241(1):172–82.
87. Oswald J, Engemann S, Lane N, et al. Active demethylation of the paternal genome in the mouse zygote. Curr Biol. 2000;10(8):475–8.
88. Wossidlo M, Arand J, Sebastiano V, et al. Dynamic link of DNA demethylation, DNA strand breaks and repair in mouse zygotes. EMBO J. 2010;29(11): 1877–88.
89. Beaujean N, Hartshorne G, Cavilla J, et al. Non-conservation of mammalian preimplantation methylation dynamics. Curr Biol. 2004;14(7):R266–7.
90. Okada Y, Yamagata K, Hong K, Wakayama T, Zhang Y. A role for the elongator complex in zygotic paternal genome demethylation. Nature. 2010;463(7280): 554–8.
91. Reik W. Stability and flexibility of epigenetic gene regulation in mammalian development. Nature. 2007;447(7143):425–32.
92. Audebert M, Salles B, Weinfeld M, Calsou P. Involvement of polynucleotide kinase in a poly(ADP-ribose) polymerase-1-dependent DNA double-strand breaks rejoining pathway. J Mol Biol. 2006;356(2): 257–65.
93. Hajkova P, Jeffries SJ, Lee C, Miller N, Jackson SP, Surani MA. Genome-wide reprogramming in the mouse germ line entails the base excision repair pathway. Science. 2010;329(5987):78–82.
94. Hirasawa R, Chiba H, Kaneda M, et al. Maternal and zygotic Dnmt1 are necessary and sufficient for the maintenance of DNA methylation imprints during preimplantation development. Genes Dev. 2008; 22(12):1607–16.
95. Nakamura T, Arai Y, Umehara H, et al. PGC7/Stella protects against DNA demethylation in early embryogenesis. Nat Cell Biol. 2007;9(1):64–71.
96. Stitzel ML, Seydoux G. Regulation of the oocyte-to-zygote transition. Science (New York NY). 2007; 316(5823):407–8.
97. Braude P, Bolton V, Moore S. Human gene expression first occurs between the four- and eight-cell stages of preimplantation development. Nature. 1988;332(6163):459–61.
98. Li X, Ito M, Zhou F, et al. A maternal-zygotic effect gene, Zfp57, maintains both maternal and paternal imprints. Dev Cell. 2008;15(4):547–57.
99. Reese KJ, Lin S, Verona RI, Schultz RM, Bartolomei MS. Maintenance of paternal methylation and repression of the imprinted H19 gene requires MBD3. PLoS Genet. 2007;3(8):e137.
100. Terranova R, Yokobayashi S, Stadler MB, et al. Polycomb group proteins Ezh2 and Rnf2 direct genomic contraction and imprinted repression in early mouse embryos. Dev Cell. 2008;15(5):668–79.
101. Market-Velker BA, Zhang L, Magri LS, Bonvissuto AC, Mann MR. Dual effects of superovulation: loss of maternal and paternal imprinted methylation in a dose-dependent manner. Hum Mol Genet. 2010; 19(1):36–51.
102. Amor DJ, Halliday J. A review of known imprinting syndromes and their association with assisted reproduction technologies. Hum Reprod (Oxford, England). 2008;23(12):2826–34.
103. Chandley AC. On the parental origin of de novo mutation in man. J Med Genet. 1991;28(4):217–23.
104. Warburton D. De novo balanced chromosome rearrangements and extra marker chromosomes identified at prenatal diagnosis: clinical significance and distribution of breakpoints. Am J Hum Genet. 1991;49(5):995–1013.
105. Suganuma R, Yanagimachi R, Meistrich ML. Decline in fertility of mouse sperm with abnormal chromatin during epididymal passage as revealed by ICSI. Hum Reprod (Oxford, England). 2005;20(11):3101–8.
106. de Boer P, Ramos L, de Vries M, Gochhait S. Memoirs of an insult: sperm as a possible source of transgenerational epimutations and genetic instability. Mol Hum Reprod. 2010;16(1):48–56.
107. Lemaitre JM, Danis E, Pasero P, Vassetzky Y, Mechali M. Mitotic remodeling of the replicon and chromosome structure. Cell. 2005;123(5):787–801.
108. Courbet S, Gay S, Arnoult N, et al. Replication fork movement sets chromatin loop size and origin choice in mammalian cells. Nature. 2008;455(7212):557–60.
109. de Mateo S, Ramos L, van der Vlag J, de Boer P, Oliva R. Improvement in chromatin maturity of human spermatozoa selected through density gradient centrifugation. Int J Androl. 20 June, 2010.
110. Steger K, Failing K, Klonisch T, et al. Round spermatids from infertile men exhibit decreased protamine-1 and -2 mRNA. Hum Reprod (Oxford, England). 2001;16(4):709–16.

111. Depa-Martynow M, Kempisty B, Lianeri M, Jagodzinski PP, Jedrzejczak P. Association between fertilin beta, protamines 1 and 2 and spermatid-specific linker histone H1-like protein mRNA levels, fertilization ability of human spermatozoa, and quality of preimplantation embryos. Folia Histochem Cytobiol. 2007;45 (Suppl) 1:S79–85.
112. de Mateo S, Gazquez C, Guimera M, et al. Protamine 2 precursors (Pre-P2), protamine 1 to protamine 2 ratio (P1/P2), and assisted reproduction outcome. Fertil Steril. 2009;91(3):715–22.
113. Oliva R. Protamines and male infertility. Hum Reprod Update. 2006;12(4):417–35.
114. Aoki VW, Liu L, Carrell DT. Identification and evaluation of a novel sperm protamine abnormality in a population of infertile males. Hum Reprod (Oxford, England). 2005;20(5):1298–306.
115. Aoki VW, Emery BR, Liu L, Carrell DT. Protamine levels vary between individual sperm cells of infertile human males and correlate with viability and DNA integrity. J Androl. 2006;27(6):890–8.
116. Carrell DT, Emery BR, Hammoud S. Altered protamine expression and diminished spermatogenesis: what is the link? Hum Reprod Update. 2007;13(3):313–27.
117. Aoki VW, Liu L, Jones KP, et al. Sperm protamine 1/protamine 2 ratios are related to in vitro fertilization pregnancy rates and predictive of fertilization ability. Fertil Steril. 2006;86(5):1408–15.
118. Torregrosa N, Dominguez-Fandos D, Camejo MI, et al. Protamine 2 precursors, protamine 1/protamine 2 ratio, DNA integrity and other sperm parameters in infertile patients. Hum Reprod (Oxford England). 2006;21(8):2084–9.
119. Aoki VW, Moskovtsev SI, Willis J, Liu L, Mullen JB, Carrell DT. DNA integrity is compromised in protamine-deficient human sperm. J Androl. 2005;26(6):741–8.
120. Hammoud S, Liu L, Carrell DT. Protamine ratio and the level of histone retention in sperm selected from a density gradient preparation. Andrologia. 2009;41(2):88–94.
121. Tesarik J, Greco E, Mendoza C. Late, but not early, paternal effect on human embryo development is related to sperm DNA fragmentation. Hum Reprod (Oxford, England). 2004;19(3):611–5.
122. Toyoshima M. Analysis of p53 dependent damage response in sperm-irradiated mouse embryos. J Radiat Res. 2009;50(1):11–7.
123. Marchetti F, Bishop JB, Cosentino L, Moore II D, Wyrobek AJ. Paternally transmitted chromosomal aberrations in mouse zygotes determine their embryonic fate. Biol Reprod. 2004;70(3):616–24.
124. Fatehi AN, Bevers MM, Schoevers E, Roelen BA, Colenbrander B, Gadella BM. DNA damage in bovine sperm does not block fertilization and early embryonic development but induces apoptosis after the first cleavages. J Androl. 2006;27(2):176–88.
125. Ahmadi A, Ng SC. Developmental capacity of damaged spermatozoa. Hum Reprod (Oxford, England). 1999;14(9):2279–85.
126. Shimura T, Inoue M, Taga M, et al. p53-dependent S-phase damage checkpoint and pronuclear cross talk in mouse zygotes with X-irradiated sperm. Mol Cell Biol. 2002;22(7):2220–8.
127. Aitken RJ, De Iuliis GN. Origins and consequences of DNA damage in male germ cells. Reprod Biomed Online. 2007;14(6):727–33.
128. Aitken RJ, De Iuliis GN. On the possible origins of DNA damage in human spermatozoa. Mol Hum Reprod. 2010;16(1):3–13.
129. Zini A, Boman JM, Belzile E, Ciampi A. Sperm DNA damage is associated with an increased risk of pregnancy loss after IVF and ICSI: systematic review and meta-analysis. Hum Reprod (Oxford, England). 2008;23(12):2663–8.
130. Greco E, Scarselli F, Iacobelli M, et al. Efficient treatment of infertility due to sperm DNA damage by ICSI with testicular spermatozoa. Hum Reprod (Oxford, England). 2005;20(1):226–30.
131. Meseguer M, Martinez-Conejero JA, O'Connor JE, Pellicer A, Remohi J, Garrido N. The significance of sperm DNA oxidation in embryo development and reproductive outcome in an oocyte donation program: a new model to study a male infertility prognostic factor. Fertil Steril. 2008;89(5):1191–9.
132. Barroso G, Valdespin C, Vega E, et al. Developmental sperm contributions: fertilization and beyond. Fertil Steril. 2009;92(3):835–48.
133. Scott L, Finn A, O'Leary T, McLellan S, Hill J. Morphologic parameters of early cleavage-stage embryos that correlate with fetal development and delivery: prospective and applied data for increased pregnancy rates. Hum Reprod (Oxford, England). 2007;22(1):230–40.
134. Ciray HN, Karagenc L, Ulug U, Bener F, Bahceci M. Use of both early cleavage and day 2 mononucleation to predict embryos with high implantation potential in intracytoplasmic sperm injection cycles. Fertil Steril. 2005;84(5):1411–6.
135. Tsai YC, Chung MT, Sung YH, Tsai TF, Tsai YT, Lin LY. Clinical value of early cleavage embryo. Int J Gynaecol Obstet. 2002;76(3):293–7.
136. Van Montfoort AP, Dumoulin JC, Kester AD, Evers JL. Early cleavage is a valuable addition to existing embryo selection parameters: a study using single embryo transfers. Hum Reprod (Oxford, England). 2004;19(9):2103–8.
137. Fu J, Wang XJ, Wang YW, Sun J, Gemzell-Danielsson K, Sun XX. The influence of early cleavage on embryo developmental potential and IVF/ICSI outcome. J Assist Reprod Genet. 2009;26(8):437–41.
138. Fenwick J, Platteau P, Murdoch AP, Herbert M. Time from insemination to first cleavage predicts

developmental competence of human preimplantation embryos in vitro. Hum Reprod (Oxford England). 2002;17(2):407–12.

139. Sakkas D, Percival G, D'Arcy Y, Sharif K, Afnan M. Assessment of early cleaving in vitro fertilized human embryos at the 2-cell stage before transfer improves embryo selection. Fertil Steril. 2001;76(6):1150–6.
140. Lundin K, Bergh C, Hardarson T. Early embryo cleavage is a strong indicator of embryo quality in human IVF. Hum Reprod (Oxford, England). 2001;16(12):2652–7.
141. Lemmen JG, Agerholm I, Ziebe S. Kinetic markers of human embryo quality using time-lapse recordings of IVF/ICSI-fertilized oocytes. Reprod Biomed Online. 2008;17(3):385–91.
142. Barros A, Sousa M, Oliveira C, Silva J, Almeida V, Beires J. Pregnancy and birth after intracytoplasmic sperm injection with totally immotile sperm recovered from the ejaculate. Fertil Steril. 1997;67(6):1091–4.
143. McKenzie LJ, Kovanci E, Amato P, Cisneros P, Lamb D, Carson SA. Pregnancy outcome of in vitro fertilization/intracytoplasmic sperm injection with profound teratospermia. Fertil Steril. 2004;82(4):847–9.
144. Tejera A, Molla M, Muriel L, Remohi J, Pellicer A, De Pablo JL. Successful pregnancy and childbirth after intracytoplasmic sperm injection with calcium ionophore oocyte activation in a globozoospermic patient. Fertil Steril. 2008;90(4):1202.e1–5.
145. Gandini L, Lombardo F, Paoli D, et al. Full-term pregnancies achieved with ICSI despite high levels of sperm chromatin damage. Hum Reprod (Oxford, England). 2004;19(6):1409–17.
146. Filkowski JN, Ilnytskyy Y, Tamminga J, et al. Hypomethylation and genome instability in the germline of exposed parents and their progeny is associated with altered miRNA expression. Carcinogenesis. 2010;31(6):1110–5.
147. Wyrobek AJ, Eskenazi B, Young S, et al. Advancing age has differential effects on DNA damage, chromatin integrity, gene mutations, and aneuploidies in sperm. Proc Natl Acad Sci USA. 2006;103(25):9601–6.
148. Ferreira RC, Braga DP, Bonetti TC, Pasqualotto FF, Iaconelli Jr A, Borges Jr E. Negative influence of paternal age on clinical intracytoplasmic sperm injection cycle outcomes in oligozoospermic patients. Fertil Steril. 2010;93(6):1870–4.
149. Frattarelli JL, Miller KA, Miller BT, Elkind-Hirsch K, Scott Jr RT. Male age negatively impacts embryo development and reproductive outcome in donor oocyte assisted reproductive technology cycles. Fertil Steril. 2008;90(1):97–103.
150. Woldringh GH, Janssen IM, Hehir-Kwa JY, et al. Constitutional DNA copy number changes in ICSI children. Hum Reprod (Oxford, England). 2009; 24(1):233–40.
151. Ceelen M, van Weissenbruch MM, Prein J, et al. Growth during infancy and early childhood in relation to blood pressure and body fat measures at age 8-18 years of IVF children and spontaneously conceived controls born to subfertile parents. Hum Reprod (Oxford, England). 2009;24(11): 2788–95.
152. Ceelen M, van Weissenbruch MM, Vermeiden JP, van Leeuwen FE, Delemarre-van de Waal HA. Cardiometabolic differences in children born after in vitro fertilization: follow-up study. J Clin Endocrinol Metab. 2008;93(5):1682–8.

Proteomic/Metabolomic Analysis of Embryos: Current Status for Use in ART

17

Mandy G. Katz-Jaffe and Susanna McReynolds

Abstract

The selection of embryos for transfer is currently based on morphological indices; though successful, the field of assisted reproductive technologies (ART) would benefit from a noninvasive quantitative method of embryo assessment. Omics technologies, including proteomics and metabolomics, have already begun providing evidence that viable embryos possess unique molecular profiles with potential biomarkers that could be utilized for selection purposes. Of particular interest in ART is the secretome (extracellular proteins and metabolites) that are present in the surrounding environment of the embryo, the microdrop of culture media. Defining the human embryonic secretome has the potential to expand our knowledge of embryonic cellular processes and may also assist in identifying those embryos with the highest implantation potential. Advances in proteomic and metabolomic technologies have allowed for the noninvasive profiling of the human embryonic secretome with ongoing research focused on correlation with outcome that may result in improved IVF outcomes and routine single embryo transfers.

Keywords

Omics • Embryo • ART • Proteomics • Metabolomics • Secretome • Embryo quality • Implantation

17.1 Introduction

The assessment of embryo competence is a crucial component of assisted reproductive technologies (ART). Current selection methods are based on detailed embryo morphology with the highest implantation rates observed following detailed morphological assessment [1, 2]. Though this information contributes to the prediction of implantation potential and is relatively successful in improving pregnancy rates and reducing multiple gestations, morphology has limitations, with more than 70% of in vitro fertilization (IVF) embryos failing to implant. This failure is likely due to both the absence of developmentally competent embryos in an IVF cohort as well as our inability to select the competent

M.G. Katz-Jaffe (✉)
Colorado Center for Reproductive Medicine, Lone Tree, CO, USA
and
National Foundation for Fertility Research, Lone Tree, CO, USA
e-mail: mkatz-jaffe@colocrm.com

C. Racowsky et al. (eds.), *Biennial Review of Infertility: Volume 2*,
DOI 10.1007/978-1-4419-8456-2_17, © Springer Science+Business Media, LLC 2011

embryo(s) present. The field of human ART would benefit from more quantitative and accurate methods of embryo viability assessment. In turn, the ability to select the most viable embryo in a cohort will allow for routine single embryo transfer, while maintaining or improving pregnancy rates [3].

Recent developments in omics technologies (genomics, transcriptomics, proteomics, and metabolomics), including improvements in platform sensitivity, are highlighting the potential of these technologies to investigate diverse biological samples. In particular, proteomic and metabolomic analysis provides a snapshot of cellular physiology and function, as well as a direct link with phenotype. Both these omics technologies allow for analysis of IVF spent culture media that would represent a noninvasive minimal risk approach to assessing embryo viability [4]. In this chapter, we discuss the role of proteomics and metabolomics in examining the mammalian embryonic secretome and their applicability to the assessment of embryo viability in ART. Defining and characterizing the mammalian embryonic secretome will also expand our knowledge of early embryogenesis and advance our understanding of the embryonic role during implantation.

17.2 Noninvasive Proteomic Analysis of Embryos for ART

Knowledge of the human embryo proteome is very limited despite recent advances in proteomic technologies. The combined effect of limited template, low protein concentration, deficient platform sensitivity, and limited protein database information has contributed as the main hurdles. The human proteome is diverse and dynamic, with over one million proteins constantly changing through both internal and external interactions and stimuli. The secretome is of particular interest to researchers investigating the dynamics of a specific physiological condition or disease state and is defined as those proteins that are produced by cells and secreted at any given time [5, 6]. In ART, the secretome incorporates those proteins that are produced by embryos and secreted at any given time into the surrounding culture medium. Indeed, proteomic assessment of secreted human embryonic proteins may assist in identifying noninvasive biomarkers that reflect developmental competence and viability [7]. To date, the investigation of the human embryonic secretome and its correlation to embryo viability and outcome has been challenging, but holds promise with recent developments and increased sensitivity of both targeted and profiling proteomic approaches.

17.2.1 Noninvasive Targeted Single Protein and Molecular Analysis

The initial studies of the human embryonic secretome involved targeted analysis of individual proteins and molecules. The soluble factor, 1-*o*-alkyl-2-acetyl-sn-glycero-3-phosphocholine (PAF), was one of the first targeted molecules to be identified in the human embryonic secretome and was shown to be produced and secreted by mammalian embryos during preimplantation development [8]. PAF has been shown to act in an autocrine fashion as a survival factor, as well as influencing a range of maternal physiology alterations including platelet activation and immune function [8].

Leptin, a 16 kDa small pleotrophic peptide, has been observed in blastocyst-conditioned medium while studying the interaction between the embryo and endometrial epithelial cells (EEC) [9]. The authors showed that competent human blastocysts secreted higher leptin concentrations into the surrounding medium than arrested embryos. Leptin has been hypothesized to initiate and establish a molecular dialog with leptin receptors in the maternal endometrium during the window of implantation [10]. Another reciprocal embryo–endometrial interaction that could transform the local uterine environment impacting both embryo development and the implantation process is HOXA10 expression by epithelial endometrial cells and the unknown soluble molecule secreted by human blastocysts that modulates its regulation [11].

Human leukocyte antigen G (HLA-G) is thought to play a role at the maternal embryonic interface during implantation. HLA-G is produced by human oocytes and embryos at both the mRNA and protein level and has also been detected extracellular in embryo spent culture media [12–14]. The presence of soluble HLA-G (sHLA-G) in embryo spent culture media has been linked by several studies to successful pregnancy outcome and suggested as a noninvasive marker to predict embryo quality and implantation success, especially when used in conjunction with current morphological embryo assessment methods [15]. These results, however, have not been absolute with pregnancies established from sHLA-G negative embryos and data revealing undetectable levels of sHLA-G in embryo spent culture media [15–17].

In a multicenter study, a wide range of sHLA-G concentrations were observed across the different ART clinics, as well as differences between sHLA-G in relation to implantation. Indeed, a significant association between sHLA-G-positive embryo spent culture media and successful implantation was only established in one of the three clinics involved in the study [18]. Another recent study was unable to detect any association between sHLA-G expression and implantation rates, but concluded that miscarriage rates were significantly lower when embryos were selected based on a graduated embryo morphology score and sHLA-G levels vs. the morphology score alone [19]. In addition, no correlation has been observed between the concentration of sHLA-G in embryo spent culture media and either embryology morphology [20] or chromosome aneuploidy by FISH for up to 11 chromosomes (8, 9, 13, 15, 16, 17, 18, 21, 22, X and Y) [21].

There are numerous factors that could influence the presence of sHLA-G in embryo spent culture media including the culture system itself, the extent of cumulus removal, single vs. group embryo culture, media composition, microdrop volume, and the day of media collection [15, 16]. Most of the studies to date have investigated the expression of sHLA-G on day 3 of embryo development at the time of embryonic genome activation. It would be reasonable to conclude that in these studies sHLA-G was most likely to be maternally derived either from the oocyte or follicular environment. Perhaps the analysis of embryonic sHLA-G on day 5 of development will be more indicative of embryo developmental competence. Another explanation for the lack of reproducibility and association observed to date could be the lack of sensitivity of the current sandwich ELISA assays used for most sHLA-G analysis. Thus, it would appear that in order to determine the true importance of sHLA-G in regards to embryo development and implantation outcome, a more sensitive (picogram level), reproducible, and quantitative detection method for analysis is required to be tested on individual spent culture media samples throughout all stages of embryo development including the blastocyst, postembryonic genome activation [16].

17.2.2 Noninvasive Protein Profiling of Embryos

The targeted secretome studies described above have been focused on only a single protein or factor; however, it would be reasonable to assume that more than one molecule would be required to predict developmental competence and/or implantation potential considering the multifactorial nature of embryonic development. With the recent advances in proteomic technologies including increased sensitivity, it has become possible for more extended investigations of the proteins and peptides produced and secreted by the human embryos.

Mass Spectrometry (MS) has rapidly become an important technology in proteomics research. Searching for consistent and significant alteration in protein expression between specific groups of samples has revealed underlying mechanisms of physiological processes and disease states [22]. MS typically involves an ion source for production of a charged species in the gas phase, and an analyzer, which can separate ions by their mass-to-charge (*m/z*) ratio. Several commonly used ionization methods include electrospray ionization (ESI), matrix attenuated laser desorption/ionization (MALDI), and surface-enhanced laser desorption/ionization (SELDI). These are coupled to either time-of-flight (TOF), ion trap, or quadrupole analyzers, which can occur in tandem for peptide sequencing. For reliable and reproducible proteomic data, a consistent protocol needs to be followed during sample collection, storage, and handling due to the dynamic and sensitive nature of the human proteome. Data prejudice during processing can be controlled for by running samples in replicates, routinely performing internal and external calibrations, and including suitable control samples with every run [23].

SELDI-TOF MS, with specific surface affinity protein chips, has allowed for fast, cost-effective, high-throughput application of small sample volumes (μL range) and enables sensitivity to be in the picomole to femtomole range. The technology has been applied to a variety of biological tissues and fluids with specific focus on oncoproteomics [24]. Using SELDI, Katz-Jaffe et al. [25] were the first to successfully analyze the protein profile of individual human embryos. The authors observed distinctive protein secretome signatures at each 24 h embryonic developmental stage from the time of fertilization to the blastocyst stage. Unique proteins were observed in the human embryonic secretome after the activation of the embryonic genome. A clear association was observed between protein expression profiles and morphology, with degenerating embryos exhibiting significant up-regulation of several potential biomarkers that might be involved in apoptotic and growth-inhibiting pathways.

In addition, the secretome of developing blastocysts revealed a significantly higher expression of an 8.5 kDa protein in comparison to the secretome of degenerating embryos, potentially indicating an association between this protein and developmental competence. Tandem MS and database peptide sequence identification indicated that the best candidate for this 8.5 kDa protein was ubiquitin, a component of the ubiquitin-dependant proteosome system that is involved in a number of physiological processes including proliferation and apoptosis. Secreted ubiquitin has been shown to be upregulated in body fluids in certain disease states and this accumulation provides evidence for an increased protein turnover [26, 27]. Interestingly, ubiquitin has been implicated to play a crucial role during mammalian implantation by controlling the activities and turnover of key signaling molecules [28].

In a retrospective study by Dominguez et al. [29], protein microarrays that contained 120 targets were used to compare implanted vs. nonimplanted blastocyst-conditioned media. With a lower detection limit of only 10 pg/mL for this system, samples were pooled following single embryo transfer according to pregnancy outcome. An increased expression of the soluble TNF receptor 1 and Interleukin-10 (IL-10) and the decreased expression of MSP-α, SCF, CXCL13, TRAILR3 and MIP-1β were observed in the conditioned media compared to control media [29]. Interestingly, there were no proteins significantly increased in the conditioned media of implanted blastocysts compared to nonimplanted blastocysts. The presence of two significantly decreased proteins, CXCL13 and GM-CSF, were observed in the pooled implanted blastocyst-conditioned media indicating consumption of these proteins by the human blastocyst. These results are corroborated by studies showing that GM-CSF promotes embryo development and implantation when present in both human and mice blastocyst culture media [30].

A follow-up study comparing protein secretome profiles between the EEC coculture system and sequential microdrop culture media revealed differential protein secretome profiles [31]. Several molecules were increased in the EEC coculture profile including IL-6, PLGF, and BCL (CXCL13), while other proteins were decreased (consumed) such as FGF-4, IL-12p40, VEGF, and uPAR. IL-6 was the most secreted protein by the EEC coculture system. Using an IL-6 ELISA assay, the sequential culture media secretome of viable blastocysts displayed an increased uptake compared to blastocysts that failed to result in a pregnancy, suggesting a potential role for IL-6 in blastocyst development and implantation [31].

Current methods used to screen for chromosome aneuploidy in embryos involve biopsy procedures which are invasive and could compromise further embryo development. A noninvasive method for aneuploidy screening of human embryos would be a significant advantage to embryo selection in ART. Using SELDI-TOF MS, protein profiles of embryo spent culture media from individual blastocysts relative to the chromosomal constitution of all 23 pairs of chromosomes were investigated [4]. The secretome of individual blastocysts identified protein expression that allowed for discrimination between euploid (correct number of chromosomes) and aneuploid chromosomal constitutions [4]. A novel set of nine differentially expressed biomarkers was identified with statistical significance and was reproducible in all spent culture media samples analyzed, classifying a euploid blastocyst from an aneuploid blastocyst. Ongoing research by this group is focused on further validation to discriminate between euploid and aneuploid blastocysts and on a future blinded prospective study. The ability to noninvasively assay for the combination of developmental competence and chromosomal constitution could represent a powerful viability selection tool in ART, but to date the lack of sensitivity and the complexity of the human embryonic proteome have been limiting factors. The challenge is to discover the proteins of interest; however, once identified, immunodetection using ELISA or radioimmunoassay will allow for sensitivity, high throughput, and should be cost-effective for application in a clinical setting.

17.3 Noninvasive Metabolomic Analysis of Embryos for ART

Complementing proteomic analysis, information regarding human embryo metabolism and metabolomic profiling may also assist in the search for noninvasive methods to distinguish competent embryos in culture. During the preimplantation stage, the nutrient requirement of the human embryo changes as it travels through the reproductive tract, from relatively high levels of pyruvate and low levels of glucose in the oviduct to lower pyruvate and higher glucose concentration in the uterus [32, 33]. In addition, amino acids are essential for development acting as energy substrates, as well as contributing to protein synthesis and pH regulation [34]. The end products of embryo metabolism and cellular processes are low molecular weight molecules called metabolites (<1,000 Da) that reflect the efficiency of the processes in response to a variety of nutrient or environmental changes; these could represent potential biomarkers of embryo viability [35]. An estimated 8,500 metabolites, representing a wide dynamic and diverse range, have to date been identified in the human metabolome which is considerably fewer than the >1 million proteins in the human proteome. Noninvasive quantitative techniques assessing the metabolic parameters of the developing embryos have been under investigation for over a decade with promising advances for predicting embryo viability and pregnancy outcome. The "quiet embryo hypothesis" has been proposed in which nonviable embryos are more metabolically active than developmentally competent embryos who are more metabolically quiescent [36].

17.3.1 Pyruvate and Glucose

Pyruvate is one of the main sources of energy during the early stages of embryogenesis through to compaction on day 4, when carboxylic acid-based metabolism is predominant [32, 33]. The uptake of pyruvate by embryos in culture has been investigated as a possible marker of embryo development and viability, with inconclusive results to date. Initial studies showed a higher uptake of pyruvate by embryos that develop to the blastocyst stage [37, 38]. This was later supported by Gardner et al. [39] who reported a significantly higher pyruvate uptake on day 4 in embryos that developed to the blastocyst stage compared to embryos that arrested and failed to develop into blastocysts. In contrast, there have been other findings suggesting a lower pyruvate uptake by the early cleavage stage embryo (two to eight cells) in association with outcome [40]. It has also been observed that embryos display a wide variation in pyruvate uptake, with the lowest uptake representing embryos that successfully implant [41]. Inconsistent data regarding pyruvate uptake would indicate that it would not be a reliable candidate for embryo viability assessment.

In comparison to pyruvate, glucose uptake, which is low during the cleavage stages, increases significantly at the transition from morula to blastocyst stage and indeed appears to correlate with the developmental competence and viability of human blastocysts. Glucose uptake by human embryos on day 4 has been reported to be significantly higher in embryos that developed into blastocysts compared to those embryos that arrested prior the blastocyst stage [39]. Furthermore, this study also determined that the greatest glucose uptake belonged to higher morphological grade blastocysts. While there may be a relationship between glucose uptake and embryo quality, the technology currently used for glucose analysis on embryo spent culture media are microfluorometric enzymatic assays. These assays are technically difficult, low throughput and require technical expertise rendering them unsuitable for clinical application. Advances in microfluidics allow for high throughput and potentially more user-friendly analysis and could move glucose uptake analysis towards clinical applicability [42].

17.3.2 Amino Acids

Great attention has been devoted to the profiling of amino acids during human embryo development. Amino acids play key roles during embryo metabolism and several studies have assessed their relationship to embryo viability. High-performance liquid chromatography (HPLC) has been used to examine the amino acid turnover (depletion and/or appearance) during preimplantation embryo development. Initial studies observed a correlation between amino acid turnover and embryos that arrested in culture compared to competent embryos that developed to the blastocyst stage [43]. Leucine was the most consistently depleted amino acid and Alanine the highest secreted amino acid throughout development by embryos that formed blastocysts. Furthermore, the data also indicated that competent embryos displayed a lower amino acid turnover than those which arrest in culture, consistent with the "quiet embryo hypothesis" [44].

In a follow-up study, HPLC was used to examine the concentration of amino acids on day 2 from individual-cultured human embryos [45]. An association was observed between the turnover of three amino acids (decreased glycine and leucine levels, and increased asparagine levels) in the embryo spent culture media with clinical pregnancy and live birth. Proton nuclear magnetic resonance (H^1-NMR) has also been used to identify amino acid biomarkers. Analysis of day 3 embryo spent culture media showed that higher glutamate levels correlated with clinical pregnancy and live birth [46].

A more recent publication has indicated an association between amino acid turnover and chromosome constitution. Following the screening of six chromosomes by FISH (13, 18, 19, 21, X and Y), asparagine, glycine, and valine turnover were significantly different between euploid and aneuploid day 3 embryos, while serine, leucine, and lysine displayed differences in their profiles between these two groups on day 4 of embryo development [47].

There are several potential explanations for the amino acid differences observed in the studies outlined above including the culture system itself, type of culture media, day of analysis, and platform used for measurement. Overall, these studies suggest an association between amino acid turnover and embryos of different reproductive potential with promise for the development of noninvasive clinical assays. However, there is a need for further exploration and validation in relation to the prediction of embryo reproductive potential as well as a more user-friendly screening method that can rapidly and routinely be used in the IVF clinic.

17.3.3 Noninvasive Metabolomic Profiling of Embryos

Metabolites are compounds with diverse chemical and physical properties, found in a variety of concentrations. Since the metabolome is defined as a spectrum of these small metabolites, there is a shift away from the analysis of single or defined metabolites towards more comprehensive analysis and metabolomic profiling. Metabolomic profiling systematically analyses this wide range of diverse metabolites that represent a functional phenotype [48].

Raman, measuring the vibrations of bonds, and Near Infrared (NIR) Spectroscopy, which primarily measures overtones and combination vibrations, are two optical spectroscopy methods that have successfully been used to profile human embryo spent culture media in relation to pregnancy outcome [49]. The advantages of optical spectroscopies include no sample processing, high throughput, and rapid turnaround (<1 min/sample). However, metabolomic profiling does not identify or quantitate specific metabolites. Instead, it relies on identifying metabolites displaying an association with a specific biological phenotype. Under this circumstance, reproducibility of profiles is even more crucial for validity. It appears that the spectral regions of the metabolomic profiles most predictive of outcome corresponded to markers of oxidative stress, including –CH, –NH, and –OH groups. These findings could indicate an association between embryo developmental competence and oxidative modification.

Using a mathematical model, Seli et al. [49] generated an algorithm based on metabolomic profiling of day 3 human embryo spent culture media with known outcome to calculate viability indexes for positive vs. negative pregnancy. The mean viability score for embryos that resulted in pregnancy was significantly higher than those that failed to implant. Follow-up studies analyzing embryo spent culture media from single embryo transfers on day 2, 3, and 5 of development using NIR spectroscopy and bioinformatics consistently showed higher mean viability scores for embryos that resulted in clinical pregnancy [3]. In addition, a blinded pilot study on retrospectively collected data, using the Raman spectroscopy platform, revealed an overall diagnostic accuracy for predicting embryonic reproductive potential, either delivery or a failed implantation, at 80.5% [50].

In summary, metabolomic profiling appears to show promise for selecting viable human embryos and has also been shown to be an independent parameter to morphology [51]. However, in each study described above, there was considerable overlap between the viability index for embryos that implanted and those that failed to result in a pregnancy, with both inter-patient and inter-embryo variation. Moreover, to date, no prospective trial has proven that such a metabolomic algorithm has selective capabilities superior to morphological evaluation alone. Therefore, the question still remains unanswered as to whether metabolomic profiling will prove to be a reliable and reproducible clinical assay for human embryo viability assessment.

17.4 Conclusion

Proteomics and metabolomics are two complementary omics platforms under investigation that show promise for the development of noninvasive methods for embryo selection in the field of ART. With the ability to assay both proteins and metabolites in embryo spent culture media, generating complimentary but different molecular profiles, a combined omics contribution seems reasonable to fully characterize the human embryonic secretome. Further, taking into account the complexity and diversity of the human embryo, it is feasible to propose that embryo viability assessment may include a combination of both these omics platforms used alone or in conjunction with morphology.

Defining the embryonic secretome could result in a rapid, user-friendly, cost-effective, noninvasive, reliable, and reproducible method for quantitative embryo assessment. Recent proteomics and metabolomics research is encouraging; however, to date no technique has proven true clinical predictive value or been examined in prospective randomized control trials. However, once true efficacy is proven, a noninvasive assay for the selection of viable human embryos could lead to routine single embryo transfers, a reduction in early pregnancy losses, and increased singleton deliveries.

References

1. Ebner T, Moser M, Sommergruber M, Tews G. Selection based on morphological assessment of oocytes and embryos at different stages of preimplantation development: a review. Hum Reprod Update. 2003;9:251–62.
2. Racowsky C, Ohno-Machado L, Kim J, Biggers JD. Is there an advantage in scoring early embryos on more than one day? Hum Reprod. 2009;24:2104–13.
3. Seli E, Vergouw CG, Morita H, et al. Noninvasive metabolomic profiling as an adjunct to morphology for noninvasive embryo assessment in women undergoing single embryo transfer. Fertil Steril. 2010;94:535–42.
4. Katz-Jaffe MG, McReynolds S, Gardner DK, Schoolcraft WB. The role of proteomics in defining the human embryonic secretome. Mol Hum Reprod. 2009;15:271–7.
5. Hu S, Loo JA, Wong DT. Human body fluid proteome analysis. Proteomics. 2006;6:6326–53.
6. Kulasingam V, Diamandis EP. Proteomics analysis of conditioned media from three breast cancer cell lines: a mine for biomarkers and therapeutic targets. Mol Cell Proteomics. 2007;6:1997–2011.
7. Katz-Jaffe MG, Gardner DK. Embryology in the era of proteomics. Theriogenology. 2007;68 Suppl 1:S125–30.
8. O'Neill C. The role of paf in embryo physiology. Hum Reprod Update. 2005;11:215–28.
9. Gonzalez RR, Caballero-Campo P, Jasper M, et al. Leptin and leptin receptor are expressed in the human endometrium and endometrial leptin secretion is regulated by the human blastocyst. J Clin Endocrinol Metab. 2000;85:4883–8.
10. Cervero A, Horcajadas JA, Dominguez F, Pellicer A, Simon C. Leptin system in embryo development and implantation: a protein in search of a function. Reprod Biomed Online. 2005;10:217–23.
11. Sakkas D, Lu C, Zulfikaroglu E, Neuber E, Taylor HS. A soluble molecule secreted by human blastocysts modulates regulation of HOXA10 expression in an epithelial endometrial cell line. Fertil Steril. 2003;80:1169–74.
12. Jurisicova A, Casper RF, MacLusky NJ, Librach CL. Embryonic human leukocyte antigen-G expression: possible implications for human preimplantation development. Fertil Steril. 1996;65:997–1002.
13. Jurisicova A, Casper RF, MacLusky NJ, Mills GB, Librach CL. HLA-G expression during preimplantation human embryo development. Proc Natl Acad Sci USA. 1996;93:161–5.
14. Yao YQ, Barlow DH, Sargent IL. Differential expression of alternatively spliced transcripts of HLA-G in human preimplantation embryos and inner cell masses. J Immunol. 2005;175:8379–85.
15. Warner CM, Lampton PW, Newmark JA, Cohen J. Symposium: innovative techniques in human embryo viability assessment. Soluble human leukocyte antigen-G and pregnancy success. Reprod Biomed Online. 2008;17:470–85.
16. Vercammen M, Verloes A, Haentjens P, Van de Velde H. Can soluble human leucocyte antigen-G predict successful pregnancy in assisted reproductive technology? Curr Opin Obstet Gynecol. 2009;21:285–90.
17. Vercammen MJ, Verloes A, Van de Velde H, Haentjens P. Accuracy of soluble human leukocyte antigen-G for predicting pregnancy among women undergoing infertility treatment: meta-analysis. Hum Reprod Update. 2008;14:209–18.
18. Tabiasco J, Perrier d'Hauterive S, Thonon F, et al. Soluble HLA-G in IVF/ICSI embryo culture supernatants does not always predict implantation success: a multicentre study. Reprod Biomed Online. 2009;18:374–81.
19. Kotze DJ, Hansen P, Keskintepe L, Snowden E, Sher G, Kruger T. Embryo selection criteria based on morphology VERSUS the expression of a biochemical marker (sHLA-G) and a graduated embryo score: prediction of pregnancy outcome. J Assist Reprod Genet. 2010;27:309–16.
20. Noci I, Fuzzi B, Rizzo R, et al. Embryonic soluble HLA-G as a marker of developmental potential in embryos. Hum Reprod. 2005;20:138–46.
21. Coulam CB, Roussev RG, Lerner S, Zlatopolsky Z, Ilkevitch Y, Tur-Kaspa I. How to predict implantation? No correlation between embryonic aneuploidy and soluble human leukocyte antigen G-concentrations. Fertil Steril. 2009;91:2408–13.
22. Dominguez DC, Lopes R, Torres ML. Proteomics: clinical applications. Clin Lab Sci. 2007;20:245–8.
23. Hu J, Coombes KR, Morris JS, Baggerly KA. The importance of experimental design in proteomic mass spectrometry experiments: some cautionary tales. Brief Funct Genomic Proteomic. 2005;3:322–31.
24. Cho WC. Contribution of oncoproteomics to cancer biomarker discovery. Mol Cancer. 2007;6:25.
25. Katz-Jaffe MG, Schoolcraft WB, Gardner DK. Analysis of protein expression (secretome) by human and mouse preimplantation embryos. Fertil Steril. 2006;86:678–85.
26. Delbosc S, Haloui M, Louedec L, et al. Proteomic analysis permits the identification of new biomarkers of arterial wall remodeling in hypertension. Mol Med. 2008;14:383–94.
27. Sandoval JA, Hoelz DJ, Woodruff HA, et al. Novel peptides secreted from human neuroblastoma: useful clinical tools? J Pediatr Surg. 2006;41:245–51.
28. Wang HM, Zhang X, Qian D, et al. Effect of ubiquitin-proteasome pathway on mouse blastocyst implantation and expression of matrix metalloproteinases-2 and -9. Biol Reprod. 2004;70:481–7.
29. Dominguez F, Gadea B, Esteban FJ, Horcajadas JA, Pellicer A, Simon C. Comparative protein-profile analysis of implanted versus non-implanted human blastocysts. Hum Reprod. 2008;23:1993–2000.
30. Robertson SA. GM-CSF regulation of embryo development and pregnancy. Cytokine Growth Factor Rev. 2007;18:287–98.

31. Dominguez F, Gadea B, Mercader A, Esteban FJ, Pellicer A, Simon C. Embryologic outcome and secretome profile of implanted blastocysts obtained after coculture in human endometrial epithelial cells versus the sequential system. Fertil Steril. 2010;93: 774–82.e771.
32. Gardner DK, Lane M, Calderon I, Leeton J. Environment of the preimplantation human embryo in vivo: metabolite analysis of oviduct and uterine fluids and metabolism of cumulus cells. Fertil Steril. 1996;65:349–53.
33. Leese HJ, Tay JI, Reischl J, Downing SJ. Formation of Fallopian tubal fluid: role of a neglected epithelium. Reproduction. 2001;121:339–46.
34. Gardner DK, Lane M. Culture and selection of viable blastocysts: a feasible proposition for human IVF? Hum Reprod Update. 1997;3:367–82.
35. Singh R, Sinclair KD. Metabolomics: approaches to assessing oocyte and embryo quality. Theriogenology. 2007;68 Suppl 1:S56–62.
36. Leese HJ. Quiet please, do not disturb: a hypothesis of embryo metabolism and viability. Bioessays. 2002;24:845–9.
37. Gott AL, Hardy K, Winston RM, Leese HJ. Non-invasive measurement of pyruvate and glucose uptake and lactate production by single human preimplantation embryos. Hum Reprod. 1990;5:104–8.
38. Hardy K, Hooper MA, Handyside AH, Rutherford AJ, Winston RM, Leese HJ. Non-invasive measurement of glucose and pyruvate uptake by individual human oocytes and preimplantation embryos. Hum Reprod. 1989;4:188–91.
39. Gardner DK, Lane M, Stevens J, Schoolcraft WB. Noninvasive assessment of human embryo nutrient consumption as a measure of developmental potential. Fertil Steril. 2001;76:1175–80.
40. Conaghan J, Hardy K, Handyside AH, Winston RM, Leese HJ. Selection criteria for human embryo transfer: a comparison of pyruvate uptake and morphology. J Assist Reprod Genet. 1993;10:21–30.
41. Turner K, Martin KL, Woodward BJ, Lenton EA, Leese HJ. Comparison of pyruvate uptake by embryos derived from conception and non-conception natural cycles. Hum Reprod. 1994;9:2362–6.
42. Urbanski JP, Johnson MT, Craig DD, Potter DL, Gardner DK, Thorsen T. Noninvasive metabolic profiling using microfluidics for analysis of single preimplantation embryos. Anal Chem. 2008;80:6500–7.
43. Houghton FD, Hawkhead JA, Humpherson PG, et al. Non-invasive amino acid turnover predicts human embryo developmental capacity. Hum Reprod. 2002;17:999–1005.
44. Leese HJ, Baumann CG, Brison DR, McEvoy TG, Sturmey RG. Metabolism of the viable mammalian embryo: quietness revisited. Mol Hum Reprod. 2008; 14:667–72.
45. Brison DR, Houghton FD, Falconer D, et al. Identification of viable embryos in IVF by non-invasive measurement of amino acid turnover. Hum Reprod. 2004;19:2319–24.
46. Seli E, Botros L, Sakkas D, Burns DH. Noninvasive metabolomic profiling of embryo culture media using proton nuclear magnetic resonance correlates with reproductive potential of embryos in women undergoing in vitro fertilization. Fertil Steril. 2008;90: 2183–9.
47. Picton HM, Elder K, Houghton FD, et al. Association between amino acid turnover and chromosome aneuploidy during human preimplantation embryo development in vitro. Mol Hum Reprod. 2010;16: 557–69.
48. Botros L, Sakkas D, Seli E. Metabolomics and its application for non-invasive embryo assessment in IVF. Mol Hum Reprod. 2008;14:679–90.
49. Seli E, Sakkas D, Scott R, Kwok SC, Rosendahl SM, Burns DH. Noninvasive metabolomic profiling of embryo culture media using Raman and near-infrared spectroscopy correlates with reproductive potential of embryos in women undergoing in vitro fertilization. Fertil Steril. 2007;88:1350–7.
50. Scott R, Seli E, Miller K, Sakkas D, Scott K, Burns DH. Noninvasive metabolomic profiling of human embryo culture media using Raman spectroscopy predicts embryonic reproductive potential: a prospective blinded pilot study. Fertil Steril. 2008;90:77–83.
51. Seli E, Robert C, Sirard MA. OMICS in assisted reproduction: possibilities and pitfalls. Mol Hum Reprod. 2010;16:513–30.

Ultrasound-Guided Embryo Transfer 18

Robert L. Gustofson and William B. Schoolcraft

Abstract

The complexity of in vitro fertilization is culminated in the embryo transfer. Failure to achieve a successful transfer can negate the effort of the entire process. Any method to facilitate an easier transfer with higher pregnancy rates is considered a necessary step. Ultrasound-guided embryo transfer has become integrated in most IVF centers because of its ease of use, reassurance of proper embryo placement, and improved pregnancy rates.

Keywords

Ultrasound guidance • Embryo transfer • Pregnancy rate • ART • Catheter • Embryo

18.1 Introduction

In vitro fertilization consists of a series of mutually dependent and intricate steps. The process begins with patient selection and is followed by controlled ovarian hyperstimulation and oocyte retrieval, which leads the process into the laboratory. Within the lab, fertilization and embryo culture is accomplished. The quality of the culture media, the maintenance of proper temperature and pH regulation, and proper air quality are all critical for the production of viable embryos. Constant quality assurance and quality control is required to maintain consistent embryo quality week in and week out. The final steps in the IVF process include adequate endometrial receptivity, proper luteal support, and finally, the quality of the embryo transfer itself. The embryo transfer is the final step in this complex chain of events. Failure during embryo transfer will negate the months of careful work and sophisticated technology predating this final stage.

The variables affecting embryo transfer success have been enumerated in the literature. These include the performance of a trial of transfer [1], contamination of the catheter tip with blood [2, 3], mucus, or endometrial tissue, the presence of retained embryos, the type of catheter [4–8], the volume and type of transfer media, the presence of bacteria in the cervix or on the catheter tip [9, 10], and the utilization of ultrasound guidance during

W.B. Schoolcraft (✉)
Colorado Center for Reproductive Medicine,
Lone Tree, CO, USA
e-mail: bschoolcraft@colocrm.com

C. Racowsky et al. (eds.), *Biennial Review of Infertility: Volume 2*,
DOI 10.1007/978-1-4419-8456-2_18, © Springer Science+Business Media, LLC 2011

the transfer. It is this last variable of ultrasound guidance that will be the focus of this chapter. Since 1985 when ultrasound guidance was first described by Strickler et al. [11], technological use of ultrasound has become widely debated but now routinely incorporated by most IVF centers.

18.2 Benefits of Ultrasound Guidance

There are many potential benefits to utilizing ultrasound guidance during transfer. First, it can help the operator avoid a difficult transfer. There are several studies demonstrating that technically difficult transfers are associated with reduced pregnancy rates [12–16]. One potential link between difficult transfers and a lower implantation rate is trauma to the endometrium [17]. This can lead to uterine contractions, which negatively influence pregnancy outcome [18]. In addition, the contamination of the catheter with blood is also more common with difficult transfers and blood itself is associated with lowering of pregnancy outcome [2]. Indeed, a meta-analysis by Sallam and Sadek [19] demonstrated a lower incidence of difficult embryo transfer with the use of ultrasound guidance vs. clinical touch.

The other benefit to ultrasound guidance is that it can facilitate proper placement of the catheter tip. Several studies have shown that placement of the embryos approximately 1.5–2 cm from the fundus results in optimal implantation rates [20, 21]. In addition, placement of the catheter close to the fundus increases the rate of ectopic pregnancy [22, 23]. Ultrasound guidance avoids these complications associated with high transfers, i.e., less than 1 cm from the fundus, as well as inadvertent low transfers that fail to clear the internal cervical os. This optimal placement of the embryos minimizes the risk of endometrial trauma, minimizes the incidence of uterine contractions, and lowers the incidence of retained embryos within the catheter [24].

Ultrasound guidance also avoids placing the catheter in a subendometrial location and detects a catheter that potentially might loop upon itself, thereby directing the embryos back downwards toward the cervix. Indeed, Woolcott and Stanger [25] demonstrated that in 17% of blind transfers, the catheter actually abutted the fundal endometrium. In addition, the outer guiding cannula indented the endometrium in 25% of transfers. The catheter actually was embedded within the endometrium in 33% of cases, and in 7% of cases, ultrasound detected a catheter that was actually cannulating the fallopian tube, which would almost have guaranteed tubal placement of the embryos. A study involving hysteroscopic examination of the uterine cavity following embryo transfer resulted in visualization of significant endometrial trauma with difficult transfers as opposed to easy transfers [17].

As mentioned earlier, uterine contractions are clearly stimulated by difficult transfers, and ultrasound guidance is a means to minimize such contractions. Increased subendometrial contractions are associated with a traumatic embryo transfer. If seen prior to embryo transfer, pregnancy rates are substantially decreased [18].

18.3 Optimization of Ultrasound Guidance

With abdominal ultrasound guidance, a full bladder is necessary for optimal visualization. A full bladder itself is a benefit as demonstrated by Lewin who showed that the presence of a full bladder without ultrasound guidance was associated with improved pregnancy rates as compared to an empty bladder [26]. In addition, Abou-Setta [27] and Sundstrom et al. [28] demonstrated not only a higher pregnancy rate with full bladder but a significantly increased incidence of easy embryo transfers with such full bladders, suggesting a passive straightening of the cervicouterine angle.

Various ultrasound techniques have been evaluated to determine best application. Ultrasound location, transabdominal vs. transvaginal, has been evaluated as well and appears to be equal efficacy [29]. Transabdominal ultrasound, however, may be advantageous due to ease of use and patient comfort compared to the transvaginal approach. Further, more advanced ultrasonography with 3D/4D approach may further enhance embryo transfer to an exact location. Current studies suggest 3D/4D ultrasound-guided embryo transfer is at least equal to 2D imaging, however, may be limited by availability of 3D technology [30, 31].

18.4 Controversy: Randomized Trials vs. Meta-Analysis

Controversy still remains regarding the use of ultrasound-guided embryo transfers and its benefits to pregnancy rates. One large randomized trial involving ultrasound guidance did not show a benefit [32]. In this study of 373 patients, there was no significant difference in pregnancy or implantation rates. It should be noted, however, that there was a trend toward fewer patients with prior ART failure in the control group as compared to the study group. In addition, there were more male factor cases and less unexplained infertility in the controls, characteristics likely to favor a better success in this group. Further, the ultrasound technologists "received training" before the study as opposed to having years of experience with such techniques. Patients had no requirement for a full bladder, suggesting that visualization would not be optimal in all cases. One clinician did all transfers in both groups and was very meticulous with his technique, which might minimize the difference between ultrasound and clinical touch. Finally, the transfer depth was greater in the ultrasound group, a variable known to negatively influence outcome. In 2008, Drakeley et al. [33] performed a large, randomized trial with 2,295 embryo transfers comparing ultrasound guidance and clinical touch demonstrating no difference in pregnancy rates. In the clinical touch arm of the study, the physician could select the catheter to utilize for transfer, adding a confounding variable.

Despite these two large randomized controlled trials, several meta-analyses demonstrated that the cumulative effects of ultrasound-guided embryo transfer lead to a better IVF outcome with respect to implantation and pregnancy rates. In 2007, prior to the large study by Drakeley, Abou-Setta et al. [34] demonstrated in their meta-analysis an odds ratio (OR) of 1.5 in favor of ultrasound guidance. When the study by Drakeley was incorporated into the Cochrane Database again, Brown found there still remained an increased ongoing pregnancy rate (OR 1.38); however, there was no difference in live birth rate [35]. Several other studies [36–38] have come to similar conclusions in favor of ultrasound guidance.

18.5 Colorado Center for Reproductive Medicine Experience

At the Colorado Center for Reproductive Medicine, our protocol for embryo transfer is as follows. We prepare the patient with oral diazepam and ask her to fill her bladder about 30–40 min prior to the anticipated transfer. Ultrasound guidance is accomplished abdominally by a licensed ultrasonographer with expertise in gynecologic evaluations. Upon inserting a speculum, the cervix is washed with culture media, gently lavaged, and all excess mucus is aspirated with an 18-gauge angiocatheter outer sheath [39, 40]. A trial of transfer is then performed just to the internal os. At this point, embryos maintained in a pediatric isolette are loaded into a Wallace™ SureView Ultrasound embryo replacement catheter (Smiths-Medical International) in a 30 μL volume. The fluid used for embryo transfer is EmbryoGlue® (Vitrolife). The catheter is placed as gently as possible with manipulation of the cervix using the speculum or a ring forceps, if necessary, to negotiate the internal os. The embryo transfer catheter is loaded so that there is initially a small column of air, followed by a 30 μL column of media, and then the embryos, followed by another small column of media just before the catheter tip. By utilizing this consistent, meticulous, standardized technique, we believe it contributes to the overall success of our program.

In cases of difficult embryo transfers, often associated with cervical stenosis, pre-cycle cervical dilation can be valuable. We have found that cervical laminaria is the most effective method to achieve useful dilation along with other authors using laminaria [41], hygroscopic rods [42], or malecot catheters [43]. Approximately 1 month prior to a scheduled embryo transfer, a patient has a medium cervical laminaria placed through the internal os. This is maintained in position overnight and removed the next day. This prolonged dilatation seems to retain its benefits up to and through the time of the transfer the following month. In contrast, cervical dilatation at the time of retrieval or thereafter lowers pregnancy rates [44].

18.6 Conclusion

Ultrasound guidance provides reassurance to both the physician and the patient that the catheter is in an optimal location for embryo deposition. While not every case of embryo transfer would necessarily benefit from ultrasound guidance, it is impossible to predict such cases in advance despite trial transfers, physician experience, or prior patient transfer. Therefore, the routine use of ultrasound seems appropriate to minimize difficulty with unexpected problematic transfers. Ultrasound may also be helpful for embryo transfer training. Residents and fellows can actually perform a mock embryo transfer under ultrasound guidance at the time of intrauterine insemination and obtain excellent experience in rehearsing their technique before applying it clinically. Given its ease of use, minimal to no discomfort, and lack of known side effects or deleterious effect on pregnancy rates, it seems intuitive that ultrasound guidance should be used routinely for embryo transfer.

References

1. Mansour R, Aboulghar M, Serour G. Dummy embryo transfer: a technique that minimizes the problems of embryo transfer and improves the pregnancy rate in human in vitro fertilization. Fertil Steril. 1990;54(4): 678–81.
2. Goudas VT, Hammitt DG, Damario MA, Session DR, Singh AP, Dumesic DA. Blood on the embryo transfer catheter is associated with decreased rates of embryo implantation and clinical pregnancy with the use of in vitro fertilization-embryo transfer. Fertil Steril. 1998;70(5):878–82.
3. Sallam HN, Agameya AF, Rahman AF, Ezzeldin F, Sallam AN. Impact of technical difficulties, choice of catheter, and the presence of blood on the success of embryo transfer–experience from a single provider. J Assist Reprod Genet. 2003;20(4):135–42.
4. Abou-Setta AM, Al-Inany HG, Mansour RT, Serour GI, Aboulghar MA. Soft versus firm embryo transfer catheters for assisted reproduction: a systematic review and meta-analysis. Hum Reprod. 2005;20(11): 3114–21.
5. Buckett WM. A review and meta-analysis of prospective trials comparing different catheters used for embryo transfer. Fertil Steril. 2006;85(3):728–34.
6. Ghazzawi IM, Al-Hasani S, Karaki R, Souso S. Transfer technique and catheter choice influence the incidence of transcervical embryo expulsion and the outcome of IVF. Hum Reprod. 1999;14(3):677–82.
7. Urman B, Aksoy S, Alatas C, et al. Comparing two embryo transfer catheters. Use of a trial transfer to determine the catheter applied. J Reprod Med. 2000;45(2):135–8.
8. Saldeen P, Abou-Setta AM, Bergh T, Sundstrom P, Holte J. A prospective randomized controlled trial comparing two embryo transfer catheters in an ART program. Fertil Steril. 2008;90(3):599–603.
9. Egbase PE, al-Sharhan M, al-Othman S, al-Mutawa M, Udo EE, Grudzinskas JG. Incidence of microbial growth from the tip of the embryo transfer catheter after embryo transfer in relation to clinical pregnancy rate following in-vitro fertilization and embryo transfer. Hum Reprod. 1996;11(8):1687–9.
10. Moore DE, Soules MR, Klein NA, Fujimoto VY, Agnew KJ, Eschenbach DA. Bacteria in the transfer catheter tip influence the live-birth rate after in vitro fertilization. Fertil Steril. 2000;74(6):1118–24.
11. Strickler RC, Christianson C, Crane JP, Curato A, Knight AB, Yang V. Ultrasound guidance for human embryo transfer. Fertil Steril. 1985;43(1):54–61.
12. Visser DS, Fourie FL, Kruger HF. Multiple attempts at embryo transfer: effect on pregnancy outcome in an in vitro fertilization and embryo transfer program. J Assist Reprod Genet. 1993;10(1):37–43.
13. Lesny P, Killick SR, Robinson J, Maguiness SD. Transcervical embryo transfer as a risk factor for ectopic pregnancy. Fertil Steril. 1999;72(2):305–9.
14. Sharif K, Afnan M, Lenton W. Mock embryo transfer with a full bladder immediately before the real transfer for in-vitro fertilization treatment: the Birmingham experience of 113 cases. Hum Reprod. 1995;10(7): 1715–8.
15. Tomas C, Tikkinen K, Tuomivaara L, Tapanainen JS, Martikainen H. The degree of difficulty of embryo transfer is an independent factor for predicting pregnancy. Hum Reprod. 2002;17(10):2632–5.
16. Lass A, Abusheikha N, Brinsden P, Kovacs GT. The effect of a difficult embryo transfer on the outcome of IVF. Hum Reprod. 1999;14(9):2417.

17. Cevrioglu AS, Esinler I, Bozdag G, Yarali H. Assessment of endocervical and endometrial damage inflicted by embryo transfer trial: a hysteroscopic evaluation. Reprod Biomed Online. 2006;13(4): 523–7.
18. Fanchin R, Righini C, Olivennes F, Taylor S, de Ziegler D, Frydman R. Uterine contractions at the time of embryo transfer alter pregnancy rates after in-vitro fertilization. Hum Reprod. 1998;13(7):1968–74.
19. Sallam HN, Sadek SS. Ultrasound-guided embryo transfer: a meta-analysis of randomized controlled trials. Fertil Steril. 2003;80(4):1042–6.
20. Pope CS, Cook EK, Arny M, Novak A, Grow DR. Influence of embryo transfer depth on in vitro fertilization and embryo transfer outcomes. Fertil Steril. 2004;81(1):51–8.
21. Coroleu B, Barri PN, Carreras O, et al. The influence of the depth of embryo replacement into the uterine cavity on implantation rates after IVF: a controlled, ultrasound-guided study. Hum Reprod. 2002;17(2): 341–6.
22. Yovich JL, Turner SR, Murphy AJ. Embryo transfer technique as a cause of ectopic pregnancies in in vitro fertilization. Fertil Steril. 1985;44(3):318–21.
23. Nazari A, Askari HA, Check JH, O'Shaughnessy A. Embryo transfer technique as a cause of ectopic pregnancy in in vitro fertilization. Fertil Steril. 1993;60(5): 919–21.
24. Silberstein T, Trimarchi JR, Shackelton R, Weitzen S, Frankfurter D, Plosker S. Ultrasound-guided miduterine cavity embryo transfer is associated with a decreased incidence of retained embryos in the transfer catheter. Fertil Steril. 2005;84(5):1510–2.
25. Woolcott R, Stanger J. Potentially important variables identified by transvaginal ultrasound-guided embryo transfer. Hum Reprod. 1997;12(5):963–6.
26. Lewin A, Schenker JG, Avrech O, Shapira S, Safran A, Friedler S. The role of uterine straightening by passive bladder distension before embryo transfer in IVF cycles. J Assist Reprod Genet. 1997;14(1):32–4.
27. Abou-Setta AM. Effect of passive uterine straightening during embryo transfer: a systematic review and meta-analysis. Acta Obstet Gynecol Scand. 2007;86(5):516–22.
28. Sundstrom P, Wramsby H, Persson PH, Liedholm P. Filled bladder simplifies human embryo transfer. Br J Obstet Gynaecol. 1984;91(5):506–7.
29. Porat N, Boehnlein LM, Schouweiler CM, Kang J, Lindheim SR. Interim analysis of a randomized clinical trial comparing abdominal versus transvaginal ultrasound-guided embryo transfer. J Obstet Gynaecol Res. 2010;36(2):384–92.
30. Baba K, Ishihara O, Hayashi N, Saitoh M, Taya J, Kinoshita K. Three-dimensional ultrasound in embryo transfer. Ultrasound Obstet Gynecol. 2000;16(4):372–3.
31. Gergely RZ, DeUgarte CM, Danzer H, Surrey M, Hill D, DeCherney AH. Three dimensional/four dimensional ultrasound-guided embryo transfer using the maximal implantation potential point. Fertil Steril. 2005;84(2):500–3.
32. Kosmas IP, Janssens R, De Munck L, et al. Ultrasound-guided embryo transfer does not offer any benefit in clinical outcome: a randomized controlled trial. Hum Reprod. 2007;22(5):1327–34.
33. Drakeley AJ, Jorgensen A, Sklavounos J, et al. A randomized controlled clinical trial of 2295 ultrasound-guided embryo transfers. Hum Reprod. 2008;23(5):1101–6.
34. Abou-Setta AM, Mansour RT, Al-Inany HG, Aboulghar MM, Aboulghar MA, Serour GI. Among women undergoing embryo transfer, is the probability of pregnancy and live birth improved with ultrasound guidance over clinical touch alone? A systemic review and meta-analysis of prospective randomized trials. Fertil Steril. 2007;88(2):333–41.
35. Brown J, Buckingham K, Abou-Setta AM, Buckett W. Ultrasound versus 'clinical touch' for catheter guidance during embryo transfer in women. Cochrane Database Syst Rev. 2010(1):CD006107.
36. Ali CR, Khashan AS, Horne G, Fitzgerald CT, Nardo LG. Implantation, clinical pregnancy and miscarriage rates after introduction of ultrasound-guided embryo transfer. Reprod Biomed Online. 2008;17(1):88–93.
37. Tang OS, Ng EH, So WW, Ho PC. Ultrasound-guided embryo transfer: a prospective randomized controlled trial. Hum Reprod. 2001;16(11):2310–5.
38. Matorras R, Urquijo E, Mendoza R, Corcostegui B, Exposito A, Rodriguez-Escudero FJ. Ultrasound-guided embryo transfer improves pregnancy rates and increases the frequency of easy transfers. Hum Reprod. 2002;17(7):1762–6.
39. Eskandar MA, Abou-Setta AM, El-Amin M, Almushait MA, Sobande AA. Removal of cervical mucus prior to embryo transfer improves pregnancy rates in women undergoing assisted reproduction. Reprod Biomed Online. 2007;14(3):308–13.
40. Visschers BA, Bots RS, Peeters MF, Mol BW, van Dessel HJ. Removal of cervical mucus: effect on pregnancy rates in IVF/ICSI. Reprod Biomed Online. 2007;15(3):310–5.
41. Glatstein IZ, Pang SC, McShane PM. Successful pregnancies with the use of laminaria tents before embryo transfer for refractory cervical stenosis. Fertil Steril. 1997;67(6):1172–4.
42. Serhal P, Ranieri DM, Khadum I, Wakim RA. Cervical dilatation with hygroscopic rods prior to ovarian stimulation facilitates embryo transfer. Hum Reprod. 2003;18(12):2618–20.
43. Yanushpolsky EH, Ginsburg ES, Fox JH, Stewart EA. Transcervical placement of a Malecot catheter after hysteroscopic evaluation provides for easier entry into the endometrial cavity for women with histories of difficult intrauterine inseminations and/or embryo transfers: a prospective case series. Fertil Steril. 2000; 73(2):402–5.
44. Groutz A, Lessing JB, Wolf Y, Yovel I, Azem F, Amit A. Cervical dilatation during ovum pick-up in patients with cervical stenosis: effect on pregnancy outcome in an in vitro fertilization-embryo transfer program. Fertil Steril. 1997;67(5):909–11.

Part IV

Evolving Controversies in Contemporary Reproductive Medicine

IMSI as a Valuable Tool for Sperm Selection During ART

19

Monica Antinori, Pierre Vanderzwalmen, and Yona Barak

Abstract

Conventional semen parameters, routinely used by clinicians to assess male reproductive potential, provide little information on the real fertility status. Nevertheless, sperm morphology analyzed by strict criteria has demonstrated its prognostic value regarding the outcome of both in vivo and in vitro reproduction. However, ICSI introduction seemed to have decreased the importance of sperm morphology in assisted reproduction, since fertilization, embryo development, pregnancies, and healthy deliveries can be achieved even in case of severe morphological impairments. This visual assessment of sperm morphology, due to the limitations attributable to its low magnification (200–400×) and concomitant low resolution, overlooks minor morphologic defects potentially related to increased risk of chromosomal abnormalities in infants conceived with ICSI and decreased success rates. Thus, based on the theory that subtle sperm morphological malformations might remain unnoticed during the routine sperm selection performed prior to microinjection, negatively affecting its outcome, a new technique, termed motile sperm organellar morphology examination (MSOME), has been recently developed to perform a real-time detailed morphological evaluation of motile spermatozoa under 6,600× high magnification. When applied immediately prior the conventional ICSI technique, this new method of sperm morphological selection is defined: intracytoplasmic morphologically selected sperm injection (IMSI).

Even though a rising number of studies have reported IMSI as having remarkable clinical advantages in terms of fertilization, embryo quality, pregnancy occurrence, and prosecution until delivery, this new method continues to be debated regarding its routine application in the ART laboratory. Although IMSI has not yet been standardized and requires further validation, it can be considered one of the most promising issues in the ART field. IMSI has been introduced to increase ART success in overcoming severe male infertility.

M. Antinori (✉)
Infertility Unit, RAPRUI Day Hospital, Rome, Italy
e-mail: monica.antinori@raprui.com

C. Racowsky et al. (eds.), *Biennial Review of Infertility: Volume 2*,
DOI 10.1007/978-1-4419-8456-2_19, © Springer Science+Business Media, LLC 2011

Keywords
Sperm morphology • High magnification • Selection • MSOME • IMSI • Embryo quality

19.1 Introduction

Clinicians routinely use conventional semen parameters attempt to obtain a reliable overview on the male reproductive potential. However, in most cases little information on the fertility status is provided unless semen parameters are grossly abnormal [1, 2]. Among them the best fertilization predictor is morphology as assessed according to strict criteria [3]. Since its introduction [4], several advantages to the outcomes of conventional in vitro fertilization [3, 5], intrauterine insemination [6], and in vivo reproduction have been shown [7]. Therefore, it is clear how a spermatozoon's morphological normality reflects its function, in relation to its ability to reach, recognize, bind, penetrate, and deliver its genome to the oocyte. Differently, once the sperm is mechanically injected into the oocyte by an ICSI method, and hence has crossed both barriers of the zona pellucida and oolemma, its abnormal morphology does not seem to interfere with its fertilizing capacity. In this respect, most authors do not notice any correlation between ICSI outcomes and the strict morphology of the sperm used for microinjection [8–11]. In patients with a poor prognosis (4% normal sperm morphology) [12], and even in extreme, specific cases of total teratozoospermia [13], globozoospermia [14, 15], and megalozoospermia [16] fertilization can be achieved with ICSI. Several points of negative impact, both genetic and epigenetic, have been identified in embryos following the ICSI procedure [4, 17–19].

Nonetheless, major morphological anomalies lead to decreased rates of fertilization, pregnancy, implantation [16, 20], embryo quality [21–23], and blastocyst formation [21, 24]. Hence, during an ICSI procedure the embryologist selects a motile, normal-looking spermatozoon and discards the most distorted forms. This visual assessment of sperm morphology, limited by its low magnification (200–400×) and concomitant low resolution [21], overlooks minor morphologic defects potentially related to sperm functional impairment. At the same time, since men with oligoasthenoteratozoospermia were shown to have significantly elevated levels of sperm numerical chromosomal aberrations, and DNA chain fragmentation [25–31], and since incidence of chromosome aneuploidy in spermatozoa might be related with the severity of sperm defects [32], there is great concern regarding the increased risk of chromosomal abnormalities in infants conceived with ICSI [33–35].

Moreover, although ICSI has provided treatment for new groups of couples with male infertility who were previously untreatable by IVF, at present the resulting pregnancy rates are only between 30 and 45% [36–38] while the European average "take-home baby" rates remain similar [76] to those of a decade ago [39, 40]. The rising demand for improvement of success rates compels us to reassess male fertility potential through the development of new tests with clinical relevance for each ART procedure.

Conventional means of light microscopy cannot identify the entire variety of sperm morphological defects, especially in the head structure [41–43]. In 1999, electron microscopy (scanning electron microscopy, SEM and transmission electron microscopy, TEM) enabled Bartoov et al. [44] to correctly identify the ultra-morphological state of seven sperm subcellular organelles (acrosome, postacrosomal lamina, nucleus, neck, axoneme, mitochondrial sheath, and outer dense fibers). These subcellular organelles were found to be highly predictive factors for male fertility potential. Due to the fact that the applied technology was expensive, and often not available in conventional laboratories, its application was limited only to those cases in which the male infertility factor could not be clearly identified by routine tests or following repeated ART failures. As for conventional sperm morphology, this new evaluation turned out to be useful only in the context of a reproductive prognosis assessment, considering that the single sperm used for fertilization might not reflect the peculiarity of the analyzed sample. Moreover, since the evaluation was based on the examination of fixed and stained sperm cells, it did not provide the patient with any information about the single sperm used for ICSI. Taking all the aforementioned into consideration, a few years later a new approach was developed for a real-time detailed morphological evaluation of motile spermatozoa. The sperm analysis, termed motile sperm organellar morphology examination (MSOME), was performed using an interference phase contrast inverted, microscope, with the optics of Nomarski, that combines maximal optical magnification (100×), magnification selector (1.5×), and a video-coupled magnification to reach a final video magnification of 6,600×. This application was developed to allow the visualization of subtle sperm morphological malformations that might remain unnoticed during the routine sperm selection performed prior to microinjection. This method was introduced to improve the success of intracytoplasmic sperm injection. Of the six sperm subcellular organelles examined (acrosome, postacrosomal lamina, neck, mitochondria, tail, and nucleus), the sperm's nucleus was demonstrated to be the most important parameter affecting ICSI outcome [45] particularly in the form of large nuclear vacuoles that were proposed to reflect damages in the nuclear DNA content and organization [46, 47] (Fig. 19.1).

Presently, only a few studies have been carried out to investigate the real meaning of nuclear vacuolization and its relationship to DNA status. The opportunity to carry on additional research justifies the application of this new technique which requires specially trained personnel and can be considered extremely time-consuming and expensive, to be routinely inserted in the ART laboratory.

19.2 IMSI in Practice

Due to the usage of the optics of Nomarski, and in accordance with the current literature, carrying out of IMSI requires a (sterile) glass-bottomed dish with the following characteristics (Fig. 19.2):

– On the left side, 4 μL *observation droplets* of sperm culture medium containing between 0 and 10% polyvinyl pyrrolidone (PVP) solution. Small bays extruding from the rim of the droplets are created in order to capture

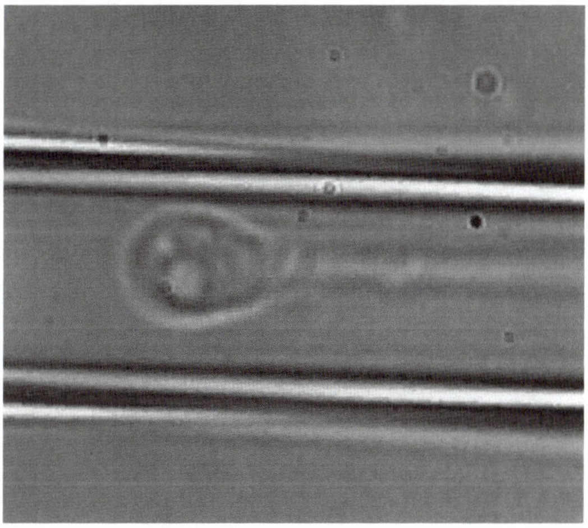

Fig. 19.1 A multivacuolated sperm clearly showing a large nuclear vacuole next to small vacuoles

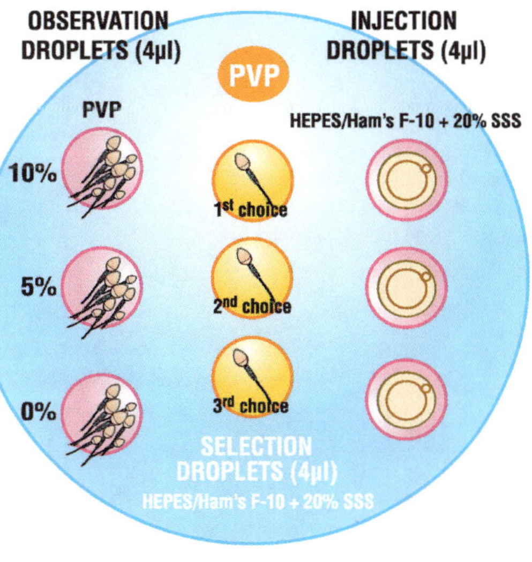

Fig. 19.2 The IMSI dish

the heads of motile spermatozoa. The temperature of the sperm sample and the PVP concentration are coordinated with the intensity of the sperm motility.

- In the middle, 4 μL *selection droplets* of sperm culture, where selected sperm cells are located after MSOME evaluation. Three distinct drops are made to host spermatozoa with different morphological features.
- On the right side, 4 μL droplets of sperm culture medium that will host the oocytes to be injected in the following ICSI procedure (*injection droplets*), one for each oocyte available for microinjection.

All microdroplets are placed under sterile liquid paraffin.

19.2.1 MSOME Criteria and Evaluation Procedure

Based on data collected by scanning and transmission electron microscopy [44], the MSOME criteria for normally shaped nuclei were defined as size (average length and width to be 4.75 ± 0.28 and 3.28 ± 0.20 μm, respectively) smoothness, symmetry, oval configuration (an extrusion or invagination of the nuclear mass was defined as a regional nuclear shape malformation, Fig. 19.3), and homogeneity of the nuclear chromatin mass containing no more than one vacuole, which occupies less than 4% of the nuclear area (0.78 ± 0.18 μm). Spermatozoa with abnormal head size are excluded by superimposing a transparent celluloid form on the motile examined gametes, representing the correct sperm size, which is calculated by the ratio of expected normal sperm size to the actual size visualized on the monitor screen. Spermatozoa with severe malformations, such as a pin, amorphous, tapered, round, or multinucleated head, which can be identified clearly even by low magnification (200–400×), are not assessed by MSOME. Spermatozoa with a doubtful determination are excluded from selection. In order to perform a correct sperm evaluation, the embryologist follows each motile single sperm cell with apparent suitability by moving the microscopic stage in the *x*, *y*, and *z* directions until also the smallest details are visualized. Actually some morphological defects, such as large vacuoles, can be revealed only during sperm movement, and therefore motility can be advantageous to the morphological observation. Furthermore, it is relevant to emphasize how a single sperm evaluation is reliable only when it is carried out on a motile sperm cell; on the other hand, static sperm images only allow evaluation of the visible part, leaving some morphological alterations undiscovered.

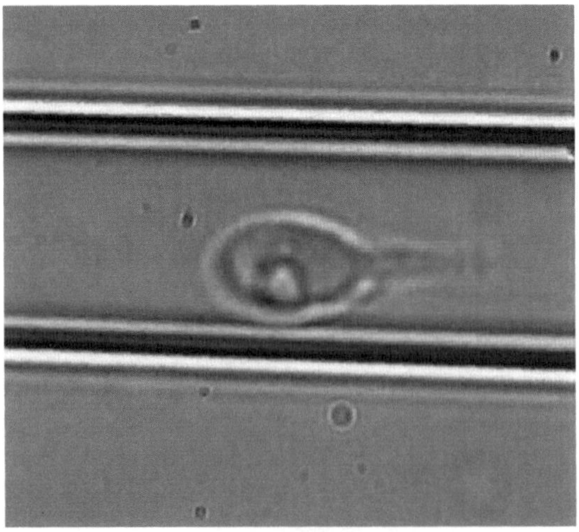

Fig. 19.3 An example of nuclear disorder, visible as a blebs protruding from the sperm head surface

Additionally, in order to minimize the subjective nature of sperm evaluation, a cooperation of two embryologists working together at the same time on the analysis of the same sample is recommended.

Finding normal-looking spermatozoa is variable according to the quality of the semen sample.

19.2.2 IMSI Step-by-Step

Freshly ejaculated semen is subjected to routine morphological selection of motile spermatozoa on the basis of a two-layer density gradient system: 1 mL of post-ejaculated liquefied semen is placed onto the gradient and centrifuged at 375 × *g* for 15 min at 25°C. The sperm cell pellet is suspended by adding 3 mL of sperm culture medium and then recentrifuged for 10 min. The supernatant is removed and replaced by sperm culture medium to bring the final concentration of motile sperm cells to about 4×10^6 spermatozoa per milliliter. In severe oligozoospermic cases with sperm density below 1×10^6 spermatozoa per ejaculate, liquefied semen is placed onto 1 mL of the low density layer only, centrifuged as previously described, and the final sperm cell pellet is resuspended in 0.1–0.2 mL of sperm culture medium.

The sperm cell suspension obtained after semen preparation is used for real-time high-magnification motile sperm organelle morphology examination (MSOME) [48] that is performed on the observation droplets by means of an inverted microscope (Olympus IX81, Tokyo, Japan) equipped with Nomarski differential interference contrast optics, an Uplan Apo ×100 oil/1.50 objective lens previously covered by a droplet of immersion oil, and a 0.55 NA condenser lens. The images are captured by a DXC-990P video camera having 1/2-in., 3-chip power HAD CCD and visualized on a color monitor screen with diagonal dimension of 355.6 mm. Calculation of the total magnification is based on four parameters: (1) objective magnification 100×; (2) magnification selector 1.5×; (3) video coupler magnification 0.99 (UPMTV X 0.3, PE X 3.3); and (4) (a) CCD chip diagonal dimension 8 mm and (b) television monitor diagonal dimension for a calculated video magnification (b/a) of 44.45. Thus, total magnification = microscope magnification (150×) X video coupler magnification (0.99×) X video magnification (44.45×) = 6,600×.

Only motile spermatozoa with morphologically normal nuclei are retrieved from the observation droplets and aspirated into a sterilized glass non-angulated pipette with a 9 μm inner diameter tip. Sperm cells are then placed into the selection droplet and finally used to be injected into the oocytes for the classical ICSI procedure [49].

This procedure is performed using a motorized micromanipulator system (TransferMan NK2, Eppendorf, Germany).

19.3 IMSI Reproductive Outcomes

A new approach for real-time motile sperm morphological evaluation (MSOME) was introduced [45]. The MSOME enabled the visualization of some morphological anomalies which conventional light microscopy cannot detect at 200–400×. Assuming that spermatozoa with severely impaired morphology show reduced fertilization, pregnancy, and implantation rates [16, 20], the study aimed to determine whether subtle morphological anomalies affect ICSI outcome and identify those that are most relevant. Having analyzed a total of 10,000 spermatozoa (100 sperm samples, 100 spermatozoa each), it was demonstrated that in routine IVF–ICSI cycles patients who exhibited less than 20% spermatozoa with normal nucleus, defined by MSOME, did not achieve any pregnancy. With respect to the ICSI fertilization rate, the morphological normalcy of the entire sperm cell, according to MSOME criteria, showed a positive and significant correlation ($r = 0.52$, $P \leq 0.01$) and a very high predictive value (area under the ROC curve, 88%), whereas no association with pregnancy outcome was found. The normalcy of the sperm nucleus (shape + chromatin content), defined by MSOME, was significantly and positively correlated with both: fertilization rate ($r = 0.42$, $P \leq 0.01$) and pregnancy occurrence ($r = 0.38$, $P \leq 0.01$). Else the predictive value of normalcy of the nucleus turned out to be significantly higher (areas under the ROC curve, 72 and 74%, respectively). Hence, the authors could conclude that sperm nucleus is the most important sperm parameter affecting ICSI outcome [45].

A further utilization of high power magnification in real-time of ICSI was applied. Using MSOME evaluation for the injected sperm in real-time was termed as intracytoplasmic morphologically selected sperm injection (IMSI) [48]. Fifty IMSI couples were compared to 50 ICSI couples in a matched control manner (e.g., couples with the similar number of previous ICSI failures). Implantation and pregnancy rates after IMSI were significantly higher, and the abortion rate was significantly lower, compared to the current ICSI trial ($F=18.0$, $P\leq0.01$; $x^2=4.4$, $P\leq0.01$; and $x^2=4.4$, $P\leq0.05$). In addition, the IMSI attempt produced a significantly higher value of top embryo percentage, compared to the current ICSI treatment ($F=6.5$, $P\leq0.01$). Moreover, the 12 cases of the unmatched IMSI group with an average of 9.1 ± 1.2 previously failed ICSI attempts achieved a 50% pregnancy rate following their first IMSI trial. The obtained results demonstrated that IMSI improves significantly the success rate in couples with at least two previous ICSI failures.

With the intention of eliminating the probability that the increased pregnancy outcome was linked to the sperm preparation technique adopted for IMSI and not to the nuclear morphology of the selected spermatozoa a comparative study was conducted. Thirty-eight transfers of embryos derived from "second best" morphologically evaluated sperm cells (negative group) following IMSI cycles took place, vs. 38 transfers derived from morphologically normal nuclei (positive group). Comparison between the groups revealed that fertilization rate, percentage of top embryos, and implantation rates were significantly higher in the positive group than in the negative group [46].

Out of six pregnancies achieved in the negative group, four turned into a first trimester abortion. Interestingly, three abortion cases occurred when microinjection was conducted with spermatozoa exhibiting large nuclear vacuoles, whereas in the other abortion case the sperm cells exhibited combined malformations: large vacuoles associated with narrow formed head shape.

A subsequent enlarged study by the same group [47] confirmed all the previous findings as follows: pregnancy rate was significantly higher and the abortion rate significantly lower following IMSI, compared with ICSI attempts ($x^2=20.1$, $P\leq0.01$; and $x^2=5.1$, $P\leq0.03$, respectively). Furthermore IMSI provided a higher percentage of top quality embryos with a better implantation rate than ICSI.

A comparison between a "best group," in which embryos were obtained from microinjection exclusively performed using spermatozoa with intact nuclei, and a "second best group" where only sperm cells with minimal impairment were used for microinjection, since no "best" sperm cells were available in those cases, demonstrated that fertilization rate, percentage of top embryos, implantation, pregnancy, and delivery rates per cycle were significantly higher, and the abortion rate was significantly lower in the "best" group than in the "second best one" ($F=10.5$, $P\leq0.01$; $F=4.6$, $P\leq0.03$; $F=23.4$, $P\leq0.01$; $x^2=15.5$, $P\leq0.05$; $x^2=19.6$, $P\leq0.01$; and $x^2=5.5$, $P\leq0.02$, respectively) [50].

These authors restricted the application of this new procedure to cases with over two previous implantation failures. Actually, according to recent publications, those couples seem to have the worst reproductive prognosis with a dramatic reduction in pregnancy and implantation rates as compared with couples who underwent 0–1 previous failed IVF attempts [51, 52]. Hence, Antinori et al. [53] designed a prospective randomized controlled protocol to assess the potential advantages of the IMSI procedure in the treatment of patients with severe oligoasthenoteratozoospermia regardless of their previous failed ICSI attempts, followed by a subgroup splitting according to the number of previous failed attempts (subgroup A: no previous attempts; subgroup B: 1 previous failed attempt; subgroup C: ≥2 previous failed attempts). The comparisons between the two different techniques were made in terms of pregnancy, abortion, and implantation rates.

Pregnancy and implantation rates resulted statistically better in IMSI than ICSI cycles (PR: 39.2 vs.26.5%; $P=0.004$) (IR: 17.3 vs. 11.3%; $P=0.007$).

However, cases with two or more failed attempts benefited most from IMSI, with a statistically significant doubling of pregnancy rate (12.9 vs. 29.8%; $P=0.017$) and a remarkable 50% reduction in the abortion rate (17 vs. 35%). Comparisons did not show any statistical difference in terms of abortions but the clinical trend was clearly in favor of the IMSI method in cases with two or more previous failed attempts.

Based on the above results, it is likely that in those couples, male factor could be featured by semen impairment, undetected by conventional diagnostic tools, thus reducing the effectiveness of previous ICSI treatments.

19.3.1 IMSI and Vacuolated Spermatozoa

Implantation and pregnancy achieved by IMSI seem associated with morphological nuclear normalcy of the sperm. Nonetheless, spermatozoa with a morphologically abnormal nucleus show low fertility potential, even if some with certain severe nuclear abnormalities may still be able to produce pregnancy following ICSI [13–16].

Some reports found that head malformations negatively correlate with DNA integrity [54–56]. Else, a clear negative association between the existence of sperm nuclear vacuoles and natural male fertility potential was reported by others [57, 58], it can be assumed that within the category of specific morphological malformations, existence of large vacuoles in the sperm nuclei indicates more damage to the nuclear DNA content and organization than nuclear shape or size impairment.

The impact of sperm with normal nuclear shape but large nuclear vacuoles on pregnancy outcome compared to those with strictly defined morphologically normal nuclei, including shape and content, was investigated by Berkovitz et al. in 2006 [47]. A lower pregnancy rate per cycle, and a higher early spontaneous abortion rate per pregnancy were observed in the study group in comparison with the same parameters in the control group (18 vs. 50%, Pearson's $x^2=6.4$, and 80 vs.7%, Pearson's $x^2=10.9$, respectively, $P=0.01$).

MSOME revealed that the ejaculates of males routinely referred for ICSI exhibit on average 30–40% spermatozoa with a vacuolated nucleus. This sperm malformation, identifiable as a pregnancy risk factor on the basis of the previous findings, can easily be missed by the standard selection prior to ICSI, and have, therefore, a chance to be chosen for microinjection of at least 30%.

In order to verify that the large nuclear vacuoles in the sperm cell reflect some underlying chromosomal or DNA defect, sperm cells with and without large vacuoles were selected from the same ejaculate and examined by different biochemical methods from an external analytic system [47].

A first step in this direction was taken by Hazout et al. [59], who compared the outcomes of 125 couples with at least two previous ICSI failures and an undetected female infertility factor that underwent conventional and high-magnification ICSI in two sequential attempts. Following sperm injection into the oocytes without nuclear alterations, a double pregnancy rate and a 50% decrease in the abortion rate were recorded as against similar cases treated by conventional ICSI. In 72 out of 125 patients involved in the study, the degree of sperm DNA fragmentation was determined by TUNEL and the outcomes of high magnification ICSI were compared in cases with different sperm DNA fragmentation degrees. However, this test was not performed directly with the sperm samples used for ICSI. A marked rise in clinical implantation and birth rates was observed in patients with both normal (<30%), moderately (30–40%) and highly (>40%) increased percentage of DNA-fragmented spermatozoa in the ejaculate.

The extent of DNA fragmentation (TUNEL assay) and the presence of denatured single-stranded or normal double-stranded DNA (acridine orange fluorescence method, AOT) in spermatozoa with large nuclear vacuoles (LNV) selected by high magnification compared to those with normal nucleus were evaluated by Franco et al. [60]. The percentage of positive DNA fragmentation was significantly higher ($P<0.0001$) in LNV spermatozoa (29.1%) than in NN spermatozoa (15.9%). Similarly, the percentage of denatured-stranded DNA was significantly higher ($P<0.0001$) in the former (67.9%) than in the latter (33.1%).

A direct correlation in DNA quality has not been tested in single selected spermatozoa. Thus, the chromatin structure (sperm DNA integrity by acridine orange; DNA fragmentation by TUNEL assay) was analyzed, in correlation to sperm aneuploidies (FISH test). The study was conducted by Garolla et al. [61] in ten patients with severe testicular damage (severe oligozoospermia) on single immotile sperm cells morphologically selected by high-magnification microscopy (13,161×). From the sample of each patient, ten spermatozoa with normal morphology and no vacuoles (group A) and ten spermatozoa with normal morphology and at least one large head-vacuole (group B) were selected. Single cells from group A showed a more physiological status of DNA integrity and DNA fragmentation than cells from group B. Furthermore, FISH analysis showed that no chromosomal alteration was present in cells from group A. Moreover, the authors reported that taking into consideration spermatozoa with normal morphology and both presence or absence of large head-vacuoles, the mean results (data not shown) from all tests were significantly better with respect to those of unselected cells performed in the first part of the study (all $P<0.001$).

Based on technical limits of the differential interference contrast (DIC), which doesn't allow intracellular evaluation [62–64], since in order to detect chromatin vacuoles the evaluation has to be performed at 20,000× magnification by electron microscopy, and because of their main localization, in the anterior part of the sperm head, the acrosomal origin of these vacuoles was theorized [65]. The first experiment of this study consisted of MSOME evaluation on immotile spermatozoa followed by acrosomal status assessment of the same spermatozoon using *Pisum sativum* agglutinin fluorescein isothiocyanate. The complete acrosome reaction corresponded in most of the cases (70.9%) to spermatozoa of regular shape with absent or slight vacuolization, whereas those sperms with incomplete or missing acrosome reaction showed 60.7% of vacuole presence. A second study comprised of ten patients whose immotile spermatozoa were analyzed according to MSOME before and after the acrosome had been induced by ionophore A23587. Vacuole-free spermatozoa increased from 41.2 to 63.8% ($P>0.005$) with a concomitant rise of the acrosome-reacted gametes from 17.4+7.8 to 36.1+12.7 ($P<0.001$). Moreover, it was possible to visualize large protruding blebs as well as a sort of invagination when seen upfront that looks like a vacuole in the following image in motile acrosome-reacted spermatozoa that were analyzed by MSOME. The authors concluded that the vacuole-free spermatozoa microinjected during IMSI are mostly acrosome-reacted spermatozoa.

19.3.2 Classification of Sperm

As was already mentioned, one of the main concerns of ICSI, for the embryologist is the aspiration of the good-quality spermatozoa for microinjection into an oocyte. It is likely that some of the injected spermatozoa do have a good developmental potential.

Else, as previously mentioned, it is accepted that the morphologic characteristics may not necessarily describe the quality of the specific single spermatozoon (in the processed sperm fraction) that was injected into the oocyte [66, 67]. However, yet, morphology, is definitely the only tool to evaluate quality of the sperm selected for oocyte injection. De Vos et al. [20] performed such a study of the individual injected sperm and the formation and development of the resultant embryo. A reduced fertilization rate following the injection of sperm cells with abnormal morphology, was observed. Nevertheless, reduced implantation rates were noted, when only "abnormal-sperm-embryos" were transferred. These investigators admitted that the low magnification (i.e., routine magnification of 400× during ICSI), and concomitant low resolution of the sperm morphology assessment on motile spermatozoa before ICSI, were a limitation of their study.

IMSI definitely overcomes these limitations; by using a high power 1,500×, inverted, light microscope with a zoom up to 6,100×, and higher, it was demonstrated that a normal spermatozoon, and more precisely, a strictly defined normal sperm nucleus, affects the fertilization rate and the occurrence of pregnancy [45–48]. Thus, the authors deemed it worthwhile to develop a tool for determining which is the preferable spermatozoon that should be injected into an oocyte.

19.3.3 Establishment of Classification Scoring Scales

In order to establish a detailed classification scoring scale to choose the individual spermatozoon with the highest predictive fertilizing and developmental potentials, in real-time, it is important to understand the correlation between the normalcy of the sperm, its fertilizability, and early embryo development and to analyze which sperm defects negatively affect the development of the embryo.

One important point is that the authors assume that the "experienced eyes" of the embryologists, omit, even under magnification of 200–400×, spermatozoa with rough morphological major abnormalities that are detectable under routine conditions. It is probable that the majority of abnormalities observed under magnification of 6,100×, are not visible using the routine conditions. Thus, it is likely that the main benefit of a scoring scale of sperm classification in IMSI is a kind of "fine tuning" and is actually more beneficial for those motile spermatozoa with normal morphological appearance, under magnification of 200–400×. This was recently confirmed when spermatozoon was first chosen for ICSI as routinely performed under conventional conditions using magnification of 400×. Thereafter, prior to injection, the spermatozoon was evaluated, inside the ICSI pipette under high magnification [67].

19.3.4 Parameters for Motile Sperm Evaluation and Classification in Real-Time

In general, it is obvious that classification parameters should be clear and will enable the embryologist to score the aspirated motile spermatozoon as fast as possible. *Normalcy of the sperm nucleus*: was first detected by Bartoov et al. [45, 47] according to the shape of sperm head. As already mentioned, normalcy of the nucleus was checked (6,000×) in the leftover sperm fraction, in 100 couples after using it for ICSI in three major IVF centers [45]. It was demonstrated that a normal spermatozoon, with a normal nuclear shape, observed under magnification of 6,000× in real-time, might increase embryo quality in terms of implantation [47]. These investigators reported that, during the IMSI procedure, spermatozoa were preselected under the magnification of 6,000× and accumulated in a droplet. Classifications of selected spermatozoa morphology have been determined as "normal" and "second" choice (one droplet for all the spermatozoa of a specific "choice"). Spermatozoa were aspirated from those accumulated motile sperm cell droplets and injected by the embryologist. One might only speculate that during IMSI when no normal head spermatozoa can be found, the only alternative then is to select those motile sperm cells that are morphologically second best. However, the parameters used by those authors to define a normal sperm nucleus, normal nuclear shape, or normal sperm, were not clearly portrayed [46, 48].

Vacuoles: The negative effect of vacuoles on fertilization and embryo development and the possible correlation with DNA integrity has previously been described. Vanderzwalmen et al. [68] classified the spermatozoa into four groups according to the presence and size of vacuoles: Grade I, normal shape and absence of vacuoles, Grade II, maximum of two small vacuoles; Grade III, more than two small vacuoles or at least one large vacuole; and Grade IV, large vacuoles in conjunction with abnormal head shapes or other abnormalities at the level of the base of the sperm head. As previously explained, it has been postulated that vacuoles of various sizes are most likely correlated to the integrity of sperm DNA and, thus, may affect the fertilization potential of the spermatozoon [53, 59, 60, 67].

However, it is not clear yet, when vacuoles are formed and why they are such important indicators of sperm quality. Nevertheless, the question whether is there a correlation with DNA damage in the sperm head is still debatable.

19.3.5 Combination of Sperm Characteristics in Real-Time

Cassuto and Barak scoring system was recently established to define more precisely the preferable spermatozoon for ICSI [67]. In the latest, each spermatozoon was initially aspirated using the routine ICSI method, i.e., magnification of 400×. Aspiration was then followed by immediate observation and scoring under magnification of 6,100×, prior to ICSI. Utilization of this method made it possible to detect each single spermatozoon in correlation to its contribution with a specific oocyte/early embryo, and to examine the effect of the morphology of an individual sperm cell. Based on the knowledge accumulated in the field of fertility [4, 14, 19, 20, 26, 45], each aspirated spermatozoon was classified into one of three classes I, II, or III taking into consideration the following characteristics: normalcy of head shape, acrosome, absence of vacuoles, normalcy of the base of sperm head, normalcy of tail, and clarity of head cytoplasm The investigators endeavour to comprehend which defect could effect the correlation between the normalcy of the sperm, fertilization, and early embryo development up to the blastocyst stage. A comparison of the fertilization rates (FR) following the injection of spermatozoa of the three various classes revealed a significant difference ($P<0.04$; $x^2=6.31$) when a pair wise comparison showed a significant difference between groups I and III ($P<0.01$; $x^2=6.3$). Moreover, a significance was noted when comparison was made between the rate of expanded blastocysts in the three groups ($P<0.03$; $x^2=6.71$). No expanded blastocyst was formed in embryos resulted following the injection of class III spermatozoa. Statistical analysis of the outcome and area under the best ROC curve revealed that: head shape, absence of vacuoles, and normalcy of head–base were the major characteristics for sperm classification. In accordance with the findings, the three classes of sperm morphology impart new information that contributes to the outcome of ICSI, in regard to fertilization and early embryo development up to the blastocyst stage. Confirmed by others (and as previously mentioned), it has clearly been shown that vacuoles in the sperm head interfere already from the first step of fertilization; a higher FR was achieved in oocytes injected with spermatozoa in which no vacuoles were observed in their heads.

Moreover, normalcy of the base appears to be a major factor, which affected embryo quality; a higher rate of "top" and "good" day 2 and 3 embryos were detected when the base of the sperm head was scored as normal. As the base of the sperm head actually contains the centrosome, and is correlated to the sperm nucleus, it does contribute to embryo quality, as has been confirmed by others [58, 69–71]. A friendly formula of a model for the classification following calculations of coefficients with: area = 0.618 of the ROC curve, was designed: Score = Head × 2 + Vacuole × 3 + Base.

Values of the major sperm criteria were scored as normal = 1 and abnormal = 0. When calculated, the range of scoring varied between 0 and 6. The recommended calculated Cassuto and Barak score for the injected spermatozoa should be 4–6 (Class I).

19.3.6 Scoring and Women's Age

Due to the data published by these investigators it seems that IMSI is more beneficial in "older oocytes" harvested from patients aged 30 years and older. Statistical analysis for the combination of the woman's age and the scored injected spermatozoa in correlation to embryo quality, distinguished between the quality of embryos resulting from oocytes of patients younger than 30 years and those which developed from oocytes originating from patients 30 years and older. A reduced rate of top D2 and D3 embryos was observed when class II and class III spermatozoa were injected to oocytes of patients between 30 and 36 years old in comparison to the injection of class II and III spermatozoa to oocytes harvested from patients <30 years (44.4 vs. 96.3%; $P<0.001$; $x^2=19.52$, respectively) [67].

The age-related decline in the quality of the oocytes, is a known phenomenon [72–74]. The outcome explains the importance of sperm scoring mainly in "older oocytes" harvested from patients aged 30 years and older. This outcome is not surprising, as the young oocyte is capable of "repairing" the DNA of the injected spermatozoon; ICSI may rescue embryos in some patients by avoiding delays in cell cycle, through a direct sperm deposition in the oocyte. The extra time helps to save maternal ribonucleic acid (mRNA) which may partially overcome epigenic defects [73–75]. Conversely, when a class I spermatozoon was injected, the age-related quality of the oocyte was neglected. This is logical, as these "top spermatozoon" does not need any reparation.

It is likely that a good scoring system would further contribute to the success rates of IMSI. In young women, it appears that scoring spermatozoa before ICSI is not crucial. However, in the older group of patients, it seems beneficial to invest time and aspirate a high-score spermatozoon using the IMSI application, for increasing fertilization rate and embryo quality.

19.4 Conclusions

The introduction of IMSI has fostered a deeper understanding of those mechanisms that interfere with male fertility potential in both natural and assisted reproduction. The lack of standardization in terms of basic techniques and morphological evaluation criteria, its routine application available in only a few ART units due to man-hours, and high costs involved, all these factors create skepticism regarding IMSI's cost-effectiveness. All things considered, the most important question is: is it ethically acceptable, according to the current literature, to not provide the infertile couple with spermatozoa of the best quality available when the technology gives you the opportunity to do so, even with the knowledge that this could compromise the ART success rate? In order to fully answer this question, it is important to first change the pervasive mindset which is limiting the full potential that could be gained by employing the most technologically advanced procedures like IMSI. ART treatments can no longer be considered mere "shots in the dark", they must become a decisive therapy with much more weight being given to the first attempt.

References

1. Dumpy BC, Neal LM, Cooke ID. The clinical value of semen analysis. Fertil Steril. 1989;51:324–9.
2. Aitkin RJ, Irvine DS, Wu FC. Prosecute analysis of sperm-oocyte fusion and reactive oxygen species generation as catena for the diagnosis of infertility. Am J Obstet Gynecol. 1991;164:542–51.
3. Vawda AI, Gunby J, Younglai EV. Semen parameters as predictors of in-vitro fertilization: the importance of strict criteria morphology. Hum Reprod. 1996;11: 1445–50.
4. Kruger TF, Menkveld R, Stander FSH, Lombard CJ, Van der Merwe JP, van Zyl JA, et al. Sperm morphologic features as a prognostic factor in vitro fertilization. Fertil Steril. 1986;46:1118–23.
5. Grow DR, Oehninger S, Seltman HJ, Toner JP, Swanson RJ, Kruger TF, et al. Sperm morphology as diagnosed by strict criteria: probing the impact of teratozoospermia on fertilization rate and pregnancy outcome in a large in vitro fertilization population. Fertil Steril. 1994;62:559–67.
6. Burr RW, Siegberg R, Flaherty SP, Wang XJ, Matthews CD. The influence of sperm morphology and the number of motile sperm inseminated on the outcome of intrauterine insemination combined with mild ovarian stimulation. Fertil Steril. 1996;65:127–32.
7. Eggert-Kruse W, Schwartz H, Rohr G, Demirakca T, Tilgen W, Runnebaum B. Sperm morphology assessment using strict criteria and male fertility under in-vivo conditions of conception. Hum Reprod. 1996;11:139–46.
8. Oehninger S, Veeck L, Lanzendorf S, Maloney M, Toner J, Muasher S. Intracytoplasmic sperm injection: achievement of high pregnancy rates in couples with severe male factor infertility is dependent primarily upon female not male factors. Fertil Steril. 1995; 64:977–81.
9. Kupker W, Schulze W, Diedrich K. Ultrastructure of gametes and intracytoplasmic sperm injection: the significance of sperm morphology. Hum Reprod. 1998;13 Suppl 1:99–106.
10. Host E, Ernst E, Lindenberg S, Smidt-Jensen S. Morphology of spermatozoa used in IVF and ICSI from oligozoospermic men. Reprod Biomed Online. 2001;3:212–5.
11. Celik-Ozenci C, Jakab A, Kovacs T, Catalanotti J, Demir R, Bray-Ward P, et al. Sperm selection for ICSI: shape properties do not predict the absence or presence of numerical chromosomal aberrations. Hum Reprod. 2004;19:2052–9.
12. Sukcharoen N, Sithipravej T, Promviengchai S, Chinpilas V, Boonkasemsanti W. Sperm morphology evaluated by computer (IVOS) cannot predict the fertilization rate in vitro after intracytoplasmic sperm injection. Fertil Steril. 1998;69:564–8.
13. Tasdemir I, Tasdemir M, Tavukcuog S, Kahraman S, Biberog K. Effect of abnormal sperm head morphology on the outcome of intracytoplasmic sperm injection in humans. Hum Reprod. 1997;12:1214–7.

14. Liu J, Nagy Z, Joris H, Tournaye H, Devroey P, Van Steirteghem A. Successful fertilization and establishment of pregnancies after intracytoplasmic sperm injection in patients with globozoospermia. Hum Reprod. 1995;10:626–9.
15. Battaglia DE, Koehler JK, Klein NA, Tucker MJ. Failure of oocyte activation after intracytoplasmic sperm injection using round-headed sperm. Fertil Steril. 1997;68:118–22.
16. Kahraman S, Akarsu C, Cengiz G, Dirican K, Sozen E, Can B, et al. Fertility of ejaculated and testicular megalohead spermatozoa with intracytoplasmic sperm injection. Hum Reprod. 1999;14:726–30.
17. Ménézo Y, Dale B. Paternal contribution to successful embryogenesis. Hum Reprod. 1994;10:1326–8.
18. Jones GM, Trouson AO, Lolatgis N, Wood C. Factors affecting the success of human blastocyst development and pregnancy following in vitro fertilization and embryo transfer. Fertil Steril. 1998; 70:1022–9.
19. Barak Y, Goldman S. Development of in vitro human embryo. In: Allahbadia G, Merchant R, editors. Contemporary perspectives on assisted reproductive technologies. New Delhi: Reed Elsevier; 2006. p. 80–8.
20. De Vos A, Van De Velde H, Joris H, Verheyen G, Devroey P, Van Steirteghem A. Influence of individual sperm morphology on fertilization, embryo morphology, and pregnancy outcome of intracytoplasmic sperm injection. Fertil Steril. 2003;79:42–8.
21. Cohen J, Alikani M, Malter H, et al. Partial zona dissection or subzonal sperm insertion: microsurgical fertilization alternatives based on evaluation of sperm and embryo morphology. Fertil Steril. 1991; 56:696–706.
22. Parinaud J, Mieusset R, Vieitez G, Labal B, Richoilley G. Influence of sperm parameters on embryo quality. Fertil Steril. 1993;60:888–92.
23. Loutradi KE, Tarlatzis BC, Goulis DG, Zepiridis L, Pagou T, Chatziioannou E, et al. The effects of sperm quality on embryo development after intracytoplasmic sperm injection. J Assist Reprod Genet. 2006;23: 69–74.
24. Miller JE, Smith TT. The effect of intracytoplasmic sperm injection and semen parameters on blastocyst development in vitro. Hum Reprod. 2001;16:918–24.
25. Huszar G, Vigue L. Incomplete development of human spermatozoa is associated with increased creatine phosphokinase concentration and abnormal head morphology. Mol Reprod Dev. 1993;34:292–8.
26. Aitken J, Krausz C, Buckingham D. Relationships between biochemical markers for residual sperm cytoplasm, reactive oxygen species generation, and the presence of leukocytes and precursor germ cells in human sperm suspensions. Mol Reprod Dev. 1994;39:268–79.
27. Bernardini L, Borini A, Preti S, Conte N, Flamigni C, Capitanio GL, et al. Study of aneuploidy in normal and abnormal germ cells from semen of fertile and infertile men. Hum Reprod. 1998;13:3406–13.
28. Rubes J, Lowe X, Moore 2nd D, Perreault S, Slott V, Evenson D, et al. Smoking cigarettes is associated with increased sperm disomy in teenage men. Fertil Steril. 1998;70:715–23.
29. Twigg JP, Irvine DS, Aitken RJ. Oxidative damage to DNA in human spermatozoa does not preclude pronucleus formation at intracytoplasmic sperm injection. Hum Reprod. 1998;13:1864–71.
30. Sakkas D, Mariethoz E, Manicardi G, Bizzaro D, Bianchi PG, Bianchi U. Origin of DNA damage in ejaculated human spermatozoa. Rev Reprod. 1999;4:31–7.
31. Griffin DK, Hyland P, Tempest HG, Homa ST. Safety issues in assisted reproduction technology: should men undergoing ICSI be screened for chromosome abnormalities in their sperm? Hum Reprod. 2003;18:229–35.
32. Carrell DT, Emery BR, Wilcox AL, Campbell B, Erickson L, Hatasaka HH, et al. Sperm chromosome aneuploidy as related to male factor infertility and some ultrastructure defects. Arch Androl. 2004;50:181–5.
33. Rubio C, Simon C, Blanco V, Vidal F, Minguez Y, Egozcue J, et al. Implications of sperm chromosome abnormalities in recurrent miscarriage. J Assist Reprod Genet. 1999;16:253–8.
34. Van Steirteghem A, Bonduelle M, Devroey P, Liebaers I. Follow up of children born after ICSI. Hum Reprod Update. 2002;8:111–6.
35. Hansen M, Kurinczuk JJ, Bower C, Webb S. The risk of major birth defects after intracytoplasmic sperm injection and in vitro fertilization. N Engl J Med. 2002;346:725–30.
36. Kuczynski W, Dhont M, Grygoruk C, Grochowski D, Wolczynski S, Szamatowicz M. The outcome of intracytoplasmic injection of fresh and cryopreserved ejaculated spermatozoa – a prospective randomized study. Hum Reprod. 2001;16:2109–13.
37. Stolwijk AM, Wetzels AM, Braat DD. Cumulative probability of achieving an ongoing pregnancy after in-vitro fertilization and intracytoplasmic sperm injection according to a woman's age, subfertility diagnosis and primary or secondary subfertility. Hum Reprod. 2000;15:203–9.
38. Olivius K, Friden B, Lundin K, Bergh C. Cumulative probability of live birth after three in vitro fertilization/intracytoplasmic sperm injection cycles. Fertil Steril. 2002;77:505–10.
39. Van Steirteghem AC, Liu J, Joris H, Nagy Z, Janssenswillen C, Tournaye H, et al. Higher success rate by intracytoplasmic sperm injection than by subzonal insemination. Report of a second series of 300 consecutive treatment cycles. Hum Reprod. 1993;8: 1055–60.
40. Harari O, Bourne H, McDonald M, Richings N, Speirs AL, Johnston WIH, et al. Intracytoplasmic sperm injection – a major advance in the management of severe male subfertility. Fertil Steril. 1995;64: 360–8.
41. Glezerman M, Bartoov B. Semen analysis. In: Insler V, Lunenfeld B, editors. Infertility: male and

female. Edinburgh: Churchill Livingstone; 1993. p. 285–315.
42. Piomboni P, Strehler E, Capitani S, Collodel G, De Santo M, Gambera L, et al. Submicroscopic mathematical evaluation of spermatozoa in assisted reproduction, in vitro fertilization (notulae seminologicae 7). J Assist Reprod Genet. 1996;13:635–46.
43. Zamboni L. The ultrastructural pathology of the spermatozoan as a course of infertility: the role of electron microscopy in the evaluation of sperm quality. Fertil Steril. 1987;48:711–34.
44. Bartoov B, Eltes F, Reichart M, Langzam J, Lederman H, Zabludovsky N. Quantitative ultramorphological analysis of human sperm: fifteen years of experience in the diagnosis and management of male factor infertility. Arch Androl. 1999;43(1):13–25.
45. Bartoov B, Berkovitz A, Eltes F, Kogosowski A, Menezo Y, Barak Y. Real-time fine morphology of motile human sperm cells is associated with IVF-ICSI outcome. J Androl. 2002;23:1–8.
46. Berkovitz A, Eltes F, Yaari S, Katz N, Barr I, Ami Fishman A, et al. The morphological normalcy of the sperm nucleus and pregnancy rate of intracytoplasmic injection with morphologically selected sperm. Hum Reprod. 2005;20:185–90.
47. Berkovitz A, Eltes F, Ellenbogen E, Peer S, Feldberg D, Bartoov B. Does the presence of nuclear vacuoles in human sperm selected for ICSI affect pregnancy outcome? Hum Reprod. 2006;21:1787–90.
48. Bartoov B, Berkovitz A, Eltes F, Kogosovsky A, Yagoda A, Lederman H, et al. Pregnancy rates are higher with intracytoplasmic morphologically selected sperm injection than with conventional intracytoplasmic injection. Fertil Steril. 2003;80:1413–9.
49. Palermo G, Joris H, Devroey P, Van Steirteghem A. Pregnancies after intracytoplasmic injection of single spermatozoon into an oocyte. Lancet. 1992;340:17.
50. Berkovitz A, Eltes F, Lederman H, Peer S, Ellenbogen A, Feldberg B, et al. 2006 How to improve IVF–ICSI outcome by sperm selection. Reprod Biomed Online. 2006;12:634–8.
51. Shapiro BS, Richter KS, Harris DC, Daneshmand ST. Dramatic declines in implantation and pregnancy rates in patients who undergo repeated cycles of in vitro fertilization with blastocyst transfer after one or more failed attempts. Fertil Steril. 2001;76:538–42.
52. Silberstein T, Trimarchi JR, Gonzalez L, Keefe D, Blazar AS. Pregnancy outcome in in vitro fertilization decreases to a plateau with repeated cycles. Fertil Steril. 2005;84:1043–5.
53. Antinori M, Licata E, Dani G, Cerusico C, Versaci C, D'Angelo D, et al. Intracytoplasmic morphologically selected sperm injection: a prospective randomized trial. Reprod Biomed Online. 2008;16:835–41.
54. Sailer BL, Jost LK, Evenson DP. Bull sperm head morphometry related to abnormal chromatin structure and fertility. Cytometry. 1996;24:167–73.
55. Virro MR, Larson-Cook KL, Evenson DP. Sperm chromatin structure assay (SCSA) parameters are related to fertilization, blastocyst development, and ongoing pregnancy in in vitro fertilization and intracytoplasmic sperm injection cycles. Fertil Steril. 2004;81:1289–95.
56. Vicari E, de Palma A, Burrello N, Longo G, Grazioso C, Barone N, et al. Effect of an abnormal sperm chromatin structural assay (SCSA) on pregnancy outcome following (IVF) with ICSI in previous IVF failures. Arch Androl. 2005;51:121–4.
57. Bartoov B, Eltes F, Pansky M, Langzam J, Reichart M, Soffer Y. Improved diagnosis of male fertility potential via a combination of quantitative ultramorphology and routine semen analyses. Hum Reprod. 1994;9:2069–75.
58. Mundy AJ, Ryder TA, Edmonds DK. A quantitative study of sperm head ultrastructure in subfertile males with excess sperm precursors. Fertil Steril. 1994;61:751–4.
59. Hazout A, Dumont-Hassan M, Junca AM, Bacrie PC, Tesarik J. High-magnification ICSI overcomes paternal effect resistant to conventional ICSI. Reprod Biomed Online. 2006;12:19–25.
60. Franco Jr JG, Baruffi RL, Mauri AL, et al. Significance of large nuclear vacuoles in human spermatozoa: implications for ICSI. Reprod Biomed Online. 2008;17:42–5.
61. Garolla A, Fortini D, Menegazzo M, et al. High-power microscopy for selecting spermatozoa for ICSI by physiological status. Reprod Biomed Online. 2008;17:610–6.
62. Hoffman R, Gross L. Reflected light differential-interference microscopy: principles, use and image interpretation. J Microsc. 1968;88:305–49.
63. Hoffman R, Gross L. Demodulation contrast microscope. Nature. 1975;254:586–8.
64. Padawer J. Denomarski interference-contrast microscope. An experimental basis for image interpretation. J R Microsc Soc. 1968;88:305–49.
65. Kacem O, Sifer C, Barraud-Lange V, Ducot B, De Ziegler D, Poirot C, et al. Sperm nuclear vacuoles, assessed by motile sperm organellar morphological examination, are mostly of acrosomal origin. Reprod Biomed Online. 2010;20:132–7.
66. Hewitson L, Dominko T, Takahashi D, Martinovich C, Ramalho-Santos J, Sutovsky P, et al. Unique checkpoints during the first cell cycle of fertilization after intracytoplasmic sperm injection in Rhesus monkeys. Nat Med. 1999;5:431–3.
67. Cassuto NG, Bouret D, Plouchart JM, Jellad S, Vanderzwalmen P, Balet R, et al. A new real-time morphology classification for human spermatozoa: a link for fertilization and improved embryo quality. Fertil Steril. 2009;92(5):1616–25.
68. Vanderzwalmen P, Hiemer A, Rubner P, Bach M, Neyer A, Stecher A, et al. Blastocyst development after sperm selection at high magnification is associated with size and number of nuclear vacuoles. Reprod Biomed Online. 2008;17:617–27.
69. Palermo GD, Colombero LT, Rosenwaks Z. The human sperm centrosome is responsible for normal

syngamy and early embryonic development. Rev Reprod. 1997;2:19–27.
70. Sathananthan AH. Paternal centrosomal dynamics in early human development and infertility. J Assist Reprod Genet. 1998;15:129–39.
71. Rawe VY, Galaverna GD, Nodar FN, Brugo-Olmedo S, Vitullo AD. Cellular events during fertilization failure in humans. Fertil Steril. 2001;76:375–6.
72. Piette C, de Mouzon J, Bachelot A, Spira A. In-vitro fertilization: influence of women's age on pregnancy rates. Hum Reprod. 1990;5:56–9.
73. Janny L, Menezo YJ. Maternal age effect on early human embryonic development and blastocyst formation. Mol Reprod Dev. 1996;45:31–7.
74. Ménézo Y, Barak Y. Comparison between day-2 embryos obtained either from ICSI or resulting from short insemination IVF: influence of maternal age. Hum Reprod. 2000;15:1776–80.
75. Menezo Y. Paternal and maternal factors in preimplantation embryogenesis: interaction with the biochemical environment. Reprod Biomed Online. 2006; 12:616–21.
76. European IVF-monitoring programme (EIM), for the European Society of Human Reproduction and Embryology (ESHRE) 2002 Assisted reproductive technology in Europe, 2002, Results generated from European registers by ESHRE. Human Reproduction 21 1680–1697.

Thoughts on IMSI

20

Gianpiero D. Palermo, Jennifer C.Y. Hu, Laura Rienzi, Roberta Maggiulli, Takumi Takeuchi, Atsumi Yoshida, Atsushi Tanaka, Hiroshi Kusunoki, Seiji Watanabe, Queenie V. Neri, and Zev Rosenwaks

Abstract

ICSI achieves consistently high fertilization and pregnancy rates regardless of sperm characteristics and even azoospermic patients have fathered children by ICSI where spermatozoa were surgically retrieved. In this review, we report multicenter study results after the use of IMSI in patients with compromised semen parameters or in patients with previous ART failure using sibling oocytes. These studies, based on higher magnification screening for sperm surface irregularities, did not seem to benefit the patients' clinical outcome in independent investigations. We conclude from these collaborative studies, IMSI does not bring any advantage in the quest to find spermatozoa devoid of surface irregularities and that it significantly lengthens the search time required.

Keywords

ICSI • IMSI • MSOME • Nuclear vacuoles • Spermiogenesis • Embryo quality

20.1 Introduction

Classically, sperm morphology has been a valuable diagnostic tool [1] and has played an important role in predicting the fertility potential of infertile men attempting IVF [2]. The introduction of ICSI [3] rendered these basic semen parameters obsolete where this technique was used because of their inability to predict fertilization and pregnancy outcomes [4]. ICSI achieves consistently high fertilization and pregnancy rates regardless of sperm characteristics and even azoospermic patients have fathered children by ICSI where spermatozoa were surgically retrieved [5–7].

Notwithstanding these outcomes, several studies have shown that suboptimal sperm morphology is often associated with aneuploidy, nuclear DNA damage, and at times an impaired ICSI outcome [8–12] .

Not surprisingly, abnormalities of the male gametes may be a harbinger of developmental problems in embryos [13, 14]. Such effects, can be separated into early and late events. Among the early effects, failed fertilization, abnormal

G.D. Palermo (✉)
The Ronald O. Perelman and Claudia Cohen Center for Reproductive Medicine, Weill Cornell Medical College, New York, NY, USA
e-mail: gdpalerm@med.cornell.edu

C. Racowsky et al. (eds.), *Biennial Review of Infertility: Volume 2*,
DOI 10.1007/978-1-4419-8456-2_20, © Springer Science+Business Media, LLC 2011

zygote morphology, impaired cleavage arising from centrosome dysfunction or lack of oocyte activating factors are most obvious. Late paternal effects include sperm aneuploidy, DNA damage, or abnormal chromatin condensation and are considered responsible for repeated implantation failures [13]. Of those factors, sperm DNA damage has been the most extensively investigated utilizing various methods considered to predict the ART outcome [15–19].

Sperm DNA integrity is currently assessed by destructive methods such as TUNEL, COMET, sperm chromatin dispersion (SCD) test, or by a sperm chromatin structural assay (SCSA). However, all of these require fixation and so destruction of the sperm being assessed [15]. Therefore, we have explored the methods that may be able to select sperm with a competent genome in a noninvasive manner to improve ART outcome.

One particular issue of interest in this context are vacuoles in the sperm nucleus. In contrast to those of other mammals, nuclear vacuoles are a very common feature of human sperm, and are considered by some to reflect the presence of DNA damage [20, 21] that may compromise the development of zygotes [16, 22, 23]. It has been speculated that the presence of nuclear vacuoles is associated also with other aspects of sperm quality, such as a lower mitochondrial membrane potential, a higher incidence of chromosomal abnormalities, and greater DNA damage [20, 21, 24]. It has also been suggested that the absence of nuclear vacuoles is indicative of completion of the acrosome reaction [25]. This conclusion posits that spermatozoa devoid of vacuoles have likely undergone the acrosome reaction and are able to induce oocyte activation more effectively [26, 27]. In addition, deformities of the midpiece section of the spermatozoon assessed under high magnification microscopy has been linked to centrosomal dysfunction [28].

A technique called "motile sperm organellar morphology examination" (MSOME) has been proposed to assess living sperm morphology under high magnification [29]. In this case, screening is used to select a spermatozoon for ICSI with an optimal shape. The procedure is called "intracytoplasmic morphologically selected sperm injection" (IMSI), and its use is claimed to result in a higher pregnancy rate than with conventional ICSI [29, 30]. The beneficial effect of IMSI has been demonstrated in a series of studies in which the clinical outcome of patients treated by this procedure was compared with that of patients treated by conventional ICSI [31–34].

The early ultrastructural studies of human sperm in the 1950s and 1960s, revealed that vacuoles in the sperm nucleus have been seen in the large majority of human spermatozoa regardless of the fertility of the donors. Therefore, vacuoles in human sperm have been considered as a physiologic finding devoid of consequence on fertility potential [35]. From this there is the need to revisit whether the presence of nuclear vacuoles portend to sperm DNA defects with consequent impaired developmental competence of the spermatozoon.

In this chapter, we revisit the actual definition, origin, and possible significance of human sperm nuclear vacuoles. We report multicenter results after the use of IMSI in patients with compromised semen parameters or in patients with previous ART failure using sibling oocytes. A detailed relative quantification of sperm surface defects in ejaculated or surgically retrieved sperm was made by high magnification light microscopy, scanning, and transmission electron microscopy (TEM) as well confocal microscopy. In addition, the developmental competence of the embryo was assessed according to the presence or absence of vacuoles in their paternal sperm. Finally, an assessment was made on the relationship between sperm surface irregularities and genomic integrity in terms of the incidence of sperm chromatin fragmentation and karyotyping.

20.2 What Are Sperm Vacuoles?

The interest towards the male gamete began in the seventeenth century and together with the concurrent refinement of new microscopic techniques have sparked the continued interest of scientists wordwide towards this fascinating highly specialized cell. Structural analysis of the

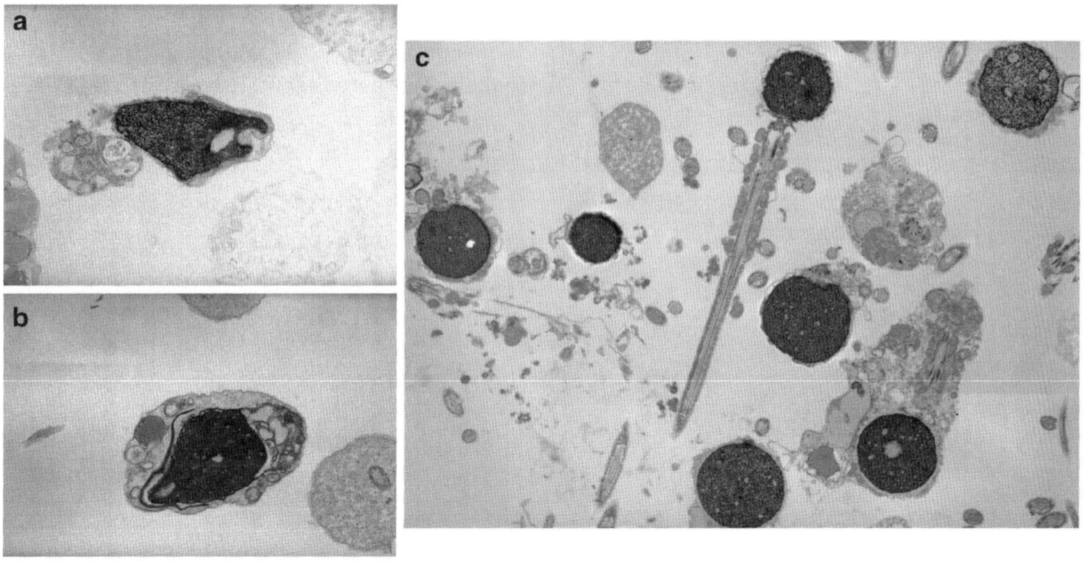

Fig. 20.1 Examples of nuclear vacuoles under transmission electron microscopy in normospermic (**a**, **b**) and globozoospermic specimens (**c**)

mammalian spermatozoon has been studied further than most of the any other differentiated cell type, yet the molecular mechanisms of motility, sperm activation, zona penetration, syngamy, and chromatin decondensation still elude us.

In the majority of species, the uniformity of the product of spermatogenesis is remarkable; hundreds of millions of sperm are produced each day with very little variation in head shape and with a surprisingly small percentage of nuclear anomalies. However, human spermatozoa display considerable structural heterogeneity even after their maturation and transit through the epididymis [36].

Shaping of the nucleus takes place in late spermiogenesis as its chromatin is undergoing a remarkable condensation that renders the sperm transcriptionally inert and highly resistant to digestion. Following the morphological transformation of the nucleus in the testis, as sperm pass through the epididymis there occurs a stabilization of the chromatin through establishment of disulfide bonds between the thiol-rich protamines [37]. The human sperm nucleus is composed also of the DNA condensing core and linker histones that have been partially replaced by protamines, thus changing the configuration of the sperm head to reach a more compact and hydrodynamic shape favorable for cell motility and penetration through the egg vestments [38, 39].

Vacuoles occur commonly in human sperm nuclei [35] but are generally observable only with TEM. Nuclear vacuoles are irregular entities in the condensed chromatin and are not limited by a membrane (Fig. 20.1a-c). These vacuoles are due to variably localized aberrations of nuclear decondensation during the histones-to-protamine exchange [37]. In an extreme example, it appears that the large majority of the round-headed (globozoospermic) sperm nuclei produced by some men have vacuoles verisimilarly related to incomplete chromatin condensation (Fig. 20.1c) and their nuclei are characterized by DNA packing anomalies related to the reduced protamine content.

Another way to assess sperm nuclear vacuoles without the use of TEM would be to perform a decondensation assay [36] in which sperm are exposed to sodium dodecyl sulfate (SDS) + dithiothreitol (DTT) that cleave weak and covalent –S-S– bonds, respectively. In other mammals except man, sperm display a uniform rate of

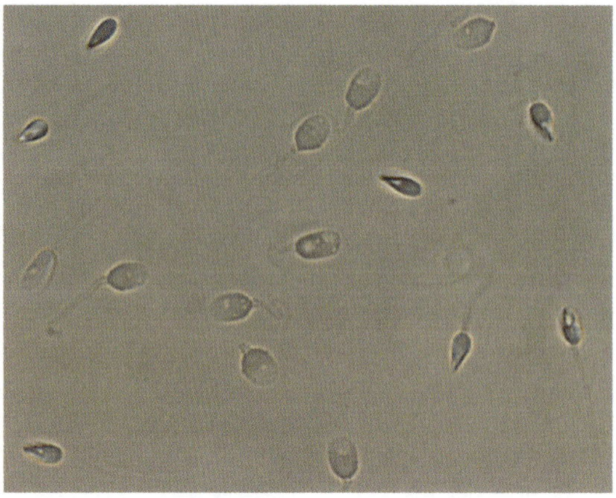

Fig. 20.2 Selected spermatozoa devoid of surface irregularities following exposure to sodium dodecyl sulfate+dithiothreitol. Spermatozoa displayed several vacuole-like structures visible at 200, 400, and 1,000×

decondensation. In the case of the human sperm, however, some decondense rapidly after treatment while others hardly react at all. Motile spermatozoa with regularly shaped heads following exposure to a nuclear decondensing agent, displayed multiple vacuole-like structures becoming visible under light microscopy (Fig. 20.2). The heterogeneity of human sperm nucleus decondensation may reflect variation in the degree of –S-S– cross-linking during nuclear compaction. It is also possible that this may be the result of an unusually variable rate of epididymal transit by individual spermatozoa that is characteristic of man. For in humans, the rate of sperm passage from the testis to the ejaculate, averages 12 days and ranges from 1–2 to 21 days. On the basis of their quasi-universal presence in human sperm heads, the intranuclear vacuoles cannot be considered as degenerative structures [35, 40].

A different type of sperm head irregularity is a surface "vacuole" or indentations, craters, dents, or hollows on the surface. In such cases, during sperm morphogenesis, the outer acrosomal membrane misforms and generates what appears to be a vacuole [41]. These vacuole-like structures disappear as the spermatozoon matures in the epididymis or at the time of the acrosome reaction [25]. In other circumstances, however, they seem to increase with temperature (37°C) and incubation time (>2 h) [42], most probably due to the plication/vacuolization of the rostral plasmalemma during capacitation. As noted later in the chapter, these vacuole-like structures or craters appear in over 90% of spermatozoa from fertile donors with normal semen parameters [43, 44].

20.3 Application of MSOME in Men with Compromised Semen Parameters

In a prospective randomized study in a single center, patients with compromised semen parameters ($<5\times10^6$/mL concentration and normal sperm morphology of <4% according to Kruger's strict criteria) were allocated 1:1 to either the ICSI and the IMSI approach. In both groups, three MII oocytes were inseminated per cycle in accordance with the Italian Law on Assisted Reproductive Technology. Accurate sperm selection for ICSI was performed in both groups (at 400×; Fig. 20.3a) and the morphology of the selected spermatozoa in the IMSI group (Fig. 20.3b) was recorded in detail. For IMSI, spermatozoa were placed in a glass bottom dish and observed at 1,000× under mineral oil with Nomarski's differential contrast (DIC) optics. The magnification was further increased by a digital imaging system in order to obtain a final magnification of 6,600× [29]. In both groups, spermatozoa were first evaluated and when selected were immobilized, and then placed in a clean PVP drop before ICSI was performed. The mean time employed to collect normal appearing spermatozoa (according to MSOME criteria) was 7.7 ± 3.1 min for ICSI and 108.3 ± 29.9 min for IMSI ($P<0.001$). Oocytes were selected as previously described [45] and all viable embryos obtained were transferred on day 2, again as required by Italian law [46]. The primary aim was to evaluate the delivery rate per transfer procedure and live births per transferred embryos, while secondary outcomes were related to fertilization rates and day 2 embryo development.

For this study, 33 couples were recruited – 16 assigned to ICSI and 17 to the IMSI approach (Table 20.1). The maternal age was comparable in both groups as were the fertilization rates and

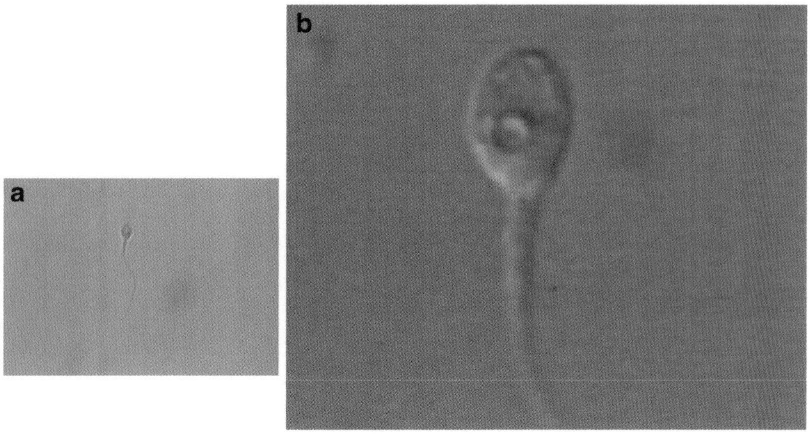

Fig. 20.3 Visualization of a spermatozoon at 400× (**a**) and at 6,600× (**b**)

Table 20.1 Benefits of MSOME in oligoasthenoteratozoospermic couples

No. of (%)	ICSI	IMSI
Cycles	16	17
Maternal age (M years ± SD)	34.9 ± 3	35.2 ± 3
2PN	40/48 (83.3)	42/49 (85.7)
Top quality day 2 embryos	27/40 (67.7)	29/42 (68.2)
Embryos transferred (M ± SD)	2.5 ± 0.8	2.5 ± 0.5
Delivery	6 (37.5)	5 (29.4)
Live birth	8/40 (20.0)	7/42 (16.7)

the number of embryos transferred. There was a trend towards higher pregnancy (37.5 vs. 29.4%) and implantation (20.0 vs. 17.6%) following ICSI indicating that IMSI did not yield any benefit over ICSI in regards to fertilization, pregnancy, and implantation rates. This analysis indicated that higher magnification microscopy did not enhance the ability to select "good looking" spermatozoa for injection while lengthening the procedure.

20.4 ICSI Versus IMSI in Sibling Oocytes

In order to limit confounding factors, only women less than 40 years of age were selected for this study. Ejaculated spermatozoa were used in patients that had at least five metaphase II (MII) oocytes, half of them being injected using IMSI and the other half by ICSI. Patients were grouped according to whether this was their first ART cycle or was a repeat following prior failed attempts. Repeat attempts were undertaken on the basis of the rationale that the ART failure was due to an incompetent male genome regardless of the adequate semen parameters. In order to compare the rates of implantation, clinical pregnancy, and delivery in relation to the sperm selection method, only embryos deriving from one procedure or other were transferred to any one patient. Briefly, oocyte-cumulus-complexes were retrieved from ovaries stimulated with exogenous gonadotropins after pituitary suppression with GnRH agonists or antagonists. Embryo transfers were performed under abdominal ultrasound guidance on day 5 following oocyte retrieval.

For IMSI, sperm selection was carried out under an inverted microscope equipped with Nomarski's DIC enhanced by digital imaging [24, 33]. Motile spermatozoa with the best available morphology, devoid of or displaying only a small vacuole occupying <4% of the nuclear area, were selected for IMSI. Conventional ICSI was performed as described by Palermo et al. [47].

A total of 276 consenting couples with male infertility were included in this study using ejaculated spermatozoa. In the group for which this was

Table 20.2 High magnification ICSI in ART couples at their first attempt

No. of (%)	ICSI	IMSI
Women	214	
Injected MII oocytes	1110	1119
2PN	718 (64.7)	694 (62.0)
Day 3 embryos	409 (56.5)	400 (57.6)
Blastocyst development	235 (32.7)	233/610 (33.6)
Embryo replacements	107	107
Transferred embryos (M ± SD)	122(1.1 ± 0.3)	120(1.1 ± 0.3)
Clinical pregnancy (+FHB)	45 (42.1)	39 (36.4)
Implantation	51 (41.8)	45 (37.5)
Deliveries or ongoing	44 (41.1)	39 (36.4)

Table 20.3 High magnification ICSI in couples with previous ART failure

No. of (%)	ICSI	IMSI
Women	62	
Injected MII oocytes	376	359
2PN	235 (62.5)	216 (60.2)
Day 3 embryos	119 (50.6)	120 (55.6)
Blastocyst development	46 (19.6)[a]	61 (28.2)[a]
Embryo replacements	26	36
Transferred embryos (M ± SD)	37 (1.5 ± 0.5)	58 (1.6 ± 0.5)
Clinical pregnancy (+FHB)	8 (30.8)	17 (47.2)
Implantation	9 (24.3)	22 (37.9)
Delivered or ongoing	8 (30.8)	17 (47.2)

[a] $P = 0.04$

the first ART attempt ($n = 214$), the mean maternal age was 33.4 ± 3 years and the paternal age was 37.0 ± 6 years. The men had an average concentration of 56.7 ± 57 × 10^6/mL with 36.4 ± 19% motility, and Kruger's morphology of 2.9 ± 2%. In this cohort, the rate of fertilization and embryo development were comparable between the two insemination methods (Table 20.2). After embryo transfer, clinical pregnancies after ICSI (42.1%) did not differ from IMSI (36.4%).

In cases with previous failed ART attempts, the average age of the women and men was 34.9 ± 3 years and 37.2 ± 4 years, respectively. The semen parameters were 48.8 ± 42 × 10^6/mL, 34.0 ± 18% motility, with a Kruger's morphology of 3.2 ± 3%. In this multiple ART failure group, fertilization rates again were comparable between ICSI and IMSI, however, the frequency of full blastocyst development was somewhat higher after IMSI ($P = 0.04$) (Table 20.3). Nonetheless, this did not translate to a superior pregnancy outcome in comparison to ICSI. This indicates that utilization of sperm void of surface irregularities does not grant a male genome with higher developmental competence.

In order to establish whether repeat treatment with ICSI would have any impact on clinical outcome, we assessed patients at Cornell of comparable age (≤40 years) that failed to achieve a clinical pregnancy with ejaculated spermatozoa at a first ICSI attempt ($n = 3{,}018$). Upon their return and subsequent treatment with ICSI, a clinical pregnancy rate of 44.2% (1,166/2,640) was achieved.

This finding suggested that an ART failures are multifactorial and cannot be simply blamed on the spermatozoon. Even if the male genome would be at fault, these findings confirmed that the genotype of the gamete cannot be simply predicted by its phenotype.

20.5 Qualitative Assessment of Sperm Nuclear Defects and Embryo Development

To determine whether "vacuoles" or "craters" on a human sperm head have any physiological significance, their incidence and size were recorded at 1,000× in ejaculated (Fig. 20.4a–c), epididymal (Fig. 20.4d), and testicular (Fig. 20.4e) spermatozoa as well as in spermatids (Fig. 20.4f). Samples obtained from consenting men included either testicular (from non-obstructive), epididymal (obstructive azoospermic), or ejaculated spermatozoa. In addition, spermatids of varying stages were also assessed.

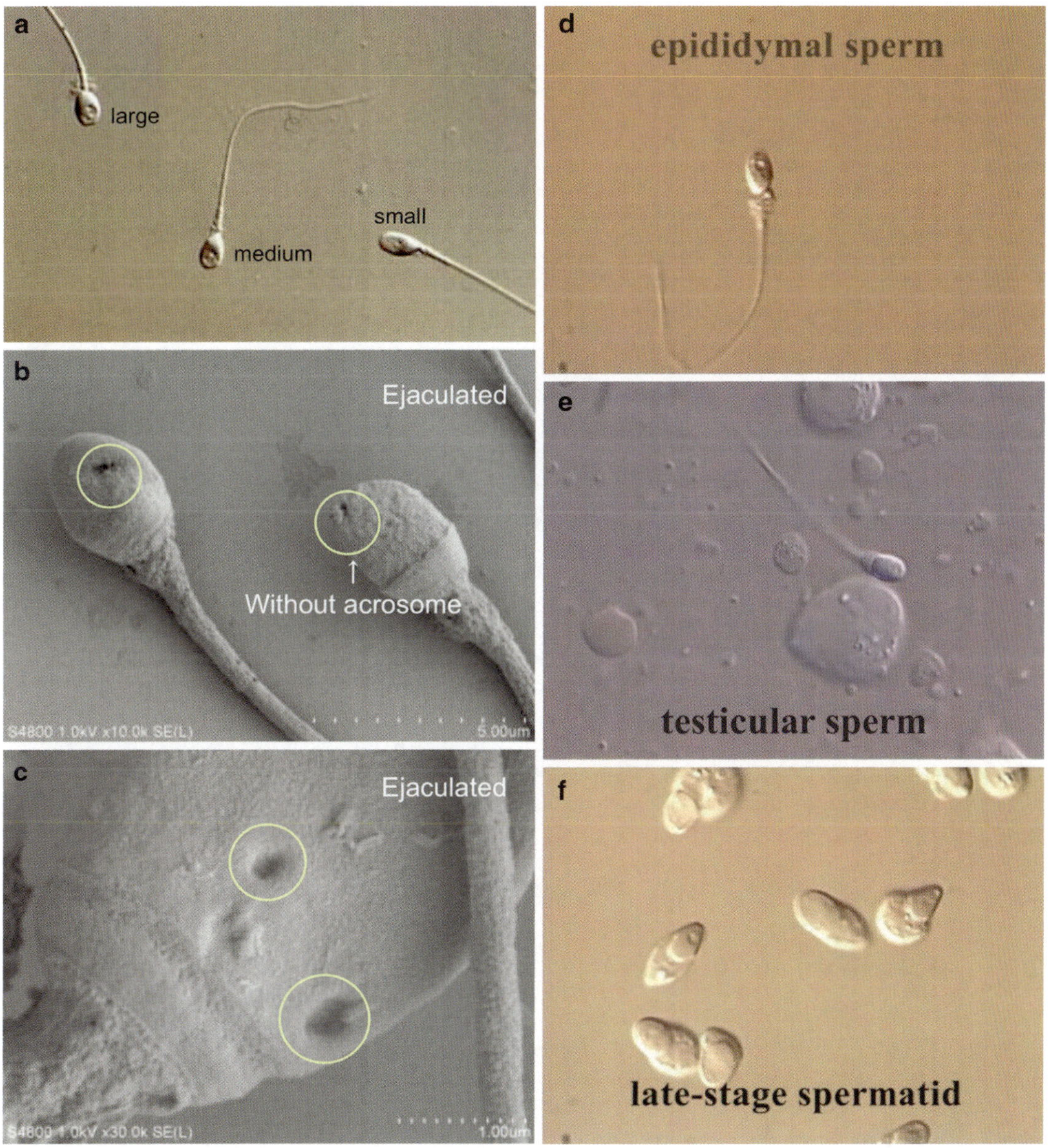

Fig. 20.4 Sperm craters under optic microscroscopy (**a**, **d–f**) and scanning electron microscopy (**b**, **c**) evidencing craters in ejaculated (**a–c**), epididymal (**d**), testicular (**e**) spermatozoa, and spermatids (**d**). SEM images (**b**, **c**) confirmed the presence of hollows in spermatozoa with and without acrosome (**b**)

Table 20.4 Full embryo development according to crater size

No. of (%)	Crater characterization for IMSI			
	Large	Small	None	ICSI
Oocytes injected	23	63	20	256
Fertilization	14 (60.9)[a]	54 (85.7)[a]	16 (80.0)[a]	167 (70.8)[a]
Blastocyst development	7 (50.0)	28 (54.9)	4 (25.0)	85 (51.0)

[a]$P = 0.008$

Regardless of the semen source, the large majority of spermatozoa had one or more craters of various sizes. Ejaculated samples had the highest proportion, the frequency ranging from 87.5 to 97.7%, while early spermatids displayed the largest craters. In the shaping of the nucleus during spermiogenesis, the number of craters increased while their size diminished as cells moved through the epididymis.

Fertilization of MII oocytes following IMSI was compared to ICSI cases (Table 20.4). IMSI using small cratered spermatozoa yielded comparable fertilization rates to sperm without such craters, whereas large craters appeared to compromise fertilization. When compared to ICSI, oocytes inseminated by IMSI with sperm having small vacuoles resulted in a higher fertilization (85.7 vs. 70.8%; $P = 0.003$). Interestingly, spermatozoa selected by MSOME was judged as being devoid of craters and generated the lowest blastocyst rate (4/16). In addition, when DNA integrity was assessed by TUNEL on large cratered sperm isolated by MSOME, there was no evidence of chromatin damage (0/21). This implies that craters do not reflect abnormalities of the sperm head genome, but may as well be common physiological variations occurring during human spermiogenesis which unlike that in animals may be partially affected by the higher temperature brought by clothing [48].

20.6 Frequency and Possible Significance of Sperm Nuclear Abnormality

A further study investigated the possibility of an association between sperm nuclear vacuoles, DNA fragmentation, and chromosomal abnormalities. For this, sperm samples were obtained from 17 infertile patients (15 IVF and 2 ICSI) and three fertile donors.

Morphologically, normal spermatozoa were assessed for nuclear vacuoles with DIC optics at 1,000× (Fig. 20.5a). The sperm samples were classified according to the presence, the size, and the localization of vacuoles as visualized by confocal microscopy (Fig. 20.5b). Nuclear vacuoles were observed in over 90% of normally shaped spermatozoa from infertile and donor males alike. In fact, regularly shaped sperm without vacuole-like structures were extremely rare (2.4%). When confocal microscopy was employed, the vacuole-like structures appeared more as surface craters.

Sperm chromosomal analysis was performed by injecting such classified spermatozoa into mouse oocytes, while DNA fragmentation was evaluated by TUNEL assay. In terms of chromosomal abnormalities, there was no difference between the spermatozoa with large nuclear vacuoles and those without. In addition, we found no correlation between the incidence of chromosomal aberrations and the size or the location of "nuclear vacuoles." Moreover, the incidence of spermatozoa with DNA fragmentation detected by TUNEL was consistently low (3.1–3.5%) regardless of the presence of large vacuoles (Fig. 20.5c). Therefore, it appears that nuclear vacuoles are not an indicator of sperm nuclear chromosomal aberrations or of sperm nuclear damage such as nicks and breaks.

20.7 Relationship Between Phenotypic and Genomic Sperm Anomalies of the Sperm Nucleus

MSOME, often requested by patients, entails the live scanning of highly magnified spermatozoa for irregularities that may compromise the ability to fertilize and support embryo development. As aforementioned, it has been claimed that genomic integrity is impaired in spermatozoa displaying

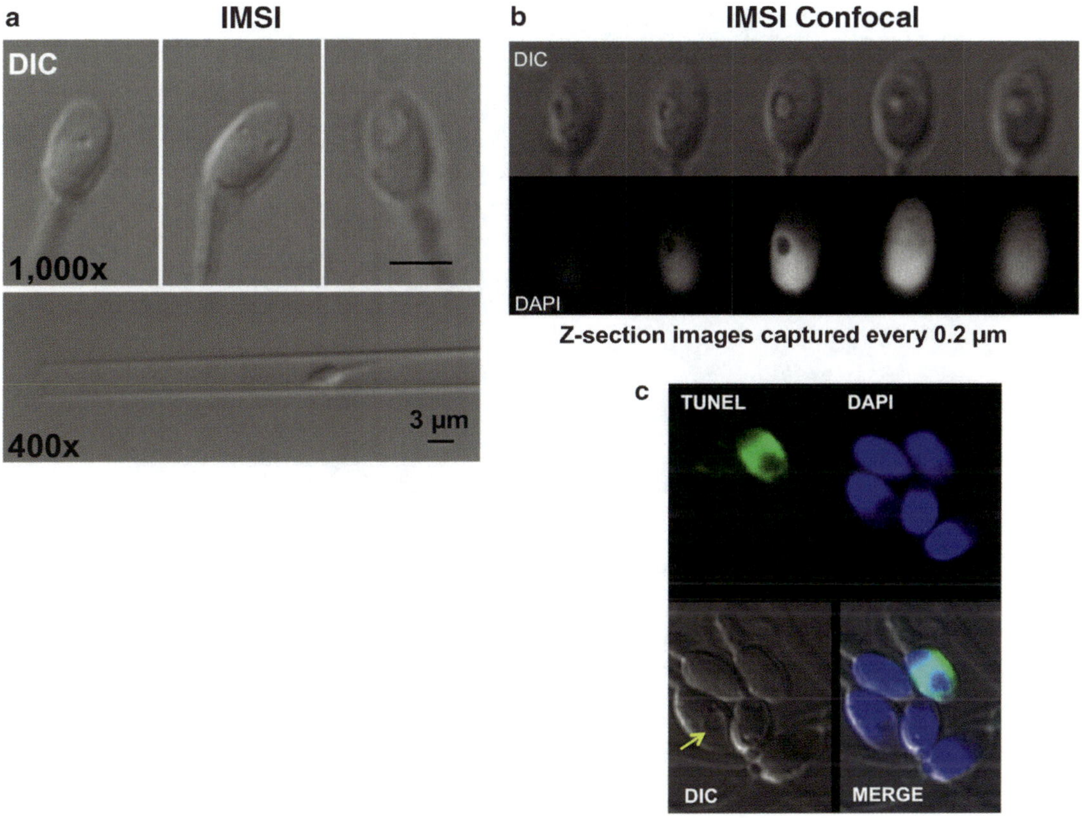

Fig. 20.5 Sperm surface irregularities under high magnification DIC (**a**) and confocal microscopy (**b**). TUNEL assay performed on spermatozoa with and without vacuole-like structures (*yellow arrow*) (**c**)

vacuoles or surface irregularities. However, the bearing of chromatin fragmentation on the health of the conceptus and its ability to implant has not been confirmed, nor has any link been demonstrated between sperm head surface defects and genomic competence. Therefore, we aimed to assess the genomic and epigenetic implications for male gametes exhibiting surface irregularities and "vacuoles."

At least 100 motile spermatozoa showing head dysmorphism (with "vacuole") were selected at 1,000× by micromanipulation, retrieved individually, and placed on pre-coated slides (Fig. 20.6). Motile sperm of normal morphology selected individually served as controls. Sperm DNA fragmentation was assessed by the Sperm Chromatin Dispersion Test (Halosperm® kit, INDAS laboratories) and TUNEL assay (APO-BrdU™ TUNEL assay kit, Invitrogen). To determine their ploidy status, fixed spermatozoa were decondensed and hybridized with locus specific probes for chromosomes X, Y, 13, 15, 16, 17, 18, 21, 22 (MultiVysion™ PB probe mixture, Abbott; OligoFISH™ probe kit, One Cell System).

The study cohort consisted of 35 men with an average age of 38.4±4 years. A total of 7,350 spermatozoa were evaluated for DNA fragmentation and ploidy status, 3,890 of which had visible surface defects and 3,460 were without. The assessment of sperm ploidy status revealed a comparable proportion of chromosomal abnormalities in the two groups (Fig. 20.7). The total fragmentation rate detected by SCD assay was 2.1% for vacuolated spermatozoa and 2.4% for the control (Fig. 20.8). When the fragmentation was assessed by TUNEL assay, 5.5% of spermatozoa with head defects displayed DNA fragmentation versus 5.6% observed in the controls (Fig. 20.9).

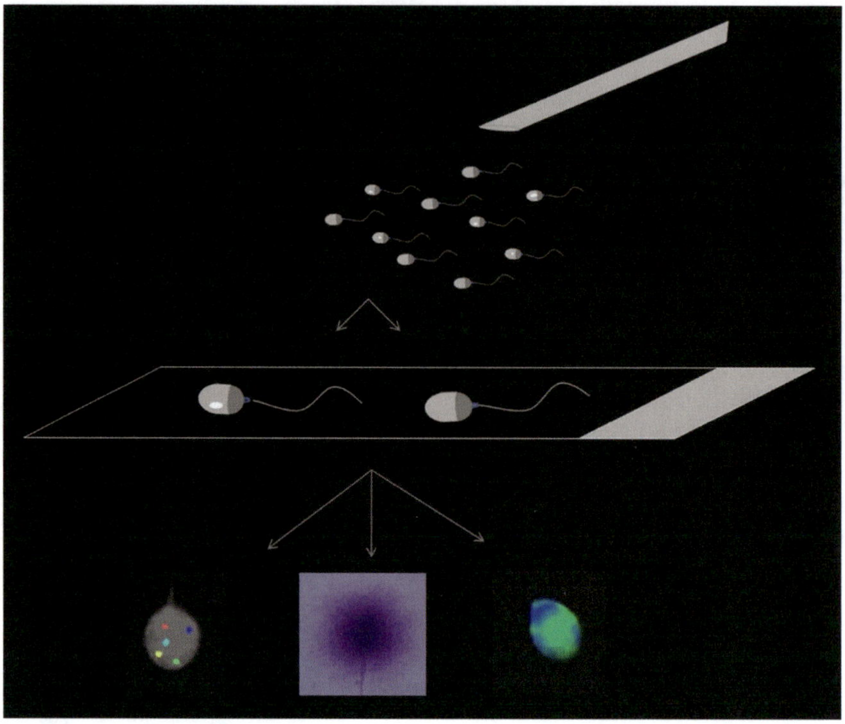

Fig. 20.6 Study design

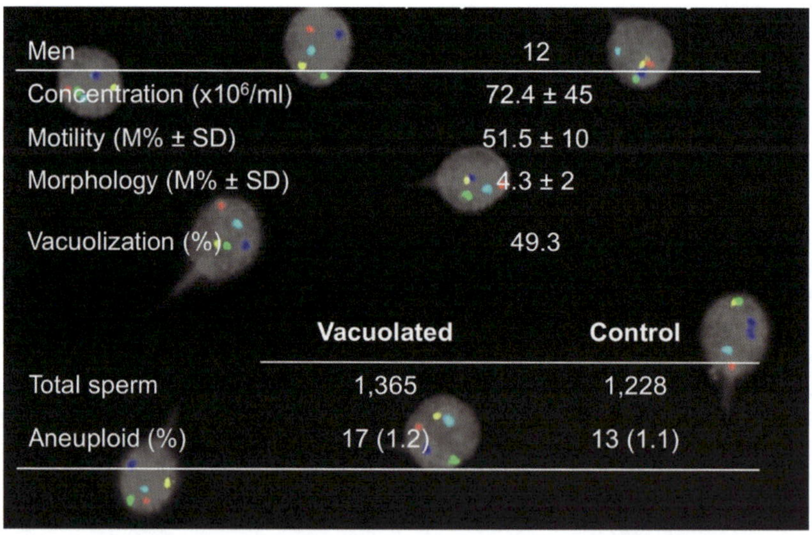

Men	12
Concentration (x10^6/ml)	72.4 ± 45
Motility (M% ± SD)	51.5 ± 10
Morphology (M% ± SD)	4.3 ± 2
Vacuolization (%)	49.3

	Vacuolated	Control
Total sperm	1,365	1,228
Aneuploid (%)	17 (1.2)	13 (1.1)

Fig. 20.7 Semen characteristics and ploidy status assessed by FISH

In conclusion, the presence of sperm nuclear defects assessed by high magnification microscopy did not appear to correlate with the ploidy or status of the sperm chromatin. Thus, defects such as nuclear vacuoles and other head abnormalities do not appear to directly reflect chromosomal imbalances or presence of DNA breakage.

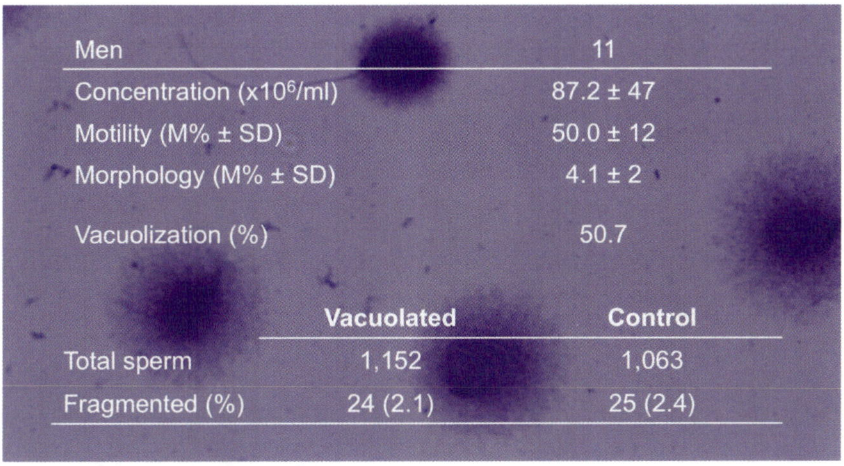

Men	11
Concentration (x10⁶/ml)	87.2 ± 47
Motility (M% ± SD)	50.0 ± 12
Morphology (M% ± SD)	4.1 ± 2
Vacuolization (%)	50.7

	Vacuolated	Control
Total sperm	1,152	1,063
Fragmented (%)	24 (2.1)	25 (2.4)

Fig. 20.8 Semen characteristics and DNA fragmentation assessed by SCD test

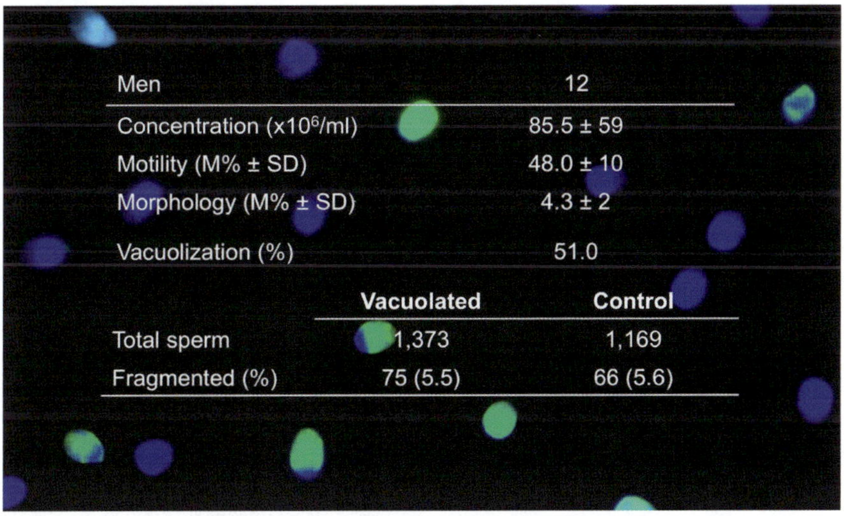

Men	12
Concentration (x10⁶/ml)	85.5 ± 59
Motility (M% ± SD)	48.0 ± 10
Morphology (M% ± SD)	4.3 ± 2
Vacuolization (%)	51.0

	Vacuolated	Control
Total sperm	1,373	1,169
Fragmented (%)	75 (5.5)	66 (5.6)

Fig. 20.9 Semen characteristics and DNA fragmentation as assessed by TUNEL assay

20.8 Conclusions

Since the development of ICSI, it has been suggested that more attention be paid to the selection of sperm while they are swimming in slow motion in a viscous medium in order to select the "best looking" spermatozoon. By selecting individual sperm cells, at the highest magnification possible, ICSI has enabled even couples with severe male factor to achieve conception.

Higher magnification screening for sperm surface irregularities did not seem to benefit the patients' clinical outcome in independent investigations. This was true for patients with compromised semen parameters and for those either undergoing first or repeated ART attempts. More detailed morphological observations indicated that in human sperm heads visible irregularities or vacuoles are almost ubiquitous, and appear to be a paraphysiologic finding. Analyses of spermatozoa from different sources, ejaculated or surgically retrieved, also revealed the varying presence and size of vacuoles that develop during the dynamic processes of spermiogenesis and maturation. This surface irregularity did not relate to the incidence of DNA fragmentation or aneuploidy, nor to the ability of vacuolated spermatozoa to generate zygotes capable of developing to blastocysts. Moreover, the safety of IMSI on how it is currently performed need to be confirmed. In fact, it has been reported that infants born after IMSI have a higher risk of low birth weight (<2500 g) [49].

Even in light of the ability of the ooplasm to overcome certain sperm genomic anomalies, it should be kept in mind that the factors contributing to impaired embryo developmental competence cannot conveniently be identified in the simple analysis of the surface irregularities of the sperm, particularly when we refer to chromosomal status or centrosomal function.

We conclude from these collaborative studies, that a 16× factor magnification does not bring any advantage in the quest to find spermatozoa devoid of surface irregularities, and significantly lengthens the search time required. The presence of vacuoles does not flag spermatozoa with fragmented DNA or aneuploidy. Finally, the putative correlation between vacuolar size and genomic integrity was not confirmed.

Acknowledgement We are grateful to all the contributors for their efforts in allowing this endeavor to be accomplished. We are thankful to Dr. J. Michael Bedford for his critical review and Justin Kocent for his technical assistance. Queenie V. Neri was funded by the grant ULI RR024996 of the Clinical and Translational Science Center at Weill Cornell Medical College.

References

1. MacLeod J, Wang Y. Male fertility potential in terms of semen quality: a review of the past, a study of the present. Fertil Steril. 1979;31(2):103–16.
2. Kruger TF, Menkveld R, Stander FS, et al. Sperm morphologic features as a prognostic factor in in vitro fertilization. Fertil Steril. 1986;46(6):1118–23.
3. Palermo G, Joris H, Devroey P, Van Steirteghem AC. Pregnancies after intracytoplasmic injection of single spermatozoon into an oocyte. Lancet. 1992;340(8810):17–8.
4. Nagy ZP, Liu J, Joris H, et al. The result of intracytoplasmic sperm injection is not related to any of the three basic sperm parameters. Hum Reprod. 1995;10(5):1123–9.
5. Palermo GD, Schlegel PN, Hariprashad JJ, et al. Fertilization and pregnancy outcome with intracytoplasmic sperm injection for azoospermic men. Hum Reprod. 1999;14(3):741–8.
6. Tournaye H, Devroey P, Liu J, Nagy Z, Lissens W, Van Steirteghem A. Microsurgical epididymal sperm aspiration and intracytoplasmic sperm injection: a new effective approach to infertility as a result of congenital bilateral absence of the vas deferens. Fertil Steril. 1994;61(6):1045–51.
7. Schoysman R, Vanderzwalmen P, Nijs M, et al. Pregnancy after fertilisation with human testicular spermatozoa. Lancet. 1993;342(8881):1237.
8. Tang SS, Gao H, Zhao Y, Ma S. Aneuploidy and DNA fragmentation in morphologically abnormal sperm. Int J Androl. 2010;33(1):e163–79.
9. De Vos A, Van De Velde H, Joris H, Verheyen G, Devroey P, Van Steirteghem A. Influence of individual sperm morphology on fertilization, embryo morphology, and pregnancy outcome of intracytoplasmic sperm injection. Fertil Steril. 2003;79(1):42–8.
10. Templado C, Hoang T, Greene C, Rademaker A, Chernos J, Martin R. Aneuploid spermatozoa in infertile men: teratozoospermia. Mol Reprod Dev. 2002;61(2):200–4.
11. Harkonen K, Suominen J, Lahdetie J. Aneuploidy in spermatozoa of infertile men with teratozoospermia. Int J Androl. 2001;24(4):197–205.
12. Tasdemir I, Tasdemir M, Tavukcuoglu S, Kahraman S, Biberoglu K. Effect of abnormal sperm head morphology on the outcome of intracytoplasmic sperm injection in humans. Hum Reprod. 1997;12(6):1214–7.
13. Tesarik J, Greco E, Mendoza C. Late, but not early, paternal effect on human embryo development is related to sperm DNA fragmentation. Hum Reprod. 2004;19(3):611–5.
14. Tesarik J, Mendoza C, Greco E. Paternal effects acting during the first cell cycle of human preimplantation development after ICSI. Hum Reprod. 2002;17(1):184–9.
15. Zini A, Sigman M. Are tests of sperm DNA damage clinically useful? Pros cons J Androl. 2009;30(3):219–29.
16. Bungum M, Humaidan P, Spano M, Jepson K, Bungum L, Giwercman A. The predictive value of sperm chromatin structure assay (SCSA) parameters for the outcome of intrauterine insemination, IVF and ICSI. Hum Reprod. 2004;19(6):1401–8.
17. Sakkas D, Manicardi GC, Bizzaro D. Sperm nuclear DNA damage in the human. Adv Exp Med Biol. 2003;518:73–84.
18. Evenson DP, Larson KL, Jost LK. Sperm chromatin structure assay: its clinical use for detecting sperm DNA fragmentation in male infertility and comparisons with other techniques. J Androl. 2002;23(1):25–43.

19. Twigg JP, Irvine DS, Aitken RJ. Oxidative damage to DNA in human spermatozoa does not preclude pronucleus formation at intracytoplasmic sperm injection. Hum Reprod. 1998;13(7):1864–71.
20. Franco Jr JG, Baruffi RL, Mauri AL, Petersen CG, Oliveira JB, Vagnini L. Significance of large nuclear vacuoles in human spermatozoa: implications for ICSI. Reprod Biomed Online. 2008;17(1):42–5.
21. Garolla A, Fortini D, Menegazzo M, et al. High-power microscopy for selecting spermatozoa for ICSI by physiological status. Reprod Biomed Online. 2008;17(5):610–6.
22. Fernandez-Gonzalez R, Moreira PN, Perez-Crespo M, et al. Long-term effects of mouse intracytoplasmic sperm injection with DNA-fragmented sperm on health and behavior of adult offspring. Biol Reprod. 2008;78(4):761–72.
23. Evenson D, Jost L. Sperm chromatin structure assay is useful for fertility assessment. Methods Cell Sci. 2000;22(2–3):169–89.
24. Vanderzwalmen P, Hiemer A, Rubner P, et al. Blastocyst development after sperm selection at high magnification is associated with size and number of nuclear vacuoles. Reprod Biomed Online. 2008;17(5):617–27.
25. Kacem O, Sifer C, Barraud-Lange V, et al. Sperm nuclear vacuoles, as assessed by motile sperm organellar morphological examination, are mostly of acrosomal origin. Reprod Biomed Online. 2010;20(1):132–7.
26. Morozumi K, Shikano T, Miyazaki S, Yanagimachi R. Simultaneous removal of sperm plasma membrane and acrosome before intracytoplasmic sperm injection improves oocyte activation/embryonic development. Proc Natl Acad Sci USA. 2006;103(47):17661–6.
27. Takeuchi T, Colombero LT, Neri QV, Rosenwaks Z, Palermo GD. Does ICSI require acrosomal disruption? An ultrastructural study. Hum Reprod. 2004; 19(1):114–7.
28. Ugajin T, Terada Y, Hasegawa H, Nabeshima H, Suzuki K, Yaegashi N. The shape of the sperm midpiece in intracytoplasmic morphologically selected sperm injection relates sperm centrosomal function. J Assist Reprod Genet. 2010;27(2–3):75–81.
29. Bartoov B, Berkovitz A, Eltes F, Kogosowski A, Menezo Y, Barak Y. Real-time fine morphology of motile human sperm cells is associated with IVF-ICSI outcome. J Androl. 2002;23(1):1–8.
30. Bartoov B, Berkovitz A, Eltes F. Selection of spermatozoa with normal nuclei to improve the pregnancy rate with intracytoplasmic sperm injection. N Engl J Med. 2001;345(14):1067–8.
31. Antinori M, Licata E, Dani G, et al. Intracytoplasmic morphologically selected sperm injection: a prospective randomized trial. Reprod Biomed Online. 2008;16(6):835–41.
32. Hazout A, Dumont-Hassan M, Junca AM, Cohen Bacrie P, Tesarik J. High-magnification ICSI overcomes paternal effect resistant to conventional ICSI. Reprod Biomed Online. 2006;12(1):19–25.
33. Berkovitz A, Eltes F, Yaari S, et al. The morphological normalcy of the sperm nucleus and pregnancy rate of intracytoplasmic injection with morphologically selected sperm. Hum Reprod. 2005;20(1):185–90.
34. Bartoov B, Berkovitz A, Eltes F, et al. Pregnancy rates are higher with intracytoplasmic morphologically selected sperm injection than with conventional intracytoplasmic injection. Fertil Steril. 2003;80(6): 1413–9.
35. Fawcett DW. The structure of the mammalian spermatozoon. Int Rev Cytol. 1958;7:195–234.
36. Bedford JM, Bent MJ, Calvin H. Variations in the structural character and stability of the nuclear chromatin in morphologically normal human spermatozoa. J Reprod Fertil. 1973;33(1):19–29.
37. Calvin HI, Bedford JM. Formation of disulphide bonds in the nucleus and accessory structures of mammalian spermatozoa during maturation in the epididymis. J Reprod Fertil Suppl. 1971;13 Suppl 13:65–75.
38. Brewer L, Corzett M, Balhorn R. Condensation of DNA by spermatid basic nuclear proteins. J Biol Chem. 2002;277(41):38895–900.
39. Dadoune JP. Expression of mammalian spermatozoal nucleoproteins. Microsc Res Tech. 2003;61(1): 56–75.
40. Chrzanowski S. Ultrastucture of human spermatozoon. Pol Med J. 1966;5(2):482–91.
41. Baccetti B, Burrini AG, Collodel G, et al. Crater defect in human spermatozoa. Gamete Res. 1989; 22(3):249–55.
42. Peer S, Eltes F, Berkovitz A, Yehuda R, Itsykson P, Bartoov B. Is fine morphology of the human sperm nuclei affected by in vitro incubation at 37 degrees C? Fertil Steril. 2007;88(6):1589–94.
43. Tanaka A, Nagayoshi M, Awata S, Tanaka I, Kusunoki H, Watanabe S. Are crater defects in human sperm heads physiological changes during spermiogenesis? Fertil Steril. 2009;92(3):S165.
44. Watanabe S, Tanaka A, Fujii S, Misunuma H. No relationship between chromosome aberrations and vacuole-like structures on human sperm head. Hum Reprod. 2009;24 Suppl 1:i94–6.
45. Rienzi L, Ubaldi FM, Iacobelli M, et al. Significance of metaphase II human oocyte morphology on ICSI outcome. Fertil Steril. 2008;90(5):1692–700.
46. Rienzi L, Ubaldi F, Iacobelli M, Minasi MG, Romano S, Greco E. Meiotic spindle visualization in living human oocytes. Reprod Biomed Online. 2005;10(2): 192–8.
47. Palermo GD, Cohen J, Alikani M, Adler A, Rosenwaks Z. Intracytoplasmic sperm injection: a novel treatment for all forms of male factor infertility. Fertil Steril. 1995;63(6):1231–40.
48. Bedford JM. Effects of elevated temperature on the epididymis and testis: experimental studies. Adv Exp Med Biol. 1991;286:19–32.
49. Junca AM, Dumont M, Cornet D, Douard S, De Mounzon J, Prisant N. Is intracytoplasmic morphologically selected sperm injection (IMSI) detrimental for pregnancy outcome? Fertil Steril. 2010;94: S31.

Index

A

Acridine orange test (AOT), 161
Agouti viable yellow (A^{vy}) allele, 187
Amino levulanic acid (ALA) synthase enzyme, 139
Angelmann syndrome (AS), 200–201
Anti-Müllerian hormone (AMH)
  aromatase, 22, 23
  ART (*see* Assisted reproduction technologies)
  clinical applications, 24
  corpus luteum, 23
  follicle-stimulating hormone, 22, 23
  gene and protein, 21
  intra-follicular concentrations, 22
  menstrual cycle, 23
  OHSS, 17
  ovarian granulosa cells, 21
  ovarian physiology, 20
  ovarian response, COH, 66, 67
  PCOS (*see* Polycystic ovary syndrome)
  sensitivity and specificity, 67, 68
  sertoli cell maturation, 21
  serum concentration, 21, 22
  steroidogenesis, 23
  testosterone, 21, 22
Antinuclear antibodies, 6
Antiovarian antibodies, 6
Antiphospholipid syndrome, 4
Antisperm antibodies, 6–7
Antithyroid antibodies, 5–6
Antral follicle count (AFC), 27, 66
Aromatase inhibitors, 15
Assisted reproductive technologies (ART)
  complications, 198–199
  controlled ovarian hyperstimulation, 26–27
  embryo assessment (*see* Embryo assessment)
  epigenetic disturbances
    agouti viable mouse, 202
    cardiovascular and metabolic dysfunction, 202
    chronic metabolic disorders, 203
    DOHAD hypothesis, 201
    global genomic hypomethylation and hypermethylation, 202
    IAP methylation, 202
  epigenetic regulation, 199–200
  gametes/embryos cryopreservation, 206
  gametogenesis, 203
  gonadotropins, 204
  hormonal superovulation, 203–204
  ICSI, 198, 204–205
  immature sperm extraction and injection, 204
  imprinting disorder, 200–201
  in vitro culture, preimplantation embryos, 205–206
  in vitro fertilization, 197
  IUI, 165, 167
  IVF and ICSI, 167–168
  male and female pronucleus, 203
  monozygotic twinning and perinatal outcomes, 92
  oocytes, 203–204
  oocytes IVG and IVM, 204
  ovarian hyperstimulation syndrome, 27–28
  ovarian-stimulated cycles, 44
  ovulation induction, 26
  PGC, 203
  PGD, 198
  sperm from infertile men, 204
  therapeutic modality, 197–198
  uterus and embryo, asynchrony, 204
Asthenozoospermia, 141
ATRX syndrome, 202
Autoimmunity and female infertility
  blastocyst, 4
  implantation, 4
  pregnancy failure
    antinuclear and antiovarian antibodies, 6
    antiphospholipid antibodies, 4–5
    antisperm antibodies, 6–7
    antithyroid antibodies, 5–6

B

Beckwith–Wiedemann syndrome (BWS), 182, 201
Bisphenol A (BPA), 138
Body mass index (BMI), 36, 142
Bone morphogenetic proteins (BMP), 21

C

Cadmium, 139
Carbendazim, 140
Chlorpyrifos, 140
Chromatin immuno precipitation (CHIP), 230

C. Racowsky et al. (eds.), *Biennial Review of Infertility: Volume 2*,
DOI 10.1007/978-1-4419-8456-2,

Chromomycin A_3 (CMA_3)
fluorochrome, 215
staining, 162
Chronic zinc deficiency, 139
Clomiphene citrate, 26
Colorado Center for Reproductive Medicine (CCRM), 257–258
Creatine phosphokinase (CK), 212, 214
Cryopreservation, 120

D
Developmental origin of health and disease (DOHAD), 201
Diamniotic pregnancies, 104
Dichorionic, diamniotic (DC/DA) twins, 94–95
Dichorionic twin pregnancies, 103–105
Diepoxybutane (DEB), 229
Differential interference contrast (DIC), 270
Di (2-ethyhexyl) phthalate (DEHP), 139
DNA and chromosomal aberrations, 128
DNA fragmentation index (DFI), 156, 172
Donor egg/recipient cycles, 86–87

E
Eight-oxoguanine (8-oxoG), 237
Embryo assessment
implantation potential, 245
mammalian embryonic secretome, 246
non-invasive metabolomic analysis
amino acids, 250
non-invasive metabolomic profiling, 250–251
protein synthesis and pH regulation, 249
pyruvate and glucose, 249–250
quiet embryo hypothesis, 249
non-invasive proteomic analysis
human embryonic proteins, 246
non-invasive protein profiling, 247–249
single protein and molecular analysis, 246–247
omics technologies, 246
EmbryoGlue®, 257
Endocrine and metabolic environment, 38–39
Environmental insults, spermatogenesis
epigenetics, 145–146
gametes production, 134
male reproductive neuroendocrine function, 134
maternal and perinatal exposure
maternal smoking and obesity, 135
medullary region, 134
offspring infertility, 135
organochlorines, 136
quinones, 137
TDS hypothesis, 135
xenobiotics, 136, 137
mature testis
agriculture fertilizers, pesticides and herbicides, 140
alcohol consumption and drugs, 141–142
cell phone and ionizing radiation, 144–145
diet and obesity, 142–143
epididymis, 137
haploid spermatids, 137
heavy metal toxicity, 139–140
hypothalamus-pituitary-gonadal axis, 138
plastic industry chemicals, 138–139
psychological and noise stress, 143
PUFA, 138
scrotal heat stress, 143–144
smoking, 141
solvents, 140
Western lifestyle, diet and exercise, 138
testicular cancer and cryptorchidism, 134
toxins and xenobiotics, 134

F
Follicle stimulating hormone (FSH)
environmental insults, spermatogenesis, 135
follicular activation and growth, 23
follicular sensitivity, 59
gonadotropins, 26
menstrual cycle or cycle disturbances, 63
ovarian activity, 61
ovarian hyperstimulation, 26–27
ovarian response, 66
serum levels, 64
sperm, cancer therapies, 118–119
steroidogenesis, 60
Follicular flushing, 16

G
Gene ontology (GO), 51
Gonadotrophin-releasing hormone (GnRH), 47

H
Homologous recombination repair (HRR), 235
Human chorionic gonadotropin (hCG), 24, 80
Human leukocyte antigen G (HLA-G), 247
Hyperinsulinemia, 25
Hypogonadotropic hypogonadism, 142

I
ICF, ATRX and Rubinstein–Taybi syndromes, 202
Immunotech-Beckman assay, 60
Imprinting centers (ICs), 187
Intracytoplasmic morphologically selected sperm injection (IMSI), 221
acrosome reaction, 278
"best group," 268
classification scoring scale, 271
DNA damage, 278
electron microscopy, 264
embryo development and sperm nuclear defects, 283–284
fertility potential, 278
ICSI, 264, 277

implantation and pregnancy rates, 267
male gametes abnormalities, 277
microdroplets, 266
motile sperm evaluation, 271
MSOME (*see* Motile sperm organellar morphology examination)
application, compromised semen parameters, 280–281
high magnification, 278
nuclear DNA content and organization damages, 265
oligoasthenoteratozoospermia, 264, 268
optics of Nomarski, 265
phenotypic and genomic sperm anomalies, 284–287
reproductive prognosis assessment, 265
scoring and women's age, 272–273
semen impairment, 268
semen parameters, 264
sibling oocytes, 278
spermatozoon's morphology, 264
sperm characteristics, 271–272
sperm classification, 270
sperm DNA integrity, 278
sperm morphology, 277
sperm nuclear abnormality, 284
sperm preparation technique, 268
sperm vacuoles, 279–280
subcellular organelles, 264, 265
vacuolated spermatozoa
DIC, 270
DNA integrity, 268
female infertility factor, 269
FISH analysis, 270
morphological nuclear normalcy, 269
PSA-FITC, 270
sperm DNA fragmentation, 269
TUNEL assay, 269
zona pellucida and oolemma, 264
Intracytoplasmic sperm injection (ICSI), 120, 167–168, 198, 204–205
Intramuscular progesterone, 81–83
Intrauterine insemination (IUI), 167
In vitro fertilization (IVF), 27, 120
adoption of, 12–13
ART, 167–168
classification and terminology, 12
fertility treatment cost, 16–17
follicular flushing, 16
mild IVF
aromatase inhibitors, 15
clomiphene and gonadotropins, 15
GnRH antagonist, 12, 15
ovulation induction, 14
modified natural cycle
clomiphene stimulation, 13
exogenous hormones, 12
follicular scan, 13
GnRH antagonists, 14
hCG injection, 13
indomethacin, 13
LH surge and oocyte retrieval methods, 13
predictive marker
qualitative ovarian response prediction, 70–71
quantitative ovarian response prediction (*see* Quantitative ovarian response prediction)
progesterone
age and ovarian reserve, 82
bioadhesive gel preparation, 82
crinone, 82–83
endometrial maturation, 81
estradiol to progesterone, luteal phase, 87–88
follicular estrogen production and corpus luteum, 80
frozen embryo transfer and donor oocyte recipient cycles, 84, 86–87
GnRH downregulation protocol, 83
GnRH modulators, 80
intramuscular injections, 81
intravaginal *vs.* intramuscular progesterone, 81–82
luteal phase, 81
odds ratio, 83
optimal timing, 84, 85
pregnancy rates, 81
retrospective studies, 80–81
serum levels monitoring, 86
vaginal gel, 82–83
vaginal progesterone, 84–85
single embryo transfer, 15–16
In vitro growth (IVG), 204
In vitro maturation (IVM), 204
IVF. *See* In vitro fertilization

L

Lindane, 140
Lipofuscin, 143
Luteinizing hormone (LH), 118–119

M

Male chromatin remodeling
artificial reproductive techniques, 228
cytoplasmic and nuclear fusion, 228
DNA repair
dsDNA repair, 232
gammaHAX foci, 231–232
H2AX, 231, 232
monopronuclear and tripronuclear, 232
MPF, 231
NHEJ, 232, 233
thymidine, 232
imprinting maintenance, zygote, 234
male germline preparation, 228–229
oocyte, embryonic development, 236–237
paternal DNA demethylation, zygotic G1, 233
paternal *vs.* maternal histones, 230–231
zygotic S-phase, 234–235
Malonyldialdehide (MDA), 214
Mass spectrometry (MS), 247
Matrix associated regions (MARs), 231, 235

Matrix attenuated laser desorption/ionization (MALDI), 247
Maturation promoting factor (MPF), 231
Microsomal ethanol-oxidizing system (MEOS), 141
MIS. *See* Mullerian inhibiting substance
Monoamniotic pregnancy, 104, 105
Monochorionic, monoamniotic (MC/MA) twins, 100
Monochorionic twin pregnancies, 103–105
Mono (2-ethylhexyl) phthalate (MEHP), 139
Monozygotic twinning and perinatal outcomes
  ART, 92
  DC/DA twins, 94–95
  determining amnionicity/chorionicity, 93–94
  embryology, 92–93
  monochorionic, diamniotic (MC/DA) twins
    anomalous cofetus, 99–100
    clinical management, 95
    MC/MA twins, 100
    risk assessment, 95
    sIUGR, 97–98
    TRAP sequence, 98–99
    TTTS (*see* Twin-twin transfusion syndrome)
  perinatal risks, 93
  triplet and higher order multiple gestations, 92, 93
  twin gestations, 92
Motile sperm organellar morphology examination (MSOME)
  application, compromised semen parameters, 280–281
  criteria and evaluation procedure, 266
  morphological anomalies visualization, 267
  regional nuclear shape malformation, 266
  sperm analysis, 265
  spermatozoa, 266
  sperm evaluation, 266
  sperm nucleus normalcy, 267
Mullerian inhibiting substance (MIS)
  clinical diagnostic marker, 71
  GnRH agonist treatment, 72
  heteromeric receptor system, 58
  homodimeric disulfide-linked glycoprotein, 58
  IVF predictive marker (*see* In vitro fertilization, predictive marker)
  ovarian ageing, 64–66
  ovarian dysfunction (*see* Ovarian dysfunction)
  ovarian folliculogenesis, 58–60
  ovarian reserve markers, 72
  ovarian stimulation regimens, 72
  type I & II receptor, 58
  women circulating
    current assays, 60
    factors modulating serum, 60–62
Multiple pregnancy
  chorionicity and amnionicity
    diamniotic pregnancies, 104
    intertwin vascular anastomoses, 104
    monoamniotic pregnancy, 104, 105
    monozygotic and dizygotic twins, 104
    spontaneous twin pregnancies, 103
    zygosity, 104
  early embryonic loss, 105–106
  "vanishing twin" syndrome
    definition, 106
    embryo reduction, 110–111
    incidence in ART, 106–107
    perinatal results, 108–110
    symptoms, 108
    trisomy 21 screening, 110
    ultrasound diagnosis, 107–108

N

Non homologous end joining (NHEJ), 232, 233
Nucleoplasmin 2 (NPM2), 230
Nucleotide excision repair (NER), 232, 233

O

1-*o*-alkyl–2-acetyl-sn-glycero–3-phosphocholine (PAF), 246
Obesity
  ART therapy, 39
  chronic disease, 36
  definitions, 36
  diet and adverse reproductive outcomes, 38
  endometrial *vs.* oocyte factors, 38–39
  prenatal growth and PCOS, 38
  reproductive health
    female, 37–38
    male, 36–37
  reproductive spectrum, 36
Odds ratio, 83
OHSS. *See* Ovarian hyperstimulation syndrome
Oligozoospermia, 142
Ovarian dysfunction
  autoimmune process, 62, 63
  clomiphene citrate, 64
  follicular ovarian pool, 62
  hypogonadotropic amenorrhea, 62
  oligomenorrheic women, 64
  PCOS, 63–64
  POI, 62
  polycystic ovaries, 63
Ovarian folliculogenesis, 58–59
Ovarian hyperstimulation syndrome (OHSS), 17, 69–70
Ovarian-stimulated cycles
  endometrial fluid, 44
  endometrial receptivity
    biopsies, 50, 51
    embryonic implantation, 51
    gene expression, 50
    gene ontology, 51
    menstrual cycle, 51, 52
    primary cell culture, 53
    stromal cells, 53
  glandular and luminal epithelium, 44
  hormonal regulation, 45–46
  human endometrium
    agonists *vs.* antagonists, 48–49

natural cycles, 46–47
stimulated cycles, 47
human uterus, 44
oocyte, 44
pseudostratification, 45
stromal edema, 45

P

Persistent Müllerian duct syndrome, 58
Phthalate esters, 139–140
Pisum sativum agglutinin-Fluorescein isothiocyanate (PSA-FITC), 270
Polycystic ovarian syndrome (PCOS)
androgen concentrations, 25
antithyroid antibodies, 6
gonadotropins, 26
insulin resistance, 25–26
pathophysiology, 24
serum concentrations, 24–25
Polymerase chain reaction (PCR), 47
Polyunsaturated fatty acids (PUFA), 138, 139
Post translational modification (PTM), 230, 231, 234
Preimplantation embryos, 188–189
Preimplantation genetic diagnosis (PGD), 198
Premature ovarian insufficiency (POI), 62
Primordial germ cells (PGCs), 188–189, 203
PTM. *See* Post translational modification

R

Radiofrequency electromagnetic waves (RF-EMW), 144–145
Reactive oxygen species (ROS), 158–159
Receiver operating characteristic (ROC) curves, 66
Recombinant follicle stimulating hormone (rFSH), 48
Reproductive autoimmune failure syndrome, 4
Retinoblastoma (RB), 201
Ring finger 8 (RNF8), 184
Rubinstein-Taybi syndrome, 202

S

SCSA. *See* Sperm Chromatin Structure Assay
Selective intrauterine growth restriction (sIUGR), 97–98
Sertoli and Leydig cells, 135
Single embryo transfer, 15–16
Singleton pregnancy, 105
Smads, 21
Soluble HLA-G (sHLA-G), 247
Sperm, cancer therapies
chemotherapy, 123–125
fertility
after cancer treatment, 126
biologic and psychosocial consideration, 127
congenital malformation, 128
ethical considerations, 128–129
post-treatment options, 127–128
pre-treatment options, 127
germ cells, 122
gonadal function, 120
gonadotoxic effects, 118
hematologic malignancies, 120
interleukins and tumor necrosis factor, 120
IVF and ICSI, 128
leukemia, 122
Leydig cells, 122
lymphoma, 121–122
multimodal therapy, 125–126
radiation therapy, 125
semen and endocrine parameters, 118
solid tumors, 122
spermatogenesis
definition, 118
downregulation, 127
intratesticular testosterone, 119
LH and FSH, 118–119
Sertoli-cell function, 119
Type A and Type B spermatogonia, 118
surgery, 123
testicular cancer, 120–121
Sperm chromatin dispersion (SCD) test, 161
Sperm chromatin structure assay (SCSA), 156, 160–161
Sperm DNA damage
abortive apoptosis, 158
andrological examination, Adam, 156
assessment methods
annexin V binding ability assay, 162
anti-/pro-apoptotic proteins evaluation, 162
AOT, 161
CMA_3, 162
COMET assay, 160
oxidized deoxynucleoside, 162
SCD test, 161
SCSA, 156, 160–161
TdT and TUNEL, 160
tolouidine blue test, 161
caspases and endonucleases activation, 159
chromatin modelling, spermiogenesis process, 158
DFI, 156, 172
hormonal status and tubal patency, Linda, 156
human sperm chromatin, 157–158
lifestyle and environmental factors, 169
ROS, 158–159
semen quality assessment, 156–157
sperm DNA integrity
and cancer, 169
chance of spontaneous pregnancy, 164–165
clinical threshold values, 172
human spermatozoa, 172
intra-individual variation, 168–169
Molecular Human Reproduction, 172
Practice Committee of the American Society for Reproductive Medicine, 172
SCSA testing, 172
testing and ART, 165–168

Sperm epigenome
cellular epigenome, 181–182
chromatin remodeling, spermatogenesis
BRDT, 184
CDY and HAT, 184
cell cycle *vs.* developmental transcription factors, 185
H2A/H2B ubiquination, 182
histone-protamine transition, 182
H3K4me and H3k27me, 185
IVF/ICSI, 184
nucleosomes, 186
P1/P2 ratio, 184
reprogramming efficiency, 185
RNF8, 184
spermatids, 182
spermatogonial stem cell, 186
zygotic transcription, 186
DNA methylation, germline, 186
genome-wide reprogramming, 188
imprinted genes, 187
Sperm selection
excessive semen ROS production, 215–216
hyaluronic acid binding
biochemical sperm markers and diminished sperm function, 212–213
chromosomal aneuploidies, 217
dysmature spermatozoa, 218
high DNA integrity, 219
"physiologic" sperm selection, 218
solid state HA, 218–219
sperm dysmaturity and persistent histones, 219
Tygerberg normal sperm, 218
ICSI, 212
IMSI, 221
infertility definition, 212
SCSA issues and usefulness, 213–214
semen analysis, 212
source, assisted reproduction, 216
spermatozoa de-selection, apoptotic marker proteins, 217
sperm biochemical markers, 212–213
sperm charge properties, 220–221
sperm chromatin maturation, 216–217
sperm nuclear DNA integrity, 213
sperm preparation, gradient centrifugation, 214–215
Steroidogenic cell autoimmunity, 62
Surface-enhanced laser desorption/ionization (SELDI), 248

T
TdT-mediated 2'-deoxyuridine 5'-triphosphate-nick end labelling (TUNEL) assay, 160
Teratozoospermia, 141
Terminal deoxynucleotidyl transferase (TdT), 160
Testicular dysgenesis syndrome (TDS), 135
Testicular sperm extraction (TESE), 127
Time-of-flight (TOF), 248
Tolouidine blue (TB) test, 161
Topoisomerase II (TopoII), 229
Tripronuclear (3PN) zygotes, 230
Turner syndrome, 63
Twin reversed arterial perfusion (TRAP) sequence, 98–99
Twin-twin transfusion syndrome (TTTS)
birthweights and neonatal hemoglobin, 96
clinical management, 97
donor and recipient twins, 96
MC/DA twin pregnancies, 95
pathophysiology, 96–97
Quintero staging system, 96
ultrasound criteria, 96

U
Ultrasound-guided embryo transfer
catheter placement, 256
CCRM experience, 257–258
ectopic pregnancy, 256
fundal endometrium, 256
in vitro fertilization, 255–256
optimization, 256–257
ovarian hyperstimulation, 255
pregnancy rates, 256
randomized trials *vs.* meta-analysis, 257

V
Vitamin C, 141, 142
Vitamin E, 141, 142

W
Window of implantation (WOI), 47, 48
World Health Organization, 36

X
Xylene, 140